Recent Advances in Signal Transduction Research and Therapy

(Volume 1)

Edited by

Manoj K. Pandey

Department of Biomedical Sciences
Cooper Medical School of Rowan University
Camden, NJ 08103
USA

&

Vijay P. Kale

Translational Safety And Bioanalytical Sciences
Amgen Inc.
South San Francisco, CA 94080
USA

Recent Advances in Signal Transduction Research and Therapy

Volume # 1

Advances in Cancer Signal Transduction and Therapy

Editors: Manoj K. Pandey & Vijay P. Kale

ISSN (Online): 2737-4432

ISSN (Print): 2737-4424

ISBN (Online): 978-981-14-5811-8

ISBN (Print): 978-981-14-5809-5

ISBN (Paperback): 978-981-14-5810-1

need for a court order if at any point you breach any terms of this License Agreement. In no event will any delay or failure by Bentham Science Publishers in enforcing your compliance with this License Agreement constitute a waiver of any of its rights.

3. You acknowledge that you have read this License Agreement, and agree to be bound by its terms and conditions. To the extent that any other terms and conditions presented on any website of Bentham Science Publishers conflict with, or are inconsistent with, the terms and conditions set out in this License Agreement, you acknowledge that the terms and conditions set out in this License Agreement shall prevail.

Bentham Science Publishers Pte. Ltd.
80 Robinson Road #02-00
Singapore 068898
Singapore
Email: subscriptions@benthamscience.net

**BENTHAM
SCIENCE**

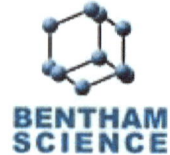

CONTENTS

PREFACE

Every year, almost 10 million people succumb to death around the world due to one or the other type of cancers. Hundreds of laboratories with thousands of scientists are trying to understand the ever-enigmatic biology of cancer cells, which is the basis for developing new therapies for cancer. Discovery of antifolates aminopterin in 1947 and methotrexate (aka amethopterin) in 1948 as potential anticancer agents by Drs. Yellapragada Subbarow and Sydney Farber not only initiated the era of chemotherapy but the discovery of these synthetic agents also infused the hope that cancers can be treated with synthetic chemicals. In the past more than seven decades, we have witnessed the journey of cancer therapy that started from nonspecific chemotherapy (*e.g.* antifolates) to targeted biologic agents (*e.g.* monoclonal antibodies) and now the era of personalized treatment (*e.g.* CART cells) and immunotherapy. However, deeper understanding of the signal transduction within the cancer cells, and between cancer cells and their surrounding tumor microenvironment has remained central to the development of therapies.

In the present volume 1 titled **'Advances in Cancer Signal Transduction and Therapy'** of the book series 'Recent advances in signal transduction research and therapy', we attempted to review recent advances in select cancer signal transduction pathways that have been targeted or could be potential targets for developing therapeutics for cancers. It would be too exhaustive to cover all the signaling pathways in all cancer types and we do not intend to do so, and due to the very rapidly progressing research on cancer signaling and therapy, we have no doubt that new discoveries will have been made by the time this book is published.

In the first chapter of this book, **Fultang *et al.*,** dive into the role of Wingless and Int-1 (Wnt) signaling in breast cancer oncogenesis. Moreover, the authors also review the current inhibitors of Wnt signaling that are under investigation. The C-X-C chemokine receptor type 4 (CXCR4) signaling is critical in hematological malignancies, while its role in breast cancer is still unraveling. In the second chapter **Raman *et al.*,** explain the intersection of CXCR4 signaling with other signaling pathways such as Phosphoinositide 3-kinase (PI3K), mitogen-activated protein kinase (MAPK), cellular Src (c-Src) and Janus kinases-signal transducer and activator of transcription proteins (JAK-STAT) in breast cancer progression and metastasis. A key role of epidermal growth factor receptor (EGFR) signaling in cell proliferation and survival in various cancers is now well known. Here in the third chapter, **Meena *et al.*,** discuss the role of EGFR in colon cancer and its prospective importance as a target for colon cancer therapy. The critical role of PI3K/AKT (protein kinase B)/mammalian target of rapamycin (mTOR) signaling pathway in various cancers has attracted cancer researchers for a long time. **Yadav and Mishra** elucidate the PI3K/AKT/mTOR signaling in hepatocellular carcinoma and review the various drugs under investigations that target this pathway in the fourth chapter. The MAPK pathway is one of the key survival pathways that have been targeted to develop cancer therapeutics. In chapter 5, **Prasad and Srivastava** review MAPK signaling in pancreatic cancer and therapeutic agents under investigation. Aberrant regulation and activation of nuclear factor kappa-light-chain-enhancer of activated B cells (NF-κB) has been implicated in several cancers, inflammatory and autoimmune disorders, and erroneous immune system development. In chapter 6, **Arora *et al.*,** summarize the role of NF-κB activation specifically in multiple myeloma and various strategies developed for its potential pharmacological intervention to abrogate the process of cancer cell proliferation. Recently, small-molecule inhibitors of Bruton's tyrosine kinase (BTK) such as ibrutinib have shown an impressive anti-tumor activity in clinical studies in patients with various B cell malignancies. BTK is crucial in B lymphocyte development, differentiation and oncogenic signaling. In chapter 7, **Gowda *et al.*,** elucidate the role of BTK in B cell malignancies and highlight the current progress in the discovery of small molecule BTK inhibitors. Finally, in the last chapter of this book, **Pathania** *et al.*, discuss the interconnection between exosomes, tumor microenvironment and cMyc transcription factor, and therapeutic strategies to break that nexus.

We sincerely hope that you will enjoy diving into this book.

Manoj K. Pandey
Department of Biomedical Sciences,
Cooper Medical School of Rowan University,
Camden, NJ 08103,
USA

&

Vijay P. Kale
Translational Safety And Bioanalytical Sciences
Amgen Inc.
South San Francisco, CA 94080
USA

LIST OF CONTRIBUTORS

Alan Prem Kumar Department of Pharmacology, Yong Loo Lin School of Medicine, National University of Singapore, Singapore

Anup S. Pathania Department of Biochemistry and Molecular Biology & The Fred and Pamela Buffett Cancer Center, University of Nebraska Medical Center, Omaha, USA

Augustus M.C. Tilley Department of Cancer Biology, University of Toledo Health Science Campus, Toledo, USA

Avtar S. Meena Department of Pure and Applied Physics, CSIR-Centre for Cellular and Molecular Biology (CCMB) Habsiguda, Hyderabad, India

Bela Peethambaran Department of Biological Sciences, University of the Sciences, Philadelphia, USA

Cory M. Howard Department of Cancer Biology, University of Toledo Health Science Campus, Toledo, USA

Dayanidhi Raman Department of Cancer Biology, University of Toledo Health Science Campus, Toledo, USA

Frank Arfuso Stem Cell and Cancer Biology Laboratory, School of Pharmacy and Biomedical Sciences, Curtin Health Innovation Research Institute, Perth, Australia

Gautam Sethi Department of Pharmacology, Yong Loo Lin School of Medicine, National University of Singapore, Singapore

Jennifer Dang Department of Biomedical Sciences, Cooper Medical School of Rowan University, Camden, USA

Krishne Gowda Department of Pharmacology, Penn State College of Medicine, Hershey, USA

Kishore B. Challagundla The Children's Health Research Institute, University of Nebraska Medical Center, Omaha, USA

Kuntal Bhowmick Department of Biomedical Sciences, Cooper Medical School of Rowan University, Camden, USA

Loukik Arora Department of Pharmacology, Yong Loo Lin School of Medicine. National University of Singapore, Singapore

Manoj K. Pandey Department of Biomedical Sciences, Cooper Medical School of Rowan University, Camden, USA

Max Von Suskil Department of Biomedical Sciences, Cooper Medical School of Rowan University, Camden, USA

Neelam Yadav Department of Biochemistry, Rammanohar Lohia Avadh University, Faizabad, India

Norman Fultang Department of Biological Sciences, University of the Sciences, Philadelphia, USA

Omar Al-Adat Department of Biomedical Sciences, Cooper Medical School of Rowan University, Camden, USA

Prachi S. Narayan Department of Biomedical Sciences, Cooper Medical School of Rowan University, Camden, USA

Pradeep K. Shukla   Department of Physiology, University of Tennessee Health Science Center, Memphis, USA

Rachel Weber   Department of Biochemistry and Molecular Biology, University of Nebraska Medical Center, Omaha, USA

Sahdeo Prasad   Department of Immunotherapeutics and Biotechnology, and Center for Tumor Immunology and Targeted Cancer Therapy, Texas Tech University Health Sciences Center, Abilene, USA

Sangita Sridharan   Department of Cancer Biology, University of Toledo Health Science Campus, Toledo, USA

Sanjay K. Srivastava   Department of Immunotherapeutics and Biotechnology, and Center for Tumor Immunology and Targeted Cancer Therapy, Texas Tech University Health Sciences Center, Abilene, USA

Shantu G Amin   Department of Pharmacology, Penn State College of Medicine, Hershey, USA

Vijay P. Kale   Translational Safety And Bioanalytical Sciences, Amgen Inc., South San Francisco, CA 94080, USA

Yoganchal Mishra   Department of Biochemistry, Rammanohar Lohia Avadh University, Faizabad, India

CHAPTER 1

Wnt Signaling in Breast Cancer Oncogenesis, Development and Progression

Norman Fultang and **Bela Peethambaran**[*]

Department of Biological Sciences, University of the Sciences, Philadelphia, PA, USA

Abstract: Wnt signaling regulates several cellular processes, including differentiation, proliferation, and stem cell pluripotency. Mutations in Wnt signaling are known to lead to tumor initiation and progression. Wnt/ β-catenin signaling is dysregulated in breast cancer, where it has been shown to mediate oncogenic progression. In this review, the canonical and non-canonical pathways of Wnt/ β-catenin signaling, and their regulation of breast cancer oncogenesis and progression are described. During the last decade, several small molecules and natural compounds have shown to interfere with Wnt signaling and demonstrate potential as Wnt-targeting therapeutic agents. This review also highlights these molecules, some of which are in clinical trials. Finally, strategies of using these molecules in combination therapies with other drug agents are discussed.

Keywords: β-catenin, Breast cancer, Canonical and Non-canonical pathways, Mutations, Oncogenesis, Proliferation, Stem cell pluripotency, Wnt signaling.

INTRODUCTION

Overview

The Wnt/β-catenin pathway is a crucial and highly conserved pathway governing the processes of growth, development, and cell fate [1]. An ever-increasing body of evidence suggests a vital role for Wnt/β-catenin signaling in the oncogenesis, development and progression of cancer [2]. This review will summarize recent findings on the role of this pathway in breast cancer and discuss the emerging therapeutic approaches targeting Wnt signaling.

The Wnt signaling cascade is an evolutionarily conserved pathway. It was first discovered to be responsible for spontaneous mammary hyperplasia and tumor formation in mice after pro-viral insertion in the int-1 locus [3]. A few years later,

---

[*] **Corresponding author Bela Peethambaran:** Department of Biological Sciences, University of the Sciences, Philadelphia, PA, USA; Tel: 215-596-8923; Fax: 215-596-8710; E-mail: b.peethambaran@usciences.edu

Manoj K. Pandey & Vijay P. Kale (Eds.)

the Wingless gene responsible for segment polarity in *Drosophila melanogaster* was found to be a homolog of int-1. Hence the int/Wingless family was named *Wnt* [4, 5]. Wnt proteins are encoded by 19 different Wnt genes with sequences sharing a high degree of homology [6]. These proteins are known to bind to cellular receptors during embryonic development and mediate several processes, such as cell proliferation, survival, migration, polarity, cell fate, and self-renewal [7]. Wnt can activate distinct signaling pathways, which include a β-catenin dependent or canonical pathway, and a β-catenin independent or non-canonical pathway [4, 7]. Wnt ligands bind primarily to multiple Frizzled (Fzd) receptors [8], but other Wnt co-receptors include members of the low density lipo-protein related protein 5 and 6 (LRP5/6), receptor-like tyrosine kinase (RYK) and receptor tyrosine-kinase like orphan receptors (ROR) 1 and 2 [8, 9]. These co-receptors are important to regulate downstream signaling either through LRP5/6 co-receptors for the β-catenin dependent or through RYK/ROR1/2 for the β-catenin independent pathway.

Wnt Biosynthesis and Regulation

During its synthesis, Wnt has to undergo a palmitoylation step catalyzed by Porcupine (PORCN), which belongs to the membrane-associated O-acyltransferase family [10, 11]. This step is required for the interaction with Fzd receptors and promotes interaction with the multi-pass transmembrane protein, Wntless, which transports Wnt to the plasma membrane. Since PORCN is required for Wnt secretion, several small molecules have been developed to target it. There are 10 Wnt antagonists that also help mediate Wnt signaling. These antagonists include the secreted Fzd-related proteins (SFRPs), Wnt-inhibitory factor 1 (WIF-1), Wise/SOST, Dickkopf proteins (DKKs), insulin-like growth factor binding protein 4 (IGFBP4), Cereberus, Shisa, Wnt-activated inhibitory factor 1 (Waifl/5 T4), adenomatosis polypsosis coli down regulated 1 (APCDD1) and Tikil [9, 12]. Several of these regulatory factors have potential as therapeutic targets, but so far, only DKK1 has been evaluated clinically for drug development [13]. The challenge in using these regulatory proteins as targets is that they often regulate the activity of other important cellular pathways. For instance, SFRPs and WIF-1 can bind to Wnt in both canonical and non-canonical signaling depending on the cellular need. SFRPS, however, also regulates the Notch and Bone Morphogenic Protein (BMP) signaling cascade, a key developmental pathway [12, 14].

TYPES OF PATHWAYS

The Canonical Wnt Signaling Pathway in Breast Cancer

Canonical Wnt signaling plays an important role in cell fate decisions in early embryogenesis during the development of organs, such as the lungs, kidney, skin, and bone [8]. This pathway is also critical in neural patterning and stem cell renewal [15]. Canonical Wnt signaling is also called the β-catenin dependent pathway as it results in an accumulation of cytoplasmic β-catenin followed by the latter's translocation to the nucleus [8, 15, 16]. Genetic and biochemical evidence suggests that Wnt binds to Fzd receptors, which have seven transmembrane receptors with a cysteine-rich domain at the N-terminal. Fzd is required for multiple Wnt pathways, but another single-pass transmembrane receptor, LRP6/5 is specifically required for the Wnt/β-catenin canonical pathway [17].

Canonical Wnt signaling results in stabilization and nuclear translocation of ß-catenin [18, 19], which is degraded by a destruction complex consisting of AXIN, Protein phosphatase 2A (PP2A), Casein Kinase 1α (CK1α), and Glycogen synthase kinase 3 (GSK3) [19, 20]. In the absence of Wnt, this destruction complex phosphorylates ß-catenin, tagging it for ubiquitination and subsequent degradation by the proteasome. Wnt ligands, when bound to the Fzd receptor and the LRP 5/6 transmembrane co-receptor, trigger the recruitment of Disheveled (Dvl) to the plasma membrane [8, 21 - 24]. AXIN is also recruited to the phosphorylated cytoplasmic tail of LRP5/6 [17, 25]. Dvl forms a complex with AXIN, Fzd, and LRP5/6 [26]. Recruitment of AXIN and Dvl prevents the formation of the destruction complex leading to the stabilization of cytoplasmic ß-catenin [18, 19]. Dvl proteins also assemble the signalosome that is responsible for phosphorylation of multiple motifs of LFP5/6, one of which is phosphorylated-PPPSPXS/T. P-PPPSPXS/T acts as a competitive inhibitor of GSK3 [26], a kinase that phosphorylates and tags ß-catenin for degradation. The net result of these events is the accumulation of unphosphorylated β-catenin resulting in its stabilization. The stabilized β-catenin translocates to the nucleus, where it acts as a transcriptional co-activator in combination with the T-cell factor (TCF) and the lymphoid enhancer-binding factor (LEF) family of transcription factors. This leads to the recruitment of transcriptional Kat3 co-activators p300 and CREB binding protein (CBP) to transcribe Wnt target genes (Fig. **1A**) [27]. ß-catenin can also interact with other transcriptional co-activators, including BRG-1, a component of the SWI/SNF nuclear remodeling complex, Hsp90 co-chaperone Cdc37, and C-terminal-binding protein (CtBP) [28 - 31]. In the absence of Wnt signaling and nuclear ß-catenin, TCF forms a complex with Groucho proteins to recruit histone deacetylases (HDACs) and repress the transcription of Wnt target genes [32 - 34].

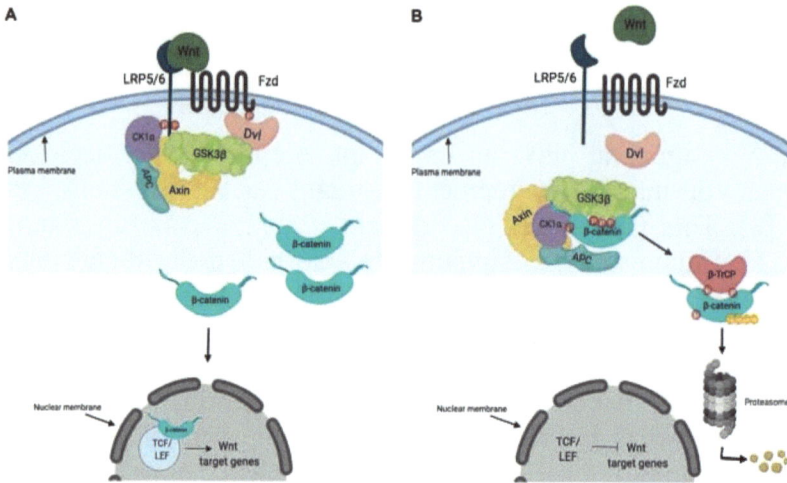

Fig. (1). A) *Wnt on.* When Wnt ligand binds to Fzd and LRP receptor, Dvl is recruited to the plasma membrane, forming a complex with Axin and other β-catenin destruction complex members resulting in β-catenin stabilization. Stabilized β-catenin then translocates to the nucleus for transcriptional activity. **B)**. *Wnt off.* In the absence of Wnt ligand bound to Fzd and LRP receptor, cytoplasmic β-catenin is phosphorylated and tagged for degradation by members of the β-catenin destruction complex. Phosphorylated β-catenin is ubiquitinated by β-TrCP and degraded by the proteasome.

In the absence of Wnt, GSK3 and CK1α, in turn, phosphorylate β-catenin. The phosphorylated β-catenin is recognized by Fbox/WD repeat protein β-TrCP, which is a ubiquitin ligase. This results in β-catenin ubiquitination and degradation in the proteasome (Fig. **1B**). A recent study identified YAP/TAZ as novel Wnt regulators. It was shown that in the absence of Wnt ligand binding, they could become part of the destruction complex and recruit β-TrCP [35]. The Hippo signaling pathway YAP/TAZ is a key oncogenic pathway that promotes stemness in breast and other cancers [36]. Recently, wnt signaling has similarly been described as a regulator of breast cancer stemness [37, 38].

Non-canonical Wnt Pathways in Breast Cancer

These pathways are characterized by Wnt-activated cellular signaling but do not result in β-catenin stabilization and transcriptional activity. The two non-canonical pathways, identified so far, are the planar cell polarity (PCP) and the Wnt/Ca^{2+} pathways [39].

The PCP pathway is an LRP5/6 and ß-catenin independent pathway that regulates cell polarity, organization, and migration through the modulation of actin cytoskeleton elements [40]. Binding of Wnt ligands to Fzd and its co-receptors ROR1/2, RYK, PTK7 or NRH1, leads to recruitment of Dvl, which in turn forms a complex with Dvl-associated activator of morphogenesis 1 (DAAM-1) [41 -

43]. DAAM1 activates G-protein Rho, which activates Rho-associated kinase, ROCK. Activated ROCK regulates the cytoskeleton and cell polarity [44]. Dvl also interacts with Rac1. Rac-1 activates c-Jun N-terminal Kinase, which can regulate actin polymerization [45]. PCP and β-catenin-dependent Wnt signaling can negatively regulate each other [46].

In the Wnt/Ca^{2+} pathway, Wnt binds to the Fzd receptors and activates G proteins, which then activate phospholipase C or cGMP-specific PDE, triggering the release of intracellular calcium [47, 48]. Calcium activates target genes, such as protein kinase C (PKC), calcineurin, and calcium/calmodulin-dependent kinase II (CaMKII), which are responsible for cell fate and migration [49].

Several non-canonical elements are aberrantly expressed in breast cancer. Overexpression of planar cell polarity protein VANGL-1, for example, correlates with increased risk of disease relapse and metastasis in breast cancer [50]. VANGL-2 is also highly expressed in breast cancer, where it contributes to increased proliferation and poorer prognosis [51]. Genome amplification of Fzd6 and its non-canonical ligands Wnt11 and Wnt5B were also observed in triple-negative breast cancer [52].

Regulators of Wnt Signaling

Wnt signaling is tightly regulated at several points to ensure proper cell function. An ever-accumulating body of evidence suggests several secreted and intracellular factors regulate various steps of Wnt signaling. As previously mentioned, extracellular factors, such as Dkk, WIF-1, SFRs, Cerberus, Frzb, Wise, SOST, IGFBP-4, and Naked cuticle, can bind to Fzd or LRP5/6 and inhibit Wnt signaling [9, 53 - 55]. These molecules constitute a regulatorily important class of Wnt antagonists. Other non-Wnt ligands can also activate Wnt signaling upon binding to Fzd. These include Norrin and members of the R-Spondin family [56, 57]. The Wnt pathways can also regulate each other: for example, the non-canonical Wnt/Ca^{2+} pathway can negatively regulate canonical Wnt/ß-catenin/TCF signaling [19, 49]. Other Wnt regulators include transmembrane E3 ubiquitin ligase ZNRF3/RNF43, which negatively regulates Wnt signaling by promoting the turnover of Fzd and LRP6 receptors [58]. R-spondins also promote Wnt signaling by binding ZNRF3, promoting its interaction with LGR4 and subsequent clearance from the plasma membrane [58].

Wnt and Breast Cancer Stem Cells

Cancer Stem Cells (CSCs) are tumor-initiating cells that possess the characteristics of self-renewal and differentiation [2, 59]. Mutations in long-term stem cells or their progeny can lead to malignancy [2]. In normal tissue, stem cells are found in organ systems, such as hematopoietic, dermal, and intestinal tissue, that regenerate and differentiate [2, 60]. Cancer stem cells similarly regenerate tumors leading to disease recurrence and relapse. Wnt has been shown to play a role in self-renewal of hematopoietic stems cells (HSC) [61, 62]. This is seen to coincide with increases in β-catenin levels with ensuing activation of TCF/LEF-1 promoter activity. Within the mammary gland, Wnt signaling plays a key role in regulating stem and progenitor cells [63]. Aberrant Wnt signaling has been linked to tumor initiation in breast cancer *via* altered regulation of mammary progenitor/stem cell populations [64, 65]. Mechanistically, key stem cell markers CD44 and ALDH1 are transcriptional targets of Wnt/ß-catenin, which might explain how aberrant Wnt hyperactivation promotes stemness [37, 66, 67].

Dysregulated Wnt signaling has also been linked with increased EMT, multidrug resistance, and immune escape in breast CSC populations contributing to tumor persistence [68 - 71]. Dysregulation of Wnt signaling was also associated with increased PD-L1 expression in triple-negative breast cancer stem cells, possibly contributing to immune evasion [72]. Wnt signaling is enriched in triple-negative breast cancer compared to other breast cancer subtypes [73]. Perhaps accordingly, triple-negative breast cancer is the most stem-like breast cancer subtype and has the worst clinical outcomes [74 - 76]. Inhibition of Wnt/ß-catenin signaling has shown promise in repressing breast cancer stemness, concurrently reducing cancer metastasis and chemoresistance [77].

Non-canonical Wnt receptor ROR1 has also been shown to promote stemness and drug resistance in breast cancer [78 - 80]. Inhibition of ROR1 with monoclonal antibodies or small molecule inhibitors repressed breast cancer stemness and potentiated chemotherapy efficacy in breast cancer [78, 79, 81].

ROLE OF WNT SIGNALING IN BREAST CANCER TUMORIGENESIS AND PROGRESSION

Several studies have shown that Wnt signaling is vital in the development of several organs, including mammary glands. A study by Van Genderen *et al.* provided evidence for LEF1 involvement in normal mammary gland development in mice [82]. LEF1 is a transcription factor of the TCF family, which associates with β-catenin to stimulate the expression of Wnt target genes. Wnt is required for mammary gland morphogenesis as was shown in a study where epithelial buds from Wnt-4 knockout mice were implanted in the post-natal mammary fat pads resulting in the reduction of lobular branching [83]. Overexpression of Wnt-4 induced pregnancy-like growth in the reconstituted mammary gland [84]. This suggests a role for Wnt in development at the bud stage. Wnt10b, also known as Wnt-12, is required for mammary bud development [85].

β-catenin is known to affect target genes, such as c-JUN, FRA-1, C-MYC, and CYCLIN D1, which are all involved in proliferation and development [86]. Consequently, overexpression or mutations in any of the Wnt pathway proteins can lead to malignant growth [87]. In breast cancer, Wnt pathways are frequently deregulated, contributing to malignancy [3]. It has been shown that treatments with Wnt ligands significantly increase breast cancer cell motility [88]. Conversely, blocking the pathway by either knocking down Wnt, Dvl, or β-catenin reduced the aggressiveness of breast cancer [89, 90]. These results have also been replicated in a mouse model of Erb2-driven tumor progression [87, 91]. Small molecule inhibition of ß-catenin as a well as knockdown of Wnt-associated transcription factor, SOX4, had similar effects repressing breast cancer proliferation and migration [92]. Blocking endogenous β-catenin by RNA interference in transgenic mice similarly showed a significant reduction in tumor cell invasion [77].

Loss of β-catenin at the membrane has been shown to be a key feature of invasive ductal carcinoma, the molecular subtype of breast cancer with the worst prognosis [93]. Expression of other components in the Wnt pathway, such as AXIN, CK1α, GSK-3β, and protein phosphatase 2A, has also been shown to be associated with breast cancer progression [94, 95]. The differential expression of co-receptors, LRP5 and LRP6, has also been shown to be associated with mammary gland tumorigenesis [96]. Silencing of these co-receptors reduced Wnt signaling, which led to decreased cancer cell proliferation and *in vivo* tumor growth. Wnt receptor Fzd7 is also upregulated in breast cancer patients, where its silencing resulted in a significant reduction in tumor growth [97].

The mutations and/or mechanisms underlying anomalous activation of Wnt pathways in breast cancer are not fully understood. Increased Wnt signaling might be a result of several factors, including mutations in ß-catenin, APC, or other members of the destruction complex or impaired activity of wnt regulatory pathways [20, 98, 99]. Modulated epigenetic regulation of several members of the Wnt pathways might also contribute to increased Wnt signaling [100].

4. ANIMAL MODELS AND CLINICAL SIGNIFICANCE OF WNT SIGNALING IN BREAST CANCER

The first Wnt transgenic mouse model was constructed by a proviral insertion of mouse mammary tumor virus (MMTV) within the int-1/Wnt1 locus leading to tumorigenesis [101]. Nusse *et al.* observed that the mice developed lobuloalveolar hyperplasia and then cancer. Other models leverage proviral activation of Wnt10B, the earliest expressed Wnt ligand, to induce hyperplasia and mammary tumors [102]. Important nodes in the Wnt pathway have also been targeted. GSK3β was repressed in a mouse model by creating a kinase inactivated GSK3ß mutant [94]. The mice were shown to have upregulated β-catenin, Cyclin-D1, and developed mammary tumors. Other GSK3ß null models with increased Wnt signaling have been used [103]. Many models targeting proteins in the destruction complex are also being used. Mice with truncated APC, for example, develop tumors with constitutively active Wnt/ß-catenin signaling [104]. Casein Kinase 2 (CK2) overexpression models that lead to mammary adenocarcinoma are also used [95, 105]– CK2 is a serine/threonine kinase, downstream of Dvl which promotes Wnt/ß-catenin signaling [106].

5. WNT SIGNALING IN TRIPLE-NEGATIVE BREAST CANCER

Triple-negative breast cancer (TNBC) is an aggressive subtype of breast cancer with poor prognosis and is characterized by the absence of estrogen receptors (ER), progesterone (PR), and Human epidermal growth factor 2 (HER2) [107, 108]. The lack of these proteins reduces the efficacy of targeted agents, such as Herceptin (targets HER2) and Tamoxifen (targets ER). Wnt signaling is highly upregulated in TNBC compared to other subtypes of breast cancer [90, 108]. It has been demonstrated that β-catenin is a marker for poor outcomes in TNBC patients [16]. Deregulated expression of components of the Wnt signaling pathway has been shown to significantly increase the risk of brain and lung metastasis in TNBC patients [109]. The gene encoding β-catenin (CTNNB1) is not mutated in TNBC patients but is seen to be over-expressed, leading to continuous activation of Wnt signaling [110, 111]. Studies have shown that β-catenin nuclear accumulation promotes cell migration and resistance to chemotherapy in TNBC cells both *in vitro* and *in vivo* [108, 112]. Dysregulation of non-canonical Wnt signaling can also promote metastasis of TNBC cells and CSCs through c-Jun N-terminal kinase activation. CSCs are thought to be responsible for the relapse of TNBC [113]. Non-canonical Wnt receptor ROR1 has also been shown to be enriched in ER-negative breast cancer compared to ER-positive breast cancer, where it interacts with CK1ε to promote cell proliferation, survival, and metastasis [80]. Other canonical and non-canonical Wnt receptors are similarly deregulated in TNBC [114].

A study by Lehmann *et al.*, based on 587 TNBC cases from 21 breast cancer data sets, identified 6 molecularly distinct sub-types of TNBC [115]. These sub-types include mesenchymal stem-like (MSL), mesenchymal (M), basal-like 1, basal-like2, immunomodulatory, and luminal androgen receptor (LAR). The LAR subtype accounts for 10% of TNBCs and has characteristic amplification of CCND1/Cyclin D1, a gene regulated by the Wnt/ β-catenin pathway [116, 117]. The basal-like subtypes have deregulated expression of Wnt associated genes CHEK1, FANCA, FANCG, MSH2, RAD21, AURKB, PLK1, CENPA, BUB1, CCNA2, MYC, NRAS and PRC1 [114, 118 - 125]. These are involved in DNA damage signaling and cell cycle regulation. In both Lehmann's M and MSL subtypes, several genes involved in Wnt/ β-catenin, such as CTNNB1, DKK2, DKK3, SFRP4, TCF4, and FZD4, are found to be up-regulated [115]. A subsequent RNA profiling analysis by Burstein *et al.* narrowed down TNBC cases to four stable, molecularly distinct subtypes [116]. These include LAR, mesenchymal, basal-like immune suppressed, and basal-like immune activated subtypes. The basal-like immune-suppressed subtypes exhibit overexpression of proliferation genes, including SOX transcription factors, which are known regulators of Wnt/ß-catenin signaling [126]. The basal-like immune-activated subtype has increased expression of CDK1, which phosphorylates and modulates Wnt regulators BCL9 and TAZ [127, 128].

NATURAL COMPOUNDS TARGETING WNT PATHWAYS AS CANCER THERAPEUTICS

Several naturally occurring molecules have been shown to modulate the activity of one or more components of the Wnt pathway (Table **1**).

Table 1. Natural products that modulate Wnt pathway activity, repressing cancer progression.

Natural Compound	Source	Mechanism of Action	Reference
Resveratol	Red grapes	Disrupts β-catenin interaction with TCF4	NCT00256334 NCT04266353 [129, 131]
Vitamin D	Fat-soluble vitamin present in some foods and produced endogenously in mammals upon skin exposure to UV light from the sun	Promotes Vitamin D receptor binding β-catenin reducing nuclear β-catenin levels	[139, 141]
Curcumin	Turmeric	Represses transcription of Wnt-responsive genes (c-myc, c-fos, c-jun, and iNOS) Represses β-catenin transcription	[145 - 147]
Retinoids	Metabolic products of Vitamin A	Promote degradation of Cyclin D1, which is regulated by GSK3	[148 - 150]

(Table 1) cont.....

Natural Compound	Source	Mechanism of Action	Reference
Genistein	Soy	Promotes transcription of SFRP2, a Wnt/β-catenin repressor	[152, 153, 156, 158, 168]
EGCG and other catechins	Tea plant/ *Camellia sinensis*	Repression of Wnt/β-catenin pathway, downregulation of β-catenin and cyclin D1 expression	[159 - 163]
Lupeol	Olives, figs, mangoes, strawberries and several other fruits	Inhibits nuclear localization of β-catenin	[166, 167]

Resveratrol - Resveratrol is a polyphenol found in red grapes [129]. Resveratrol is known for its anti-cancer properties and activity, notably in breast and colon cancer [129 - 131]. In both colon and breast cancer, it has been shown to inhibit Wnt signaling [129, 130]. It has also been shown to decrease ß-catenin nuclear localization and disrupt ß-catenin/TCF4 interaction [130, 131]. Resveratrol is a phyto-estrogen that can be both antagonistic and agonistic to the estrogen receptors contributing to its bioactivity in breast cancer [132, 133]. Resveratrol, as an inhibitor of Wnt signaling in colon cancer, was explored in a clinical trial (NCT00256334). Results suggested that resveratrol failed to significantly inhibit Wnt signaling in colon cancer tissue but was effective in inhibiting Wnt in normal colonic mucosa [134]. Resveratrol also inhibits oncogenic growth factor IGF2 [135]– IGF2 potentially inhibits ß-catenin inhibitor GSK3ß *via* activation of P13K/AKT [136, 137]. In an on-going clinical trial (NCT04266353), the inhibitory effect of resveratrol on serum IGF2 in African American women with breast cancer is being evaluated.

Vitamin D- Vitamin D was shown to suppress Wnt-signaling in breast cancer, inducing apoptosis, and promoting tamoxifen sensitivity [138]. It has also been shown to be a chemopreventive agent in breast cancer animal models [139, 140]. In colon cancer cells, vitamin D treatment resulted in vitamin D receptors binding to β-catenin, reducing its localization to the nucleus [139, 141], and in turn, reducing colon cancer proliferation and survival.

Curcumin- Curcumin (diferuloylmethane [1,7-bis(4-hydoxy-3-methoxypheyl)- 1, 6-helptadiene-3,5-dione] is a bioactive compound in turmeric [142]. Curcumin is known to affect different kinds of cancers, such as colon, breast, and skin. Curcumin inhibits breast cancer stem cells *via* inhibition of both Wnt/ß-catenin and sonic hedgehog pathways [143]. It was also shown to inhibit VEGF in breast cancer cells *via* inhibition of ß-catenin [144]. Curcumin also targets the transcription of Wnt target genes, such as c-myc, c-fos, c-jun, and iNOS in a variety of cancer cells [145]. In another study, curcumin reduced the transcription of β-catenin in colon cancer [146, 147]. Treatment with 40μM of curcumin resulted in the degradation of β-catenin and a decrease in nuclear β-catenin levels [147].

Retinoids- Vitamin A is converted to a number of metabolites called retinoids [148]. Retinoids have been demonstrated to be potent anti-cancer compounds *in vitro*, *in vivo* and in clinical trials [149]. The mechanism by which retinoids inhibit cancer cell progression is by inhibiting the activity of oncogenic AP-1 and Wnt/ β-catenin signaling [150]. Retinoids also play a key role in the degradation of Cyclin D1 in cancer cells, which is mediated by GSK3β- an important component of the Wnt/ β-catenin signaling pathway [151].

Genistein- Genistein is an isoflavone abundantly found in soy [152]. Genistein has shown potency in several cancers, where it promotes sFRP2 and GSK3ß activity and represses ß-catenin [153 - 156]. Genistein has also shown to inhibit Wnt-1 induced proliferation and repress the transcription of wnt-target genes, c-myc and Cyclin D1 [157, 158].

EGCG and other catechins- Catechins are primarily found in tea derived from *Camellia sinesis* [159, 160]. The most characterized catechins are epigallocatechin-3-gallate (EGCG), epigallocatechin, epicatechin-3-gallate, and epicatechin. Wnt/β-catenin signaling is inhibited by EGCG in breast cancer [161]. EGCG was also shown to reduce both proliferation and invasiveness of breast cancer through induction of HMG-box containing protein 1 and repression of Wnt/ β-catenin signaling [162, 163]. Extracts from green tea were also found to inhibit aberrant colonic crypts in rats and intestinal polyps in the APC-Min mouse [164]. The decrease in tumor burden was associated with the downregulation of β-catenin in the intestine and lower expression of c-jun and cyclin D1.

Lupeol-Lupeol is found in several fruits, such as olives, figs, strawberries, and mangoes [165]. Lupeol has several medicinal benefits, including activity against cancer [165, 166]. Lupeol can inhibit the growth of melanoma cells that have constitutive Wnt/ β-catenin signaling [167]. In these cells, Lupeol prevents nuclear localization of β-catenin by decreasing the latter's phosphorylation at serine 552 and serine 675, which is necessary for its translocation into the nucleus [167]. This also modulates the expression of several genes in the Wnt signaling pathway. Lupeol also modulates both NF-ƙB and P13K/Akt pathways, which interact with Wnt signaling pathways [166].

SMALL MOLECULES AND NOVEL THERAPEUTICS THAT TARGET WNT SIGNALING

Several small molecules that either inhibit or activate Wnt signaling have been identified (Table **2**). Compounds, such as IWR [169] and XAV939 [170], that impact the stability of Axin, which is regulated by tankyrase-mediated ADP-ribosylation, have been characterized. These compounds inhibit tankyrase, increasing Axin levels, and lowering β-catenin. There are also compounds that block Porcupine, the enzyme that catalyzes the acylation of Wnt proteins. These molecules are IWP2 [171], C59 [172], and LGK974 [173] (Table **2**). Acylation of Wnt is required for Wnt transport. LGK974 is currently undergoing clinical trials for a variety of solid tumors.

Table 2. Small molecules that target Wnt pathway proteins, currently in preclinical development or clinical trials.

Drug	Tumor Type	Mechanism of Action	Reference
IWR	Solid tumors Bladder carcinoma	Stabilization of Axin	[169]
XAV939	Solid tumors Hepatic cancer Neuroblastoma	Tankyrase inhibitor	[170]
LGK974	Colorectal cancer Pancreatic cancer Melanoma Triple-negative breast cancer	PORCN inhibitor	NCT01351103
IWP2, C59, LGK974	Solid tumors Gastric cancer	Inactivate PORCN Inhibit palmitoylation of Wnt	[171 - 173]
OMP-18R5	Solid tumors Pancreatic cancer Non-small cell lung carcinoma Breast cancer	Monoclonal antibody raised against Fzd receptors	[174] NCT01345201 NCT02005315 NCT01973309 NCT01957007
L807mts, Bio, CHIR, SB-216763	Neurodegenerative disorders	GSK3 regulators.	[175]
UC-961	Chronic Lymphocytic leukemia B cell lymphoma HER2 negative breast cancer	Monoclonal antibody raised against ROR1	NCT02222688 NCT03088878 NCT02776917
BKQ880	Multiple Myeloma	Monoclonal antibody raised against DKK-1	NCT00741377
Foxy-5	Metastatic Breast, Colorectal, Prostate cancers	Formylated peptide that mimics Wnt-5a	NCT02020291 [176]

Wnt signaling can also be interrupted at the receptor level. There was a recent screen for RNF43 mutations that sensitize pancreatic tumor cells to therapy and make them dependent on the Wnt ligand [177]. Several mutants found in this screen, that suppressed the RNF43 growth phenotype, were due to aberrations in FZD5, indicating that the tumor cells are dependent on Wnt-FZD signaling [177]. The growth of these tumors could be reduced by the use of antibodies against FZD (OMP-18R5), which has been shown to bind to several FZD family members [174]. Wnt protein is highly hydrophobic and because of this, it is challenging to use this as a drug. Recently soluble Wnt agonists have been shown to activate Wnt signaling *in vivo* [178]. Compounds, such as L807mts, Bio, CHIR, SB-216763, are known to interfere with Wnt signaling, specifically GSK3 [175]. A formylated 6 amino acid fragment Foxy-5, which mimics the effects of Wnt-5a by binding Fzd to impair migration in epithelial cells and Wnt-5a-low cancer cells, was recently investigated in a clinical trial for metastatic breast, colorectal, and prostate cancers (NCT02020291) [176]. A PTK7-antibody drug conjugate (PTK7-ADC) is also being used to treat metastatic and triple-negative breast cancers (NCT03243331) [179].

Perhaps the most effective therapeutic target would be the TCF/β-catenin complex. However, to date, there is no known molecule identified that could disrupt this complex. The binding affinity of these two proteins is very high, making the development of effective small molecule inhibitors of the complex, difficult [7, 180].

CONCLUSION AND FUTURE DIRECTIONS

In this review, several studies that provide a deeper understanding of the role of Wnt signaling in breast cancer are highlighted. It is well established that non-canonical Wnt signaling is similar in development and cancer but yields two distinct outcomes. Non-canonical Wnt signaling results in tissue mobility in development but metastasis in cancer. The interaction of canonical and non-canonical Wnt pathways and the mechanisms underlying their tissue-specific regulation are also highlighted. Several Wnt-targeted agents are now undergoing clinical trials Table **2**, but historically, Wnt signaling has been difficult to target clinically. Wnt signaling is a ubiquitous developmental and regulatory pathway present in several cells and tissue types in the body. This makes non-specific targeting of non-malignant tissue an issue. Another concern is Wnt's significant role in stem cell regulation and tissue/organ regeneration. Wnt inhibitors/modulators could drastically affect normal stem cell populations and be detrimental to tissue regeneration. To date, no Wnt-inhibitors have been approved by the FDA.

Wnt inhibition can also synergize with other therapies for cancer. Modulating Wnt pathway activity can increase cancer cell sensitivity to chemotherapy [68]. Novel Wnt inhibitor, OMP-18RF, when combined with paclitaxel in lung and breast cancer models showed an enhanced response [181]. Similarly, other Wnt inhibitors, such as PRI-724, in combination with gemcitabine, showed a better response in pancreatic cancer [182]. In a recent study, we showed that inhibition of non-canonical Wnt receptor, ROR1, with Strictinin, a small molecule, increases breast cancer cell sensitivity to Doxorubicin and Cisplatin [78]. ROR1 inhibition has similarly been shown to potentiate Paclitaxel efficacy in breast cancer [79]. In tumors that proliferate independently of Wnt signaling, Wnt inhibition may be able to render hematopoietic stem cells and gut epithelial cells non-proliferative. Because chemotherapeutic agents typically target hyperproliferative cells, this would protect the cells from side effects that are cell cycle-specific. Higher doses of chemotherapy could then be administered without fear of excess gastrointestinal toxicity or myelosuppression.

There is also significant immunomodulation in Wnt activated tumors [70]. It has been shown that there is an inverse relationship between CD8+ T cell function and β-catenin expression, such that the up-regulated Wnt/ β-catenin signaling is associated with T cell exhaustion, reduced infiltration, and activation [183 - 185]. Combination therapeutic approaches for cancer using Wnt inhibitors, which could concurrently potentiate immunotherapy, might be worth exploring.

In conclusion, various Wnt signaling pathways are summarized and their role in mammary development, oncogenesis and breast cancer progression is discussed. We also highlight naturally occurring Wnt inhibitors and various Wnt-targeted agents being explored in clinical trials. Several studies are currently underway unearthing new regulatory mechanisms for Wnt signaling and potential therapeutic avenues. Undoubtedly, Wnt modulators will soon become potent drug agents for a variety of human malignancies.

ABBREVIATIONS

Fzd	Frizzled receptors
LRP5/6	lipo-protein related protein 5 and 6
ROR	receptor tyrosine-kinase like orphan receptors
RYK	Related to Receptor tyrosine kinase
PORCN	Porcupine
WIF-1	Wnt-inhibitory factor 1
DKKs	Dickkopf proteins
IGFBP4	insulin-like growth-factor binding protein 4
Waif1/5 T4	Wnt-activated inhibitory factor 1

APCDD1	adenomatosis polypsosis coli down regulated 1
BMF	Bone Morphogenic Protein
SFRPS	Secreted frizzled-related proteins
PP2A	Protein phosphatase 2A
CK1α	Casein Kinase 1α
GSK3	Glycogen synthase kinase 3
TCF	T-cell factor
CBP	CREB binding protein
LEF	lymphoid enhancer-binding factor
CtBP	C-terminal-binding protein
PTK7	Tyrosine-Protein Kinase-like 7
NRH1	Neurotrophin Receptor Homolog 1
DAAM	Dvl-associated activator of morphogenesis 1
ROCK	Rho-associated kinase
PCP	Planar Cell Polarity
PKC	protein kinase C
CaMKII	calcium/calmodulin dependent kinase II
VANGL-1	planar cell polarity protein
WIF1	WNT Inhibitory Factor 1
CSC	Cancer stem cell
SOX4	Wnt-associated transcription factor
MMTV	mouse mammary tumor virus
CTNNB1	gene encoding β-catenin
MSL	mesenchymal stem-like
CHEK1	Checkpoint kinase 1
FANCA	Fanconi anaemia, complementation group A
FANCG	Fanconi anemia group G protein
MSH2	MutS homolog 2
RAD21	Double-strand-break repair protein rad21 homolog
AURKB	Aurora B kinase
PLK1	Serine/threonine-protein kinase
CENPA	Centromere protein A
BUB1	Mitotic checkpoint serine/threonine-protein kinase BUB1
CCNA2	Cyclin-A2
NRAS	Neuroblastoma RAS viral oncogene homolog

PRC1	Protein Regulator of cytokinesis 1
BCL9	B-cell CLL/lymphoma 9 protein
TAZ	Tafazzin
IGF2	Insulin Like Growth Factor 2
TNBC	Triple negative breast cancer
VEGF	vascular endothelial growth factor
EGCG	epigallocatechin-3-gallate
NF-ƙB	nuclear factor kappa-light-chain-enhancer of activated B cells

CONSENT FOR PUBLICATION

Not applicable.

CONFLICT OF INTEREST

The author declares that there is no conflict of interest in this chapter.

ACKNOWLEDGEMENTS

Declared none.

REFERENCES

[1] Gurney A, Axelrod F, Bond CJ, *et al.* Wnt pathway inhibition *via* the targeting of Frizzled receptors results in decreased growth and tumorigenicity of human tumors. Proc Natl Acad Sci USA 2012; 109(29): 11717-22.
[http://dx.doi.org/10.1073/pnas.1120068109] [PMID: 22753465]

[2] Medema JP. Cancer stem cells: the challenges ahead. Nat Cell Biol 2013; 15(4): 338-44.
[http://dx.doi.org/10.1038/ncb2717] [PMID: 23548926]

[3] Mohinta S, Wu H, Chaurasia P, Watabe K. Wnt pathway and breast cancer. Front Biosci 2007; 12: 4020-33.
[http://dx.doi.org/10.2741/2368] [PMID: 17485355]

[4] Janda CY, Waghray D, Levin AM, Thomas C, Garcia KC. Structural basis of Wnt recognition by Frizzled. Science 2012; 337(6090): 59-64.
[http://dx.doi.org/10.1126/science.1222879] [PMID: 22653731]

[5] Baker NE. Molecular cloning of sequences from wingless, a segment polarity gene in Drosophila: the spatial distribution of a transcript in embryos. EMBO J 1987; 6(6): 1765-73.
[http://dx.doi.org/10.1002/j.1460-2075.1987.tb02429.x] [PMID: 16453776]

[6] Logan CY, Nusse R. The Wnt signaling pathway in development and disease. Annu Rev Cell Dev Biol 2004; 20: 781-810.
[http://dx.doi.org/10.1146/annurev.cellbio.20.010403.113126] [PMID: 15473860]

[7] Kahn M. Can we safely target the WNT pathway? Nat Rev Drug Discov 2014; 13(7): 513-32.
[http://dx.doi.org/10.1038/nrd4233] [PMID: 24981364]

[8] Bilić J, Huang YL, Davidson G, *et al.* Wnt induces LRP6 signalosomes and promotes dishevelled-dependent LRP6 phosphorylation. Science 2007; 316(5831): 1619-22.

[http://dx.doi.org/10.1126/science.1137065] [PMID: 17569865]

[9]   Cruciat C-M, Niehrs C. Secreted and transmembrane wnt inhibitors and activators. Cold Spring Harb Perspect Biol 2013; 5(3): a015081.
[http://dx.doi.org/10.1101/cshperspect.a015081] [PMID: 23085770]

[10]   Liu J, Pan S, Hsieh MH, *et al.* Targeting Wnt-driven cancer through the inhibition of Porcupine by LGK974. Proc Natl Acad Sci USA 2013; 110(50): 20224-9.
[http://dx.doi.org/10.1073/pnas.1314239110] [PMID: 24277854]

[11]   Madan B, Ke Z, Harmston N, *et al.* Wnt addiction of genetically defined cancers reversed by PORCN inhibition. Oncogene 2016; 35(17): 2197-207.
[http://dx.doi.org/10.1038/onc.2015.280] [PMID: 26257057]

[12]   Esteve P, Sandonìs A, Cardozo M, *et al.* SFRPs act as negative modulators of ADAM10 to regulate retinal neurogenesis. Nat Neurosci 2011; 14(5): 562-9.
[http://dx.doi.org/10.1038/nn.2794] [PMID: 21478884]

[13]   Kagey MH, He X. Rationale for targeting the Wnt signalling modulator Dickkopf-1 for oncology. Br J Pharmacol 2017; 174(24): 4637-50.
[http://dx.doi.org/10.1111/bph.13894] [PMID: 28574171]

[14]   Lee HX, Ambrosio AL, Reversade B, De Robertis EM. Embryonic dorsal-ventral signaling: secreted frizzled-related proteins as inhibitors of tolloid proteinases. Cell 2006; 124(1): 147-59.
[http://dx.doi.org/10.1016/j.cell.2005.12.018] [PMID: 16413488]

[15]   Yang-Snyder J, Miller JR, Brown JD, Lai C-J, Moon RT. A frizzled homolog functions in a vertebrate Wnt signaling pathway. Curr Biol 1996; 6(10): 1302-6.
[http://dx.doi.org/10.1016/S0960-9822(02)70716-1] [PMID: 8939578]

[16]   López-Knowles E, Zardawi SJ, McNeil CM, *et al.* Cytoplasmic localization of β-catenin is a marker of poor outcome in breast cancer patients. Cancer Epidemiol Biomarkers Prev 2010; 19(1): 301-9.
[http://dx.doi.org/10.1158/1055-9965.EPI-09-0741] [PMID: 20056651]

[17]   Zeng X, Huang H, Tamai K, *et al.* Initiation of Wnt signaling: control of Wnt coreceptor Lrp6 phosphorylation/activation *via* frizzled, dishevelled and axin functions. Development 2008; 135(2): 367-75.
[http://dx.doi.org/10.1242/dev.013540] [PMID: 18077588]

[18]   Rao TP, Kühl M. An updated overview on Wnt signaling pathways: a prelude for more. Circ Res 2010; 106(12): 1798-806.
[http://dx.doi.org/10.1161/CIRCRESAHA.110.219840] [PMID: 20576942]

[19]   MacDonald BT, Tamai K, He X. Wnt/β-catenin signaling: components, mechanisms, and diseases. Dev Cell 2009; 17(1): 9-26.
[http://dx.doi.org/10.1016/j.devcel.2009.06.016] [PMID: 19619488]

[20]   Minde DP, Anvarian Z, Rüdiger SG, Maurice MM. Messing up disorder: how do missense mutations in the tumor suppressor protein APC lead to cancer? Mol Cancer 2011; 10: 101.
[http://dx.doi.org/10.1186/1476-4598-10-101] [PMID: 21859464]

[21]   Gammons MV, Renko M, Johnson CM, Rutherford TJ, Bienz M. Wnt signalosome assembly by DEP domain swapping of Dishevelled. Mol Cell 2016; 64(1): 92-104.
[http://dx.doi.org/10.1016/j.molcel.2016.08.026] [PMID: 27692984]

[22]   Gammons MV, Rutherford TJ, Steinhart Z, Angers S, Bienz M. Essential role of the dishevelled DEP domain in a Wnt-dependent human-cell-based complementation assay. J Cell Sci 2016; 129(20): 3892-902.
[http://dx.doi.org/10.1242/jcs.195685] [PMID: 27744318]

[23]   Schwarz-Romond T, Merrifield C, Nichols BJ, Bienz M. The Wnt signalling effector Dishevelled forms dynamic protein assemblies rather than stable associations with cytoplasmic vesicles. J Cell Sci 2005; 118(Pt 22): 5269-77.

[http://dx.doi.org/10.1242/jcs.02646] [PMID: 16263762]

[24]   Wong H-C, Bourdelas A, Krauss A, *et al.* Direct binding of the PDZ domain of Dishevelled to a conserved internal sequence in the C-terminal region of Frizzled. Mol Cell 2003; 12(5): 1251-60.
[http://dx.doi.org/10.1016/S1097-2765(03)00427-1] [PMID: 14636582]

[25]   Davidson G, Wu W, Shen J, *et al.* Casein kinase 1 γ couples Wnt receptor activation to cytoplasmic signal transduction. Nature 2005; 438(7069): 867-72.
[http://dx.doi.org/10.1038/nature04170] [PMID: 16341016]

[26]   Fiedler M, Mendoza-Topaz C, Rutherford TJ, Mieszczanek J, Bienz M. Dishevelled interacts with the DIX domain polymerization interface of Axin to interfere with its function in down-regulating β-catenin. Proc Natl Acad Sci USA 2011; 108(5): 1937-42.
[http://dx.doi.org/10.1073/pnas.1017063108] [PMID: 21245303]

[27]   Hecht A, Vleminckx K, Stemmler MP, van Roy F, Kemler R. The p300/CBP acetyltransferases function as transcriptional coactivators of β-catenin in vertebrates. EMBO J 2000; 19(8): 1839-50.
[http://dx.doi.org/10.1093/emboj/19.8.1839] [PMID: 10775268]

[28]   Mosimann C, Hausmann G, Basler K. Parafibromin/Hyrax activates Wnt/Wg target gene transcription by direct association with β-catenin/Armadillo. Cell 2006; 125(2): 327-41.
[http://dx.doi.org/10.1016/j.cell.2006.01.053] [PMID: 16630820]

[29]   Städeli R, Hoffmans R, Basler K. Transcription under the control of nuclear Arm/β-catenin. Curr Biol 2006; 16(10): R378-85.
[http://dx.doi.org/10.1016/j.cub.2006.04.019] [PMID: 16713950]

[30]   Kim TW, Kwak S, Shin J, *et al.* Ctbp2-mediated β-catenin regulation is required for exit from pluripotency. Exp Mol Med 2017; 49(10): e385-5.
[http://dx.doi.org/10.1038/emm.2017.147] [PMID: 29026198]

[31]   Fang M, Li J, Blauwkamp T, Bhambhani C, Campbell N, Cadigan KM. C-terminal-binding protein directly activates and represses Wnt transcriptional targets in Drosophila. EMBO J 2006; 25(12): 2735-45.
[http://dx.doi.org/10.1038/sj.emboj.7601153] [PMID: 16710294]

[32]   Kumar A, Chalamalasetty RB, Kennedy MW, *et al.* Zfp703 is a Wnt/β-catenin feedback suppressor targeting the β-catenin/Tcf1 complex. Mol Cell Biol 2016; 36(12): 1793-802.
[http://dx.doi.org/10.1128/MCB.01010-15] [PMID: 27090637]

[33]   Staal FJ, Luis TC, Tiemessen MM. WNT signalling in the immune system: WNT is spreading its wings. Nat Rev Immunol 2008; 8(8): 581-93.
[http://dx.doi.org/10.1038/nri2360] [PMID: 18617885]

[34]   Costa AMS, Pereira-Castro I, Ricardo E, Spencer F, Fisher S, da Costa LT. GRG5/AES interacts with T-cell factor 4 (TCF4) and downregulates Wnt signaling in human cells and zebrafish embryos. PLoS One 2013; 8(7): e67694.
[http://dx.doi.org/10.1371/journal.pone.0067694] [PMID: 23840876]

[35]   Azzolin L, Panciera T, Soligo S, *et al.* YAP/TAZ incorporation in the β-catenin destruction complex orchestrates the Wnt response. Cell 2014; 158(1): 157-70.
[http://dx.doi.org/10.1016/j.cell.2014.06.013] [PMID: 24976009]

[36]   Piccolo S, Dupont S, Cordenonsi M. The biology of YAP/TAZ: hippo signaling and beyond. Physiol Rev 2014; 94(4): 1287-312.
[http://dx.doi.org/10.1152/physrev.00005.2014] [PMID: 25287865]

[37]   de Sousa E Melo F, Vermeulen L. Wnt signaling in cancer stem cell biology. Cancers (Basel) 2016; 8(7): 60.
[http://dx.doi.org/10.3390/cancers8070060] [PMID: 27355964]

[38]   Braune E-B, Seshire A, Lendahl U. Notch and Wnt dysregulation and its relevance for breast cancer and tumor initiation. Biomedicines 2018; 6(4): 101.

[http://dx.doi.org/10.3390/biomedicines6040101] [PMID: 30388742]

[39] Prockop DJ, Gregory CA, Spees JL. One strategy for cell and gene therapy: harnessing the power of adult stem cells to repair tissues. Proc Natl Acad Sci USA 2003; 100 (Suppl. 1): 11917-23.
[http://dx.doi.org/10.1073/pnas.1834138100] [PMID: 13679583]

[40] Seifert JR, Mlodzik M. Frizzled/PCP signalling: a conserved mechanism regulating cell polarity and directed motility. Nat Rev Genet 2007; 8(2): 126-38.
[http://dx.doi.org/10.1038/nrg2042] [PMID: 17230199]

[41] Barrow JR. Wnt/PCP signaling: a veritable polar star in establishing patterns of polarity in embryonic tissues. Semin Cell Dev Biol 2006; 17(2): 185-93.
[http://dx.doi.org/10.1016/j.semcdb.2006.04.002] [PMID: 16765615]

[42] https://www.frontiersin.org/articles/10.3389/fcell.2020.00025/full

[43] https://www.spandidos-publications.com/10.3892/or.2019.7424

[44] Amano M, Nakayama M, Kaibuchi K. Rho-kinase/ROCK: A key regulator of the cytoskeleton and cell polarity. Cytoskeleton (Hoboken) 2010; 67(9): 545-54.
[http://dx.doi.org/10.1002/cm.20472] [PMID: 20803696]

[45] Gordon MD, Nusse R. Wnt signaling: multiple pathways, multiple receptors, and multiple transcription factors. J Biol Chem 2006; 281(32): 22429-33.
[http://dx.doi.org/10.1074/jbc.R600015200] [PMID: 16793760]

[46] Hayes M, Naito M, Daulat A, Angers S, Ciruna B. Ptk7 promotes non-canonical Wnt/PCP-mediated morphogenesis and inhibits Wnt/β-catenin-dependent cell fate decisions during vertebrate development. Development 2013; 140(8): 1807-18.
[http://dx.doi.org/10.1242/dev.090183] [PMID: 23533179]

[47] Kohn AD, Moon RT. Wnt and calcium signaling: β-catenin-independent pathways. Cell Calcium 2005; 38(3-4): 439-46.
[http://dx.doi.org/10.1016/j.ceca.2005.06.022] [PMID: 16099039]

[48] Wang H, Lee Y, Malbon CC. PDE6 is an effector for the Wnt/Ca^{2+}/cGMP-signalling pathway in development. Biochem Soc Trans 2004; 32(Pt 5): 792-6.
[http://dx.doi.org/10.1042/BST0320792] [PMID: 15494017]

[49] Komiya Y, Habas R. Wnt signal transduction pathways. Organogenesis 2008; 4(2): 68-75.
[http://dx.doi.org/10.4161/org.4.2.5851] [PMID: 19279717]

[50] Anastas JN, Biechele TL, Robitaille M, *et al.* A protein complex of SCRIB, NOS1AP and VANGL1 regulates cell polarity and migration, and is associated with breast cancer progression. Oncogene 2012; 31(32): 3696-708.
[http://dx.doi.org/10.1038/onc.2011.528] [PMID: 22179838]

[51] Puvirajesinghe TM, Bertucci F, Jain A, *et al.* Identification of p62/SQSTM1 as a component of non-canonical Wnt VANGL2-JNK signalling in breast cancer. Nat Commun 2016; 7: 10318.
[http://dx.doi.org/10.1038/ncomms10318] [PMID: 26754771]

[52] Corda G, Sala G, Lattanzio R, *et al.* Functional and prognostic significance of the genomic amplification of frizzled 6 (FZD6) in breast cancer. J Pathol 2017; 241(3): 350-61.
[http://dx.doi.org/10.1002/path.4841] [PMID: 27859262]

[53] Malinauskas T, Aricescu AR, Lu W, Siebold C, Jones EY. Modular mechanism of Wnt signaling inhibition by Wnt inhibitory factor 1. Nat Struct Mol Biol 2011; 18(8): 886-93.
[http://dx.doi.org/10.1038/nsmb.2081] [PMID: 21743455]

[54] Semënov MV, He X. Secreted antagonists/modulators of Wnt Signaling. Madame Curie Bioscience Database. Landes Bioscience 2000-2013.

[55] Zhu W, Shiojima I, Ito Y, *et al.* IGFBP-4 is an inhibitor of canonical Wnt signalling required for cardiogenesis. Nature 2008; 454(7202): 345-9.

[http://dx.doi.org/10.1038/nature07027] [PMID: 18528331]

[56]   Chen J-Z, Wang S, Tang R, *et al.* Cloning and identification of a cDNA that encodes a novel human protein with thrombospondin type I repeat domain, hPWTSR. Mol Biol Rep 2002; 29(3): 287-92.
[http://dx.doi.org/10.1023/A:1020479301379] [PMID: 12463421]

[57]   Kazanskaya O, Glinka A, del Barco Barrantes I, Stannek P, Niehrs C, Wu W. R-Spondin2 is a secreted activator of Wnt/β-catenin signaling and is required for Xenopus myogenesis. Dev Cell 2004; 7(4): 525-34.
[http://dx.doi.org/10.1016/j.devcel.2004.07.019] [PMID: 15469841]

[58]   Hao H-X, Xie Y, Zhang Y, *et al.* ZNRF3 promotes Wnt receptor turnover in an R-spondin-sensitive manner. Nature 2012; 485(7397): 195-200.
[http://dx.doi.org/10.1038/nature11019] [PMID: 22575959]

[59]   Hatina J, Fernandes MI, Hoffmann MJ, Zeimet AG. Cancer Stem Cells – Basic Biological Properties and Experimental Approaches in eLS. American Cancer Society 2013.

[60]   Weissman IL. Stem cells: units of development, units of regeneration, and units in evolution. Cell 2000; 100(1): 157-68.
[http://dx.doi.org/10.1016/S0092-8674(00)81692-X] [PMID: 10647940]

[61]   Nishita M, Yoo SK, Nomachi A, *et al.* Filopodia formation mediated by receptor tyrosine kinase Ror2 is required for Wnt5a-induced cell migration. J Cell Biol 2006; 175(4): 555-62.
[http://dx.doi.org/10.1083/jcb.200607127] [PMID: 17101698]

[62]   Adler PN. The frizzled/stan pathway and planar cell polarity in the Drosophila wing. Curr Top Dev Biol 2012; 101: 1-31.

[63]   Lindvall C, Bu W, Williams BO, Li Y. Wnt signaling, stem cells, and the cellular origin of breast cancer. Stem Cell Rev 2007; 3(2): 157-68.
[http://dx.doi.org/10.1007/s12015-007-0025-3] [PMID: 17873348]

[64]   Shackleton M, Vaillant F, Simpson KJ, *et al.* Generation of a functional mammary gland from a single stem cell. Nature 2006; 439(7072): 84-8.
[http://dx.doi.org/10.1038/nature04372] [PMID: 16397499]

[65]   Lindvall C, Evans NC, Zylstra CR, Li Y, Alexander CM, Williams BO. The Wnt signaling receptor Lrp5 is required for mammary ductal stem cell activity and Wnt1-induced tumorigenesis. J Biol Chem 2006; 281(46): 35081-7.
[http://dx.doi.org/10.1074/jbc.M607571200] [PMID: 16973609]

[66]   Ginestier C, Hur MH, Charafe-Jauffret E, *et al.* ALDH1 is a marker of normal and malignant human mammary stem cells and a predictor of poor clinical outcome. Cell Stem Cell 2007; 1(5): 555-67.
[http://dx.doi.org/10.1016/j.stem.2007.08.014] [PMID: 18371393]

[67]   Al-Hajj M, Wicha MS, Benito-Hernandez A, Morrison SJ, Clarke MF. Prospective identification of tumorigenic breast cancer cells. Proc Natl Acad Sci USA 2003; 100(7): 3983-8.
[http://dx.doi.org/10.1073/pnas.0530291100] [PMID: 12629218]

[68]   Zhang ZM, Wu JF, Luo QC, *et al.* Pygo2 activates MDR1 expression and mediates chemoresistance in breast cancer *via* the Wnt/β-catenin pathway. Oncogene 2016; 35(36): 4787-97.
[http://dx.doi.org/10.1038/onc.2016.10] [PMID: 26876203]

[69]   Spranger S, Gajewski TF. A new paradigm for tumor immune escape: β-catenin-driven immune exclusion. J Immunother Cancer 2015; 3: 43.
[http://dx.doi.org/10.1186/s40425-015-0089-6] [PMID: 26380088]

[70]   Martin-Orozco E, Sanchez-Fernandez A, Ortiz-Parra I, Ayala-San Nicolas M. WNT signaling in tumors: the way to evade drugs and immunity. Front Immunol 2019; 10: 2854.
[http://dx.doi.org/10.3389/fimmu.2019.02854] [PMID: 31921125]

[71]   Noman MZ, Van Moer K, Marani V, *et al.* CD47 is a direct target of SNAI1 and ZEB1 and its

blockade activates the phagocytosis of breast cancer cells undergoing EMT. OncoImmunology 2018; 7(4): e1345415.
[http://dx.doi.org/10.1080/2162402X.2017.1345415] [PMID: 29632713]

[72] Castagnoli L, Cancila V, Cordoba-Romero SL, *et al.* WNT signaling modulates PD-L1 expression in the stem cell compartment of triple-negative breast cancer. Oncogene 2019; 38(21): 4047-60.
[http://dx.doi.org/10.1038/s41388-019-0700-2] [PMID: 30705400]

[73] Khramtsov AI, Khramtsova GF, Tretiakova M, Huo D, Olopade OI, Goss KH. Wnt/β-catenin pathway activation is enriched in basal-like breast cancers and predicts poor outcome. Am J Pathol 2010; 176(6): 2911-20.
[http://dx.doi.org/10.2353/ajpath.2010.091125] [PMID: 20395444]

[74] Ma F, Li H, Wang H, *et al.* Enriched CD44(+)/CD24(-) population drives the aggressive phenotypes presented in triple-negative breast cancer (TNBC). Cancer Lett 2014; 353(2): 153-9.
[http://dx.doi.org/10.1016/j.canlet.2014.06.022] [PMID: 25130168]

[75] Honeth G, Bendahl PO, Ringnér M, *et al.* The CD44+/CD24- phenotype is enriched in basal-like breast tumors. Breast Cancer Res 2008; 10(3): R53.
[http://dx.doi.org/10.1186/bcr2108] [PMID: 18559090]

[76] Li H, Ma F, Wang H, *et al.* Stem cell marker aldehyde dehydrogenase 1 (ALDH1)-expressing cells are enriched in triple-negative breast cancer. Int J Biol Markers 2013; 28(4): e357-64.
[http://dx.doi.org/10.5301/JBM.5000048] [PMID: 24338721]

[77] Jang G-B, Kim JY, Cho SD, *et al.* Blockade of Wnt/β-catenin signaling suppresses breast cancer metastasis by inhibiting CSC-like phenotype. Sci Rep 2015; 5: 12465.
[http://dx.doi.org/10.1038/srep12465] [PMID: 26202299]

[78] Fultang N, Illendula A, Lin J, Pandey MK, Klase Z, Peethambaran B. ROR1 regulates chemoresistance in Breast Cancer *via* modulation of drug efflux pump ABCB1. Sci Rep 2020; 10(1): 1821.
[http://dx.doi.org/10.1038/s41598-020-58864-0] [PMID: 32020017]

[79] Zhang S, Zhang H, Ghia EM, *et al.* Inhibition of chemotherapy resistant breast cancer stem cells by a ROR1 specific antibody. Proc Natl Acad Sci USA 2019; 116(4): 1370-7.
[http://dx.doi.org/10.1073/pnas.1816262116] [PMID: 30622177]

[80] Zhang S, Chen L, Cui B, *et al.* ROR1 is expressed in human breast cancer and associated with enhanced tumor-cell growth. PLoS One 2012; 7(3): e31127.
[http://dx.doi.org/10.1371/journal.pone.0031127] [PMID: 22403610]

[81] Fultang N, Illendula A, Chen B, *et al.* Strictinin, a novel ROR1-inhibitor, represses triple negative breast cancer survival and migration *via* modulation of PI3K/AKT/GSK3ß activity. PLoS One 2019; 14(5): e0217789.
[http://dx.doi.org/10.1371/journal.pone.0217789] [PMID: 31150511]

[82] van Genderen C, Okamura RM, Fariñas I, *et al.* Development of several organs that require inductive epithelial-mesenchymal interactions is impaired in LEF-1-deficient mice. Genes Dev 1994; 8(22): 2691-703.
[http://dx.doi.org/10.1101/gad.8.22.2691] [PMID: 7958926]

[83] Brisken C, Heineman A, Chavarria T, *et al.* Essential function of Wnt-4 in mammary gland development downstream of progesterone signaling. Genes Dev 2000; 14(6): 650-4.
[PMID: 10733525]

[84] Bradbury JM, Edwards PA, Niemeyer CC, Dale TC. Wnt-4 expression induces a pregnancy-like growth pattern in reconstituted mammary glands in virgin mice. Dev Biol 1995; 170(2): 553-63.
[http://dx.doi.org/10.1006/dbio.1995.1236] [PMID: 7649383]

[85] Christiansen JH, Dennis CL, Wicking CA, Monkley SJ, Wilkinson DG, Wainwright BJ. Murine Wnt-11 and Wnt-12 have temporally and spatially restricted expression patterns during embryonic

development. Mech Dev 1995; 51(2-3): 341-50.
[http://dx.doi.org/10.1016/0925-4773(95)00383-5] [PMID: 7547479]

[86]   Sutherland RL, Musgrove EA. Cyclins and breast cancer. J Mammary Gland Biol Neoplasia 2004;
       9(1): 95-104.
       [http://dx.doi.org/10.1023/B:JOMG.0000023591.45568.77] [PMID: 15082921]

[87]   Schroeder JA, *et al.* ErbB/beta-catenin complexes are associated with human infiltrating ductal breast
       and MMTV-Wnt-1 and MMTV-c-neu transgenic carcinomas. J Biol Chem 2002; 277: 22692-8.
       [http://dx.doi.org/10.1074/jbc.M201975200] [PMID: 11950845]

[88]   Matsuda Y, Schlange T, Oakeley EJ, Boulay A, Hynes NE. WNT signaling enhances breast cancer
       cell motility and blockade of the WNT pathway by sFRP1 suppresses MDA-MB-231 xenograft
       growth. Breast Cancer Res 2009; 11(3): R32.
       [http://dx.doi.org/10.1186/bcr2317] [PMID: 19473496]

[89]   Zhu Y, Tian Y, Du J, *et al.* Dvl2-dependent activation of Daam1 and RhoA regulates Wnt5a-induced
       breast cancer cell migration. PLoS One 2012; 7(5): e37823.
       [http://dx.doi.org/10.1371/journal.pone.0037823] [PMID: 22655072]

[90]   Xu J, Prosperi JR, Choudhury N, Olopade OI, Goss KH. β-catenin is required for the tumorigenic
       behavior of triple-negative breast cancer cells. PLoS One 2015; 10(2): e0117097.
       [http://dx.doi.org/10.1371/journal.pone.0117097] [PMID: 25658419]

[91]   Schroeder JA, Troyer KL, Lee DC. Cooperative induction of mammary tumorigenesis by TGF alpha
       and Wnts. Oncogene 2000; 19(28): 3193-9.
       [http://dx.doi.org/10.1038/sj.onc.1203652] [PMID: 10918574]

[92]   Bilir B, Kucuk O, Moreno CS. Wnt signaling blockage inhibits cell proliferation and migration, and
       induces apoptosis in triple-negative breast cancer cells. J Transl Med 2013; 11: 280.
       [http://dx.doi.org/10.1186/1479-5876-11-280] [PMID: 24188694]

[93]   Sawyer EJ, Hanby AM, Rowan AJ, *et al.* The Wnt pathway, epithelial-stromal interactions, and
       malignant progression in phyllodes tumours. J Pathol 2002; 196(4): 437-44.
       [http://dx.doi.org/10.1002/path.1067] [PMID: 11920740]

[94]   Farago M, Dominguez I, Landesman-Bollag E, *et al.* Kinase-inactive glycogen synthase kinase 3β
       promotes Wnt signaling and mammary tumorigenesis. Cancer Res 2005; 65(13): 5792-801.
       [http://dx.doi.org/10.1158/0008-5472.CAN-05-1021] [PMID: 15994955]

[95]   Landesman-Bollag E, Romieu-Mourez R, Song DH, Sonenshein GE, Cardiff RD, Seldin DC. Protein
       kinase CK2 in mammary gland tumorigenesis. Oncogene 2001; 20(25): 3247-57.
       [http://dx.doi.org/10.1038/sj.onc.1204411] [PMID: 11423974]

[96]   Maubant S, Maire V, Tesson B, *et al.* The depletion of LRP5, unlike that of LRP6, promotes apoptosis
       in triple-negative breast cancer cells, making it an interesting therapeutic target. AACR 2014.

[97]   Ugolini F, Charafe-Jauffret E, Bardou VJ, *et al.* WNT pathway and mammary carcinogenesis: loss of
       expression of candidate tumor suppressor gene SFRP1 in most invasive carcinomas except of the
       medullary type. Oncogene 2001; 20(41): 5810-7.
       [http://dx.doi.org/10.1038/sj.onc.1204706] [PMID: 11593386]

[98]   Howe LR, Brown AM. Wnt signaling and breast cancer. Cancer Biol Ther 2004; 3(1): 36-41.
       [http://dx.doi.org/10.4161/cbt.3.1.561] [PMID: 14739782]

[99]   Taketo MM. Shutting down Wnt signal-activated cancer. Nat Genet 2004; 36(4): 320-2.
       [http://dx.doi.org/10.1038/ng0404-320] [PMID: 15054482]

[100] Serman L, Nikuseva Martic T, Serman A, Vranic S. Epigenetic alterations of the Wnt signaling
       pathway in cancer: a mini review. Bosn J Basic Med Sci 2014; 14(4): 191-4.
       [http://dx.doi.org/10.17305/bjbms.2014.4.205] [PMID: 25428669]

[101] Nusse R, Varmus HE. Many tumors induced by the mouse mammary tumor virus contain a provirus

integrated in the same region of the host genome. Cell 1982; 31(1): 99-109.
[http://dx.doi.org/10.1016/0092-8674(82)90409-3] [PMID: 6297757]

[102] Beghini A, Lazzaroni F. WNT10B (wingless-type MMTV integration site family). 2017.

[103] Patel S, Doble BW, MacAulay K, Sinclair EM, Drucker DJ, Woodgett JR. Tissue-specific role of glycogen synthase kinase 3β in glucose homeostasis and insulin action. Mol Cell Biol 2008; 28(20): 6314-28.
[http://dx.doi.org/10.1128/MCB.00763-08] [PMID: 18694957]

[104] Gaspar C, Franken P, Molenaar L, *et al.* A targeted constitutive mutation in the APC tumor suppressor gene underlies mammary but not intestinal tumorigenesis. PLoS Genet 2009; 5(7): e1000547.
[http://dx.doi.org/10.1371/journal.pgen.1000547] [PMID: 19578404]

[105] Landesman-Bollag E, Song DH, Romieu-Mourez R, *et al.* Protein kinase CK2: signaling and tumorigenesis in the mammary gland. Mol Cell Biochem 2001; 227(1-2): 153-65.
[http://dx.doi.org/10.1023/A:1013108822847] [PMID: 11827167]

[106] Gao Y, Wang HY. Casein kinase 2 Is activated and essential for Wnt/β-catenin signaling. J Biol Chem 2006; 281(27): 18394-400.
[http://dx.doi.org/10.1074/jbc.M601112200] [PMID: 16672224]

[107] Foulkes WD, Smith IE, Reis-Filho JS. Triple-negative breast cancer. N Engl J Med 2010; 363(20): 1938-48.
[http://dx.doi.org/10.1056/NEJMra1001389] [PMID: 21067385]

[108] Dey N, Barwick BG, Moreno CS, *et al.* Wnt signaling in triple negative breast cancer is associated with metastasis. BMC Cancer 2013; 13: 537.
[http://dx.doi.org/10.1186/1471-2407-13-537] [PMID: 24209998]

[109] Fatima I, El-Ayachi I, Playa HC, *et al.* Simultaneous Multi-Organ Metastases from Chemo-Resistant Triple-Negative Breast Cancer Are Prevented by Interfering with WNT-Signaling. Cancers (Basel) 2019; 11(12): 2039.
[http://dx.doi.org/10.3390/cancers11122039] [PMID: 31861131]

[110] King TD, Suto MJ, Li Y. The Wnt/β-catenin signaling pathway: a potential therapeutic target in the treatment of triple negative breast cancer. J Cell Biochem 2012; 113(1): 13-8.
[http://dx.doi.org/10.1002/jcb.23350] [PMID: 21898546]

[111] Geyer FC, Lacroix-Triki M, Savage K, *et al.* β-catenin pathway activation in breast cancer is associated with triple-negative phenotype but not with CTNNB1 mutation. Mod Pathol 2011; 24(2): 209-31.
[http://dx.doi.org/10.1038/modpathol.2010.205] [PMID: 21076461]

[112] Schade B, Lesurf R, Sanguin-Gendreau V, *et al.* β-catenin signaling is a critical event in ErbB2-mediated mammary tumor progression. Cancer Res 2013; 73(14): 4474-87.
[http://dx.doi.org/10.1158/0008-5472.CAN-12-3925] [PMID: 23720052]

[113] O'Brien CA, Kreso A, Jamieson CH. Cancer stem cells and self-renewal. Clin Cancer Res 2010; 16(12): 3113-20.
[http://dx.doi.org/10.1158/1078-0432.CCR-09-2824] [PMID: 20530701]

[114] Pohl S-G, Brook N, Agostino M, Arfuso F, Kumar AP, Dharmarajan A. Wnt signaling in triple-negative breast cancer. Oncogenesis 2017; 6(4): e310-0.
[http://dx.doi.org/10.1038/oncsis.2017.14] [PMID: 28368389]

[115] Lehmann BD, Bauer JA, Chen X, *et al.* Identification of human triple-negative breast cancer subtypes and preclinical models for selection of targeted therapies. J Clin Invest 2011; 121(7): 2750-67.
[http://dx.doi.org/10.1172/JCI45014] [PMID: 21633166]

[116] Burstein MD, Tsimelzon A, Poage GM, *et al.* Comprehensive genomic analysis identifies novel subtypes and targets of triple-negative breast cancer. Clin Cancer Res 2015; 21(7): 1688-98.
[http://dx.doi.org/10.1158/1078-0432.CCR-14-0432] [PMID: 25208879]

[117]   Abramson VG, Lehmann BD, Ballinger TJ, Pietenpol JA. Subtyping of triple-negative breast cancer: implications for therapy. Cancer 2015; 121(1): 8-16.
[http://dx.doi.org/10.1002/cncr.28914] [PMID: 25043972]

[118]   Huard CC, Tremblay CS, Magron A, Lévesque G, Carreau M. The Fanconi anemia pathway has a dual function in Dickkopf-1 transcriptional repression. Proc Natl Acad Sci USA 2014; 111(6): 2152-7.
[http://dx.doi.org/10.1073/pnas.1314226111] [PMID: 24469828]

[119]   Castiglia D, Bernardini S, Alvino E, *et al.* Concomitant activation of Wnt pathway and loss of mismatch repair function in human melanoma. Genes Chromosomes Cancer 2008; 47(7): 614-24.
[http://dx.doi.org/10.1002/gcc.20567] [PMID: 18384130]

[120]   Xu H, Yan Y, Deb S, *et al.* Cohesin Rad21 mediates loss of heterozygosity and is upregulated *via* Wnt promoting transcriptional dysregulation in gastrointestinal tumors. Cell Rep 2014; 9(5): 1781-97.
[http://dx.doi.org/10.1016/j.celrep.2014.10.059] [PMID: 25464844]

[121]   Huang Y-L, Anvarian Z, Döderlein G, Acebron SP, Niehrs C. Maternal Wnt/STOP signaling promotes cell division during early Xenopus embryogenesis. Proc Natl Acad Sci USA 2015; 112(18): 5732-7.
[http://dx.doi.org/10.1073/pnas.1423533112] [PMID: 25901317]

[122]   Kikuchi K, Niikura Y, Kitagawa K, Kikuchi A. Dishevelled, a Wnt signalling component, is involved in mitotic progression in cooperation with Plk1. EMBO J 2010; 29(20): 3470-83.
[http://dx.doi.org/10.1038/emboj.2010.221] [PMID: 20823832]

[123]   Chiacchiera F, Rossi A, Jammula S, *et al.* Polycomb complex PRC1 preserves intestinal stem cell identity by sustaining Wnt/β-catenin transcriptional activity. Cell Stem Cell 2016; 18(1): 91-103.
[http://dx.doi.org/10.1016/j.stem.2015.09.019] [PMID: 26526724]

[124]   He T-C, Sparks AB, Rago C, *et al.* Identification of c-MYC as a target of the APC pathway. Science 1998; 281(5382): 1509-12.
[http://dx.doi.org/10.1126/science.281.5382.1509] [PMID: 9727977]

[125]   Conrad WH, Swift RD, Biechele TL, Kulikauskas RM, Moon RT, Chien AJ. Regulating the response to targeted MEK inhibition in melanoma: enhancing apoptosis in NRAS- and BRAF-mutant melanoma cells with Wnt/β-catenin activation. Cell Cycle 2012; 11(20): 3724-30.
[http://dx.doi.org/10.4161/cc.21645] [PMID: 22895053]

[126]   Kormish JD, Sinner D, Zorn AM. Interactions between SOX factors and Wnt/β-catenin signaling in development and disease. Dev Dyn 2010; 239(1): 56-68.
[PMID: 19655378]

[127]   Zhang L, Chen X, Stauffer S, Yang S, Chen Y, Dong J. CDK1 phosphorylation of TAZ in mitosis inhibits its oncogenic activity. Oncotarget 2015; 6(31): 31399-412.
[http://dx.doi.org/10.18632/oncotarget.5189] [PMID: 26375055]

[128]   Chen J, Rajasekaran M, Xia H, *et al.* CDK1-mediated BCL9 phosphorylation inhibits clathrin to promote mitotic Wnt signalling. EMBO J 2018; 37(20): e99395.
[http://dx.doi.org/10.15252/embj.201899395] [PMID: 30217955]

[129]   Fu Y, Chang H, Peng X, *et al.* Resveratrol inhibits breast cancer stem-like cells and induces autophagy *via* suppressing Wnt/β-catenin signaling pathway. PLoS One 2014; 9(7): e102535.
[http://dx.doi.org/10.1371/journal.pone.0102535] [PMID: 25068516]

[130]   Hope C, Planutis K, Planutiene M, *et al.* Low concentrations of resveratrol inhibit Wnt signal throughput in colon-derived cells: implications for colon cancer prevention. Mol Nutr Food Res 2008; 52 (Suppl. 1): S52-61.
[http://dx.doi.org/10.1002/mnfr.200700448] [PMID: 18504708]

[131]   Chen H-J, Hsu L-S, Shia Y-T, Lin M-W, Lin C-M. The β-catenin/TCF complex as a novel target of resveratrol in the Wnt/β-catenin signaling pathway. Biochem Pharmacol 2012; 84(9): 1143-53.
[http://dx.doi.org/10.1016/j.bcp.2012.08.011] [PMID: 22935447]

[132] Bhat KP, Lantvit D, Christov K, Mehta RG, Moon RC, Pezzuto JM. Estrogenic and antiestrogenic properties of resveratrol in mammary tumor models. Cancer Res 2001; 61(20): 7456-63. [PMID: 11606380]

[133] Bowers JL, Tyulmenkov VV, Jernigan SC, Klinge CM. Resveratrol acts as a mixed agonist/antagonist for estrogen receptors alpha and beta. Endocrinology 2000; 141(10): 3657-67. [http://dx.doi.org/10.1210/endo.141.10.7721] [PMID: 11014220]

[134] Nguyen AV, Martinez M, Stamos MJ, *et al.* Results of a phase I pilot clinical trial examining the effect of plant-derived resveratrol and grape powder on Wnt pathway target gene expression in colonic mucosa and colon cancer. Cancer Manag Res 2009; 1: 25-37. [http://dx.doi.org/10.2147/CMAR.S4544] [PMID: 21188121]

[135] Vyas S, Asmerom Y, De León DD. Resveratrol regulates insulin-like growth factor-II in breast cancer cells. Endocrinology 2005; 146(10): 4224-33. [http://dx.doi.org/10.1210/en.2004-1344] [PMID: 16037384]

[136] Barroca V, Lewandowski D, Jaracz-Ros A, Hardouin S-N. Paternal Insulin-like Growth Factor 2 (Igf2) Regulates Stem Cell Activity During Adulthood. EBioMedicine 2017; 15: 150-62. [http://dx.doi.org/10.1016/j.ebiom.2016.11.035] [PMID: 28007480]

[137] L. N., OHBOSHI, S. & SOARES, M. J. Akt1 and insulin-like growth factor 2 (Igf2) regulate placentation and fetal/post-natal development. Int J Dev Biol 2012; 56: 255-61. [http://dx.doi.org/10.1387/ijdb.113407lk] [PMID: 22562201]

[138] Zheng W, Duan B, Zhang Q, *et al.* Vitamin D-induced vitamin D receptor expression induces tamoxifen sensitivity in MCF-7 stem cells *via* suppression of Wnt/β-catenin signaling. Biosci Rep 2018; 38(6): BSR20180595. [http://dx.doi.org/10.1042/BSR20180595] [PMID: 30314996]

[139] Akhter J, Chen X, Bowrey P, Bolton EJ, Morris DL. Vitamin D3 analog, EB1089, inhibits growth of subcutaneous xenografts of the human colon cancer cell line, LoVo, in a nude mouse model. Dis Colon Rectum 1997; 40(3): 317-21. [http://dx.doi.org/10.1007/BF02050422] [PMID: 9118747]

[140] Pálmer HG, González-Sancho JM, Espada J, *et al.* Vitamin D(3) promotes the differentiation of colon carcinoma cells by the induction of E-cadherin and the inhibition of β-catenin signaling. J Cell Biol 2001; 154(2): 369-87. [http://dx.doi.org/10.1083/jcb.200102028] [PMID: 11470825]

[141] VanWeelden K, Flanagan L, Binderup L, Tenniswood M, Welsh J. Apoptotic regression of MCF-7 xenografts in nude mice treated with the vitamin D3 analog, EB1089. Endocrinology 1998; 139(4): 2102-10. [http://dx.doi.org/10.1210/endo.139.4.5892] [PMID: 9528999]

[142] Narayan S. Curcumin, a multi-functional chemopreventive agent, blocks growth of colon cancer cells by targeting β-catenin-mediated transactivation and cell-cell adhesion pathways. J Mol Histol 2004; 35(3): 301-7. [http://dx.doi.org/10.1023/B:HIJO.0000032361.98815.bb] [PMID: 15339049]

[143] Li X, Wang X, Xie C, *et al.* Sonic hedgehog and Wnt/β-catenin pathways mediate curcumin inhibition of breast cancer stem cells. Anticancer Drugs 2018; 29(3): 208-15. [http://dx.doi.org/10.1097/CAD.0000000000000584] [PMID: 29356693]

[144] Lee C-K, Chung W-Y, Park K-K. Effects of xanthorrhizol, curcumin and tamoxifen on the expression of vascular endothelial growth factor through Wnt signalnig pathway in human breast cancer cells. Cancer Res 2004; 64: 727-8.

[145] Jaiswal AS, Marlow BP, Gupta N, Narayan S. β-catenin-mediated transactivation and cell-cell adhesion pathways are important in curcumin (diferuylmethane)-induced growth arrest and apoptosis in colon cancer cells. Oncogene 2002; 21(55): 8414-27.

[http://dx.doi.org/10.1038/sj.onc.1205947] [PMID: 12466962]

[146] Soprano DR, Qin P, Soprano KJ. Retinoic acid receptors and cancers. Annu Rev Nutr 2004; 24: 201-21.
[http://dx.doi.org/10.1146/annurev.nutr.24.012003.132407] [PMID: 15189119]

[147] Ryu M-J, Cho M, Song JY, *et al.* Natural derivatives of curcumin attenuate the Wnt/β-catenin pathway through down-regulation of the transcriptional coactivator p300. Biochem Biophys Res Commun 2008; 377(4): 1304-8.
[http://dx.doi.org/10.1016/j.bbrc.2008.10.171] [PMID: 19000900]

[148] Liu Y, Lee MO, Wang HG, *et al.* Retinoic acid receptor beta mediates the growth-inhibitory effect of retinoic acid by promoting apoptosis in human breast cancer cells. Mol Cell Biol 1996; 16(3): 1138-49.
[http://dx.doi.org/10.1128/MCB.16.3.1138] [PMID: 8622658]

[149] Houle B, Rochette-Egly C, Bradley WE. Tumor-suppressive effect of the retinoic acid receptor beta in human epidermoid lung cancer cells. Proc Natl Acad Sci USA 1993; 90(3): 985-9.
[http://dx.doi.org/10.1073/pnas.90.3.985] [PMID: 8381540]

[150] Easwaran V, Pishvaian M, Salimuddin , Byers S. Cross-regulation of β-catenin-LEF/TCF and retinoid signaling pathways. Curr Biol 1999; 9(23): 1415-8.
[http://dx.doi.org/10.1016/S0960-9822(00)80088-3] [PMID: 10607566]

[151] Zhou Q, Stetler-Stevenson M, Steeg PS. Inhibition of cyclin D expression in human breast carcinoma cells by retinoids *in vitro*. Oncogene 1997; 15(1): 107-15.
[http://dx.doi.org/10.1038/sj.onc.1201142] [PMID: 9233783]

[152] Badger TM, Ronis MJ, Simmen RC, Simmen FA. Soy protein isolate and protection against cancer. J Am Coll Nutr 2005; 24(2): 146S-9S.
[http://dx.doi.org/10.1080/07315724.2005.10719456] [PMID: 15798082]

[153] Zhang Y, Chen H. Genistein attenuates WNT signaling by up-regulating sFRP2 in a human colon cancer cell line. Exp Biol Med (Maywood) 2011; 236(6): 714-22.
[http://dx.doi.org/10.1258/ebm.2011.010347] [PMID: 21571909]

[154] Sarkar FH, Li Y, Wang Z, Kong D. Cellular signaling perturbation by natural products. Cell Signal 2009; 21(11): 1541-7.
[http://dx.doi.org/10.1016/j.cellsig.2009.03.009] [PMID: 19298854]

[155] Li Y, Wang Z, Kong D, Li R, Sarkar SH, Sarkar FH. Regulation of Akt/FOXO3a/GSK-3β/AR signaling network by isoflavone in prostate cancer cells. J Biol Chem 2008; 283(41): 27707-16.
[http://dx.doi.org/10.1074/jbc.M802759200] [PMID: 18687691]

[156] Zhang Y, Li Q, Zhou D, Chen H. Genistein, a soya isoflavone, prevents azoxymethane-induced up-regulation of WNT/β-catenin signalling and reduces colon pre-neoplasia in rats. Br J Nutr 2013; 109(1): 33-42.
[http://dx.doi.org/10.1017/S0007114512000876] [PMID: 22716201]

[157] Su Y, Simmen FA, Xiao R, Simmen RC. Expression profiling of rat mammary epithelial cells reveals candidate signaling pathways in dietary protection from mammary tumors. Physiol Genomics 2007; 30(1): 8-16.
[http://dx.doi.org/10.1152/physiolgenomics.00023.2007] [PMID: 17341692]

[158] Su Y, Simmen RC. Soy isoflavone genistein upregulates epithelial adhesion molecule E-cadherin expression and attenuates β-catenin signaling in mammary epithelial cells. Carcinogenesis 2009; 30(2): 331-9.
[http://dx.doi.org/10.1093/carcin/bgn279] [PMID: 19073877]

[159] Lambert JD, Elias RJ. The antioxidant and pro-oxidant activities of green tea polyphenols: a role in cancer prevention. Arch Biochem Biophys 2010; 501(1): 65-72.
[http://dx.doi.org/10.1016/j.abb.2010.06.013] [PMID: 20558130]

[160] Orner GA, Dashwood W-M, Dashwood RH. Tumor-suppressing effects of antioxidants from tea. J Nutr 2004; 134(11): 3177S-8S.
[http://dx.doi.org/10.1093/jn/134.11.3177S] [PMID: 15514295]

[161] Dashwood W-M, Orner GA, Dashwood RH. Inhibition of β-catenin/Tcf activity by white tea, green tea, and epigallocatechin-3-gallate (EGCG): minor contribution of H(2)O(2) at physiologically relevant EGCG concentrations. Biochem Biophys Res Commun 2002; 296(3): 584-8.
[http://dx.doi.org/10.1016/S0006-291X(02)00914-2] [PMID: 12176021]

[162] Kim J, Zhang X, Rieger-Christ KM, *et al.* Suppression of Wnt signaling by the green tea compound (-)-epigallocatechin 3-gallate (EGCG) in invasive breast cancer cells. Requirement of the transcriptional repressor HBP1. J Biol Chem 2006; 281(16): 10865-75.
[http://dx.doi.org/10.1074/jbc.M513378200] [PMID: 16495219]

[163] Melgarejo E, Urdiales JL, Sánchez-Jiménez F, Medina MÁ. Targeting polyamines and biogenic amines by green tea epigallocatechin-3-gallate. Amino Acids 2010; 38(2): 519-23.
[http://dx.doi.org/10.1007/s00726-009-0411-z] [PMID: 19956995]

[164] Carter O, Dashwood RH, Wang R, *et al.* Comparison of white tea, green tea, epigallocatechin--gallate, and caffeine as inhibitors of PhIP-induced colonic aberrant crypts. Nutr Cancer 2007; 58(1): 60-5.
[http://dx.doi.org/10.1080/01635580701308182] [PMID: 17571968]

[165] Saleem M. Lupeol, a novel anti-inflammatory and anti-cancer dietary triterpene. Cancer Lett 2009; 285(2): 109-15.
[http://dx.doi.org/10.1016/j.canlet.2009.04.033] [PMID: 19464787]

[166] Saleem M, Afaq F, Adhami VM, Mukhtar H. Lupeol modulates NF-kappaB and PI3K/Akt pathways and inhibits skin cancer in CD-1 mice. Oncogene 2004; 23(30): 5203-14.
[http://dx.doi.org/10.1038/sj.onc.1207641] [PMID: 15122342]

[167] Tarapore RS, Siddiqui IA, Saleem M, Adhami VM, Spiegelman VS, Mukhtar H. Specific targeting of Wnt/β-catenin signaling in human melanoma cells by a dietary triterpene lupeol. Carcinogenesis 2010; 31(10): 1844-53.
[http://dx.doi.org/10.1093/carcin/bgq169] [PMID: 20732907]

[168] Barnes S. Effect of genistein on *in vitro* and *in vivo* models of cancer. J Nutr 1995; 125(3) (Suppl.): 777S-83S.
[PMID: 7884564]

[169] Lu J, Ma Z, Hsieh JC, *et al.* Structure-activity relationship studies of small-molecule inhibitors of Wnt response. Bioorg Med Chem Lett 2009; 19(14): 3825-7.
[http://dx.doi.org/10.1016/j.bmcl.2009.04.040] [PMID: 19410457]

[170] Huang S-MA, Mishina YM, Liu S, *et al.* Tankyrase inhibition stabilizes axin and antagonizes Wnt signalling. Nature 2009; 461(7264): 614-20.
[http://dx.doi.org/10.1038/nature08356] [PMID: 19759537]

[171] Chen B, Dodge ME, Tang W, *et al.* Small molecule-mediated disruption of Wnt-dependent signaling in tissue regeneration and cancer. Nat Chem Biol 2009; 5(2): 100-7.
[http://dx.doi.org/10.1038/nchembio.137] [PMID: 19125156]

[172] Proffitt KD, Madan B, Ke Z, *et al.* Pharmacological inhibition of the Wnt acyltransferase PORCN prevents growth of WNT-driven mammary cancer. Cancer Res 2013; 73(2): 502-7.
[http://dx.doi.org/10.1158/0008-5472.CAN-12-2258] [PMID: 23188502]

[173] Kulak O, Chen H, Holohan B, *et al.* Disruption of Wnt/β-catenin signaling and telomeric shortening are inextricable consequences of tankyrase inhibition in human cells. Mol Cell Biol 2015; 35(14): 2425-35.
[http://dx.doi.org/10.1128/MCB.00392-15] [PMID: 25939383]

[174] Storm EE, Durinck S, de Sousa e Melo F, *et al.* Targeting PTPRK-RSPO3 colon tumours promotes

differentiation and loss of stem-cell function. Nature 2016; 529(7584): 97-100.
[http://dx.doi.org/10.1038/nature16466] [PMID: 26700806]

[175] Licht-Murava A, Paz R, Vaks L, *et al.* A unique type of GSK-3 inhibitor brings new opportunities to the clinic. Sci Signal 2016; 9(454): ra110-0.
[http://dx.doi.org/10.1126/scisignal.aah7102] [PMID: 27902447]

[176] Canesin G, Evans-Axelsson S, Hellsten R, *et al.* Treatment with the WNT5A-mimicking peptide Foxy-5 effectively reduces the metastatic spread of WNT5A-low prostate cancer cells in an orthotopic mouse model. PLoS One 2017; 12(9): e0184418.
[http://dx.doi.org/10.1371/journal.pone.0184418] [PMID: 28886116]

[177] Steinhart Z, Pavlovic Z, Chandrashekhar M, *et al.* Genome-wide CRISPR screens reveal a Wnt-FZD5 signaling circuit as a druggable vulnerability of RNF43-mutant pancreatic tumors. Nat Med 2017; 23(1): 60-8.
[http://dx.doi.org/10.1038/nm.4219] [PMID: 27869803]

[178] Janda CY, Dang LT, You C, *et al.* Surrogate Wnt agonists that phenocopy canonical Wnt and β-catenin signalling. Nature 2017; 545(7653): 234-7.
[http://dx.doi.org/10.1038/nature22306] [PMID: 28467818]

[179] Damelin M, Bankovich A, Bernstein J, *et al.* A PTK7-targeted antibody-drug conjugate reduces tumor-initiating cells and induces sustained tumor regressions. Sci Transl Med 2017; 9(372): eaag2611.
[http://dx.doi.org/10.1126/scitranslmed.aag2611] [PMID: 28077676]

[180] Sun J, Weis WI. Biochemical and structural characterization of β-catenin interactions with nonphosphorylated and CK2-phosphorylated Lef-1. J Mol Biol 2011; 405(2): 519-30.
[http://dx.doi.org/10.1016/j.jmb.2010.11.010] [PMID: 21075118]

[181] Le PN, McDermott JD, Jimeno A. Targeting the Wnt pathway in human cancers: therapeutic targeting with a focus on OMP-54F28. Pharmacol Ther 2015; 146: 1-11.
[http://dx.doi.org/10.1016/j.pharmthera.2014.08.005] [PMID: 25172549]

[182] Ko AH, *et al.* Final results of a phase Ib dose-escalation study of PRI-724, a CBP/beta-catenin modulator, plus gemcitabine (GEM) in patients with advanced pancreatic adenocarcinoma (APC) as second-line therapy after FOLFIRINOX or FOLFOX. American Society of Clinical Oncology 2016; 34(15)
[http://dx.doi.org/10.1200/JCO.2016.34.15_suppl.e15721]

[183] Xue J, Yu X, Xue L, Ge X, Zhao W, Peng W. Intrinsic β-catenin signaling suppresses CD8[+] T-cell infiltration in colorectal cancer. Biomed Pharmacother 2019; 115: 108921.
[http://dx.doi.org/10.1016/j.biopha.2019.108921] [PMID: 31078045]

[184] Li X, Xiang Y, Li F, Yin C, Li B, Ke X. WNT/β-catenin signaling pathway regulating T cell-inflammation in the tumor microenvironment. Front Immunol 2019; 10: 2293.
[http://dx.doi.org/10.3389/fimmu.2019.02293] [PMID: 31616443]

[185] Driessens G, Zheng Y, Locke F, Cannon JL, Gounari F, Gajewski TF. Beta-catenin inhibits T cell activation by selective interference with linker for activation of T cells-phospholipase C-γ1 phosphorylation. J Immunol 2011; 186(2): 784-90.
[http://dx.doi.org/10.4049/jimmunol.1001562] [PMID: 21149602]

CHAPTER 2

CXCR4 Signaling and its Impact on Tumor Progression and Metastasis in Breast Cancer

Dayanidhi Raman[*], **Cory M. Howard**, **Sangita Sridharan** and **Augustus M.C. Tilley**

Department of Cancer Biology, University of Toledo Health Science Campus, Toledo, OH, USA

Abstract: CXCR4 is a G_i-coupled chemokine receptor involved in chemotaxis (directed migration) of tumor and stromal cells into the primary tumor and the pro-metastatic niche that are enriched in CXCL12. In breast cancer, cell surface CXCR4 levels and activity are upregulated and play an important role in local invasion and metastasis. During cancer progression, the CXCL12-CXCR4 axis orchestrates infiltration of endothelial cells and a variety of leukocytes to drive an immuno-suppressive tumor microenvironment (TME). When CXCL12 from the TME activates plasma membrane-resident CXCR4 in tumor and stromal cells, a variety of pathways are activated involving signaling modules such as PI3K-AKT, MEK-ERK, and c-Sr--p130CAS-paxillin. This triggers a wide variety of cellular processes that drive breast cancer progression, chemoresistance, and metastasis. This provides an opportunity to intervene and target these signaling axes or nodes in clinical trials to antagonize tumor growth metastasis. Finally, careful selection of targeted therapies in combination with the standard of care therapy should be selected judiciously for each patient (precision medicine) with the aim of improving the longevity with minimal toxicity to metastatic breast cancer patients.

Keywords: Breast Cancer, CXCR4, Metastasis, Signaling, Tumor Progression.

INTRODUCTION

Longitudinal exposure to noxious agents such as non-infectious (environmental toxins, food additives, oxidative stress), infectious factors (certain bacteria and viruses), and infestations (parasites) contribute to chronic inflammation. The chronic inflammation is accompanied by the presence of pro-inflammatory cytokines such as interleukins [IL-1α/β [1], IL-6)], interferons (IFN-α), and tumor necrosis factor-α (TNF-α) [2 - 4]. These cytokines trigger the release of chemotactic cytokines or chemokines and the unresolved chronic inflammation

[*] **Corresponding author Dayanidhi Raman:** Department of Cancer Biology, University of Toledo Health Science Campus, Toledo, OH, USA; Tel: 419-383-4616, Fax: 419-383-6228 18; E-mail: dayanidhi.raman@utoledo.edu

Manoj K. Pandey & Vijay P. Kale (Eds.)

leads to the formation of a neoplastic foci. Chemokines are a family of small molecules (8-12 kDa) that have the ability to facilitate survival, proliferation, migration, local invasion, and eventually metastasis of the breast cancer cells to distant organs. This is important as it is the metastasis that is lethal and not the primary breast tumor. The intra- and inter-tumor heterogeneity observed in breast cancer supports tumor progression and facilitates metastasis. The stromal cells along with acellular matrices form the tumor microenvironment (TME) [5,6]. The stromal TME plays a key role in orchestrating tumor progression and also contributes to chemoresistance. Importantly, chemokines secreted into the TME recruits the pro-tumor stromal cells such as M2-like macrophages [7], N2 neutrophils [8 - 10], myeloid-derived suppressor cells (MDSCs) [11,12], endo-thelial progenitor cells (EPCs) [13], adipocytes, and endothelial cells [14]. The recruited and subverted stromal cells secrete many cytokines, chemokines and growth factors such as IL-6, CXCL8, CXCL12, and vascular endothelial growth factor (VEGF). They also secrete extracellular matrix proteins such as tenascin-C, collagen I, and matrix metalloproteinases (MMPs). This facilitates autocrine and paracrine signaling in the TME-resident tumor and stromal cells which recruits additional pro-tumorigenic cells to the developing TME. Carcinoma-associated fibroblasts (CAFs) are already present around the tumor cells and support tumor growth, chemoresistance, and metastasis [15 - 17]. The acellular matrix provides a desmoplastic microenvironment that makes the tumor denser and renders them more chemoresistant. Thus, the paracrine interactions between the breast cancer cells with the tumor-educated stromal cells facilitate all stages of breast cancer progression, survival, angiogenesis, and metastasis (Fig. **1**). The CXCL12-CXCR4 axis is intricately involved in many of these steps of tumorigenesis and metastasis.

CXCL12-CXCR4 AXIS

The chemokine stromal-derived factor-1α (SDF-1α) or CXCL12 is the ligand for the heterotrimeric, seven transmembrane G-protein coupled receptor (GPCR) CXCR4. There are six alternatively spliced isoforms of CXCL12 that have been identified [18]. CXCL12-α is made of 89 amino acid residues while CXCL12-β contains an additional four amino acid residues at the C-terminus [19]. The ligands, CXCL12-α and CXCL12-β, bind with comparable affinity to CXCR4 receptor (K_d of 7.5 and 13.7 nM, respectively) [20]. Four additional splice variants (CXCL12-γ, CXCL12-δ, CXCL12-ε, and CXCL12- Φ) have been identified that contain 30 additional amino acid residues at their C-termini as compared to CXCL12-α [21]. All of these isoforms are functional and have a differential tissue distribution, but CXCL12-α is the predominantly expressed form. CXCL12-γ has been detected in patients with advanced disease (stage IV) at the mRNA level

[22]. The cell migration induced by CXCL12-γ showed resistance to inhibition by common CXCR4 antagonists [22].

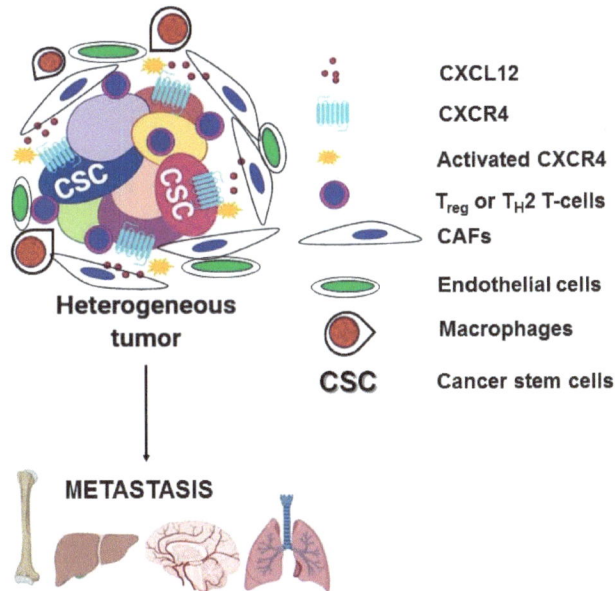

Fig. (1). Understanding the role of the heterogeneous breast tumor and the CXCL12-CXCR4 axis in the metastatic breast cancer cascade. The CXCL12 enriched microenvironment in distant organs such as the bone, lungs, liver or brain facilitates the metastatic spread of breast cancer cells expressing the cell surface CXCR4.

The CXCL12-CXCR4 axis is highly involved in primary tumor progression and metastasis in breast cancer [23 - 25]. Upon binding of CXCL12 to CXCR4, the receptor gets activated and triggers conformational changes in the heterotrimeric G-protein (Gαβγ$_i$, pertussis toxin-sensitive) initiating several divergent network of signaling pathways in breast cancer cells. Activation of CXCR4 signaling facilitates increase in intracellular calcium, cell survival and proliferation, gene transcription, cell adhesion, directional cell migration (chemotaxis), local invasion and metastasis [26 - 29]. Among them, the phosphatidylinositol 3'-kinase (PI3K), mitogen-activated protein kinase (MAPK), and c-*Src* signaling pathways tremendously contribute to tumorigenesis and subsequent metastasis [30] (Fig. **2**). CXCR4 also couples with Gα$_{13}$ to facilitate Rho GTPase-mediated transendothelial migration of basal-like breast cancer cells [31,32]

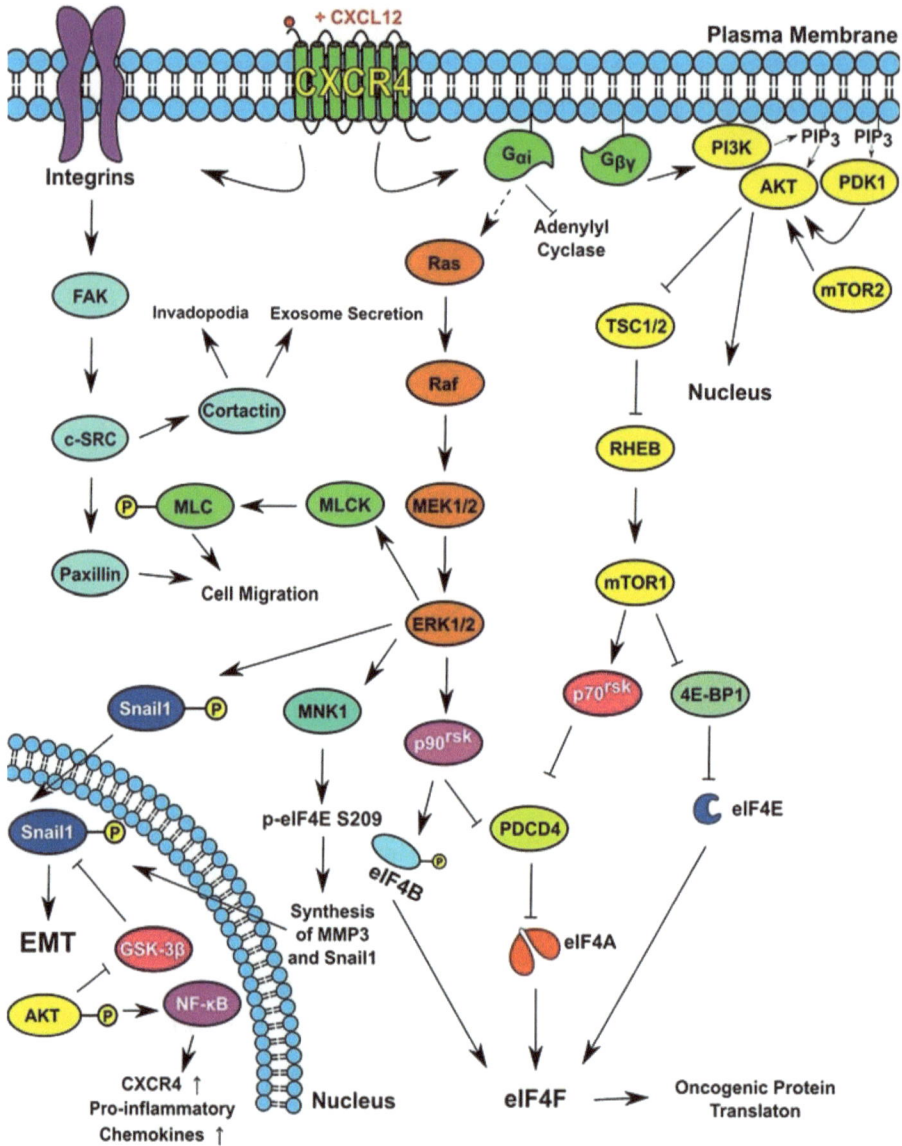

Fig. (2). CXCR4 signal transduction pathway. Activation of CXCR4 by CXCL12 transduces many cellular signaling pathways. Three major pathways include the PI3K-AKT-mTOR, MEK-ERK, FAK-Src- paxillin signaling cascade modules.

Generally, monomeric CXCR4 is capable of signaling on its own. CXCR4 can homodimerize as well as heterodimerize with CCR2, CCR5, ACKR3 or CXCR7, Na^+/H^+ exchanger regulatory factor 1 (NHERF1), CXCR3, α_1-adrenergic receptor

(AR) and the opioid receptors. Binding of different ligands to the heterodimers formed will produce variations in the adopted receptor conformations leading to differential signaling outcomes (biased agonism) [33].

CXCR4 PATHWAYS OPERATING IN BREAST CANCER

PI3K Pathway

PI3K pathway is one of the vital and crucial signaling pathways activated by the chemokine receptor CXCR4 in breast cancer cells. PI3K signaling integrates the two key signaling nodes AKT and mammalian target of rapamycin (mTOR). Activation of AKT and mTOR regulates tumor cell survival, proliferation, metabolic fitness, cell motility and invasion of the breast cancer cells [34]. Normally, PI3K is functionally regulated balance by the tumor suppressor protein, phosphatase and tensin homolog (PTEN). PTEN antagonizes the enzymatic activity of PI3K on D3-phosphoinositides. The germline deletion or mutations of PTEN is frequently observed in breast tumors. PTEN is a lipid phosphatase regulating the PI3K activity. In PTEN-null breast cancer patients, the PI3K pathway is hyperactivated. PTEN activity-compromised patients are more prone to develop breast cancer and subsequent metastasis.

PI3K is a family of lipid kinases with three classes. The class IA catalytic subunits (p110α, p110β, p110δ encoded by *PIK3CA*, *PIK3CB*, and *PIK3CD* genes) form a heterodimeric complex with p85 regulatory subunit that keeps the kinase in an inactive state in the cytoplasm. p110γ catalytic subunit encoded by *PIK3CG* gene is mainly expressed in hematopoietic cells such as neutrophils [34]. Active $G\beta\gamma_i$ subunits interact with the inactive p110-p85 complex and recruit it to the plasma membrane. This recruitment enables the interaction with its lipid substrate phosphatidylinositol 4, 5-bisphosphate (PIP_2). Activated class I PI3Ks phosphorylates PIP_2 substrate to phosphatidylinositol 3, 4, 5-trisphosphate (PIP_3) [34]. Localized accumulation of PIP_3 at the plasma membrane serves as docking sites for the pleckstrin homology (PH) domain of AKT kinase and its upstream activator 3-phosphoinositide-dependent protein kinase 1 (PDK1), thereby recruiting them to their substrates. Signal-induced production of PIP_3 can also recruit 3-phosphoinositide dependent kinase-1 (PDK1) to the big scaffold protein, IQ motif-containing GTPase-activating protein 1 (IQGAP1) [35 - 38]. This facilitates further signaling through phosphorylation events.

AKT (or Protein Kinase B) Signaling Node

Activation of CXCR4 by CXCL12 leads to stimulation of AKT which is a key effector of the CXCR4 signaling pathway [39 - 41]. AKT is a serine kinase and is a pivotal signaling node in the oncogenic activity of breast tumor cells. Treatment of breast cancer cells with CXCL12 stimulated AKT within 15 min and was sustained over 4 h [42]. Once AKT is recruited to the plasma membrane, PDK1 phosphorylates AKT at T308 leading to its partial activation. Phosphorylation of AKT at S473 by target of the rapamycin complex 2 (TORC2) kinase stimulates full activation of AKT [43 - 45] . Functionally, AKT regulates a wide variety of cellular activities. These include inhibition of apoptosis (enhanced survival), proliferation, cell migration and invasion all of which support a tumorigenic and metastatic phenotype [46 - 48] .

Akt regulates cell growth through its effects on the tuberous sclerosis complex (TSC) tumor suppressor proteins (TSC1/TSC2 complex) and mTORC signaling [49]. It regulates cell proliferation *via* phosphorylation of the endogenous cell division kinase (CDK) inhibitors such as p21 and p27. It contributes to cell survival through direct inhibition of pro-apoptotic proteins like BAD or inhibition of pro-apoptotic signals generated by Forkhead transcription factors such as FOXO. Additionally, AKT can increase cell survival by enhancing the transactivation potential of RelA / p65 (classical pathway of NF-κB) pathway by phosphorylating the RelA / p65 on S536 in the nucleus. One of the key target genes for NF-kB transcription factor is CXCR4 itself and this feedback loop would complete the vicious cycle [50]. Activated NF-kB can trigger synthesis of not only CXCR4, but also key pro-inflammatory, oncogenic chemokines by transcriptional upregulation of their mRNA. This creates a 'chemokine storm' facilitating the recruitment of the stromal cells. AKT is critically involved in the regulation of cancer cell metabolism through activation of AKT substrate of 160 kDa (AS160) which regulates the translocation of glucose transporters such as GLUT4. Increased recruitment of GLUT4 to the plasma membrane would upregulate the glucose uptake into the cancer cells. AS160 is frequently hyperphosphorylated in breast cancer [51]. The enzyme 6-phosphofructo-2-kinase/fructose-2, 6-bisphosphatase 2 (PFKFB2) is involved in regulating glycolysis (Warburg effect in cancer cells) [52]. Taken together, controlling PI3K will retard tumor progression and metastasis though the drug resistance develops eventually.

mTOR Node

AKT phosphorylates and inactivates TSC1/2 complex which in turn activates the small GTPase, Ras homolog enriched in brain (RHEB). RHEB activates mechanistic target of rapamycin (mTOR). mTORC1 is 1 MDa dimeric complex consisting of mTOR kinase, and the subunits RAPTOR and mLST8 [53]. Binding of RHEB induces global conformational changes that allosterically realign the active site residues of the mTOR kinase, thus accelerating its catalysis. The typical mTORC1 substrates are eIF4E-binding protein 1 (4EBP1) and the p70 ribosomal S6 kinase 1 (p70[rsk]). Phosphorylation of 4EBP1 and release of eIF4E from 4EBP1-eIF4E complex activates the cap-dependent translation. Phosphorylation of p70[rsk] promotes multiple aspects of protein synthesis and anabolic pathways [54]. Recently, CXCR4 has been shown to feed into eukaryotic translation initiation factor eIF4B and programmed cell death protein 4 (PDCD4) phosphorylation events through activation of p70[rsk] [55]. This was demonstrated to activate the mRNA helicase, eIF4A1, resulting in selective translation of oncogenic proteins such as survivin, MDM2, ROCK1, and cyclin D1 [55]. Treatment with the CXCR4 antagonist abolished such events indicating the specificity involved. mTORC2 has been implicated in cell migration. mTORC2 but not mTORC1 has been implicated in vascular sprouting and angiogenesis [56]. At this present time, the exact molecular mechanisms of mTORC2 in the control of breast cancer cell migration, invasion, and metastasis remains unclear.

MAPK Pathway

CXCL12-mediated activation of CXCR4 triggers the activation of the MAPK signaling pathway. This pathway is aberrantly activated in breast cancer cells. Signal amplification leads to growth, survival, migration, and local invasion of breast tumor cells. This can often contribute to chemoresistance when other upstream receptor tyrosine kinase pathways are blocked by chemotherapies. Activation of the evolutionarily conserved MAPK signaling module by CXCR4 occurs in two phases. The first phase is through CXCR4-mediated activation of G-proteins and a second one through the adaptor proteins called β-arrestins (Arrestin2 and Arrestin3) at the early endosome level. Briefly, CXCR4 signaling promotes the accumulation of Ras-GTP (active form). GTP-bound Ras triggers a kinase cascade by stimulating the serine/threonine kinase c-Raf1 through phosphorylation. c-Raf1 in turn phosphorylate and activate the dual specificity serine and tyrosine kinase called mitogen-activated protein kinase kinase 1/2 (MAP2K) or MEK1/2. MEK1/2 activates extracellular signal regulated kinases 1/2 (ERK1/2) or mitogen activated protein kinase1/2 (MAPK1/2) or p42/p44 kinases through phosphorylation of their activation loop residues T202/Y204 and T185/Y187, respectively [57 - 60]. A constitutively active form of CXCR4 has been reported to activate ERK1/2 in the absence of any stimulation by CXCL12 in breast cancer cells [61].

Oncoprotein Translation by MAPKs

Activated ERKs phosphorylate and regulate the activities of a plethora of substrates (over 160 proteins) present in the cytosol, organelles, and the nucleus

[62]. Importantly, ERK plays an active role in oncoprotein translation. ERK activates MAP kinase interacting kinase 1/2 (MNK1/2). MNK plays a key role in breast cancer [63,64]. MNK1/2 has been shown to phosphorylate the eukaryotic translation initiation factor eIF4E on S209 which is a key phosphorylation event in cap-dependent protein translation [65,66]. The generation of p-eIF4E-S209 is necessary for oncogenic transformation. In mouse mammary carcinoma models with phosphonull mutant of eIF4E that cannot be phosphorylated, the incidence of lung metastasis was reduced and the isolated cells displayed an impaired invasion [67]. Additionally, these mice had a reduced survival of prometastatic neutrophils (N2 neutrophils) *via* decreased expression of the anti-apoptotic proteins, Bcl-2 and Mcl-1 [67, 68]. Activated ERK can also phosphorylate p90 ribosomal S6 kinase 1 (p90^{rsk}) which subsequently phosphorylates programmed cell death 4 (PDCD4). PDCD4 is an endogenous inhibitor of the mRNA helicase eIF4A1. The phospho-PDCD4 releases bound eIF4A1 which can then form the eIF4F complex and enable cap-dependent translation of oncogenic mRNAs. Released eIF4A1 can processively unwind oncogenic mRNAs with classical secondary or stem-loo--structure (SLS) at their 5'-leader sequence. Phosphorylation of eIF4B (a cofactor that augments the mRNA helicase eIF4A1) at Ser422 by p90^{rsk} reportedly increases the rate of protein translation. The pS422-eIF4B also increases its interaction with eukaryotic translation initiation factor 3 (eIF3) [69, 70]. This potentiates the synthesis of key oncogenic proteins such as survivin, murine double minute 2 (MDM2), Rho kinase 1 (ROCK1), and cyclin D1/D3 that play vital roles in breast cancer [55]. The transcription factor Elk-1 is a key nuclear target for ERK1/2 [71].

Epithelial-mesenchymal Transition (EMT) and Cell Migration

ERK2 has been reported to directly phosphorylate Snail1, a transcription factor involved in EMT. Phosphorylation of Snail1 induces the nuclear translocation and stabilization of Snail1. Active Snail1 can promote breast cancer cell migration and invasion *in vitro* [72]. Thus, active ERK2 can sustain an EMT phenotype through this mechanism in tumor cells. ERK has also been demonstrated to contribute to cell migration by activating myosin light chain kinase (MLCK). MLCK phosphorylates myosin light chain subsequently on S19 residue [73 - 75]. This phosphorylation event induces the contractility of the cytoskeleton of the tumor cells. ERK signaling pathway has also been proposed to regulate cell migration through the expression of Fra-1 and c-Jun both of which are necessary for cell migration [76].

Inactivation of ERK1/2

p44/42 kinases are negatively regulated by a family of dual-specificity (T/Y)

MAPK phosphatases or dual specificity protein phosphatases (DUSPs) [77]. Sustained activation of ERK pathway has been reported due to the loss of the specific MAPK phosphatase DUSP4 in basal-like breast cancer. Loss of DUSP4 has been correlated with the promotion of breast cancer stemness [78]. Interestingly, DUSP4 deficiency has been related to drug resistance and minimal residual disease (MRD) [79]. Analysis of the phosphatases revealed that DUSP4 is a critical regulator of growth and invasion in breast cancer, if the expression is not low or deleted [80]. Interleukin-4 (IL-4) has been reported to increase the aggressiveness of the breast cancer *via* the suppression of DUSP4 [81]. Therefore, the MEK pathway can be strategically targeted in breast cancer patients with low DUSP4 expression [82].

C-*SRC* Pathway

Activation of CXCR4 stimulates integrin activation which in turn activates focal adhesion kinase (FAK) through its tyrosine phosphorylation. Activated FAK phosphorylates c-*Src* which is a proto-oncogene and a cytosolic tyrosine kinase. Phosphorylated and activated c-*Src* will further regulate p130Cas and paxillin phosphorylation which plays a role in cell migration [83, 84]. The released $G\beta\gamma_i$ subunit following the activation of CXCR4 can also directly activate c-*Src*. Activation of CXCR4 also enhanced the secretion of matrix metalloprotease 2 and 9 (MMP2 and MMP9). The c-*Src*-cortactin axis plays a vital role in breast tumorigenesis and metastasis. Activation of c-*Src* also phosphorylates and recruits cortactin to the plasma membrane. This recruitment was shown to be important for activation of ERK pathway and chemotaxis [85]. Cortactin plays a major role in invadopodia and proteolysis of the extracellular matrices by metalloproteases and is involved in tumor progression [86 - 89]. Tyrosine phosphorylated cortactin has also been demonstrated to recruit Vav2 guanine nucleotide exchange factor that activates Rac3 and promote invadopodial function in invasive breast cancer cells [90]. Cortactin was also shown to potentiate metastasis of the breast cancer cells to the bone [91]. Interestingly, cortactin was shown to be a pivotal protein for the secretion of the exosomes to the cell exterior. This is vital for co-opting the stromal cells to be pro-tumor in nature. In addition, the tyrosine phosphorylation of annexin A2 (Anxa2) by *c-Src* in the Anxa2/receptor for activated C-kinase 1 (RACK1) complex correlated with drug resistance and invasive / metastatic potential of breast cancer cells [92].

JAK-STAT Pathway

The Janus kinase / signal transducer and activator of transcription (JAK-STAT) signaling complex is a key effector in breast cancer. CXCL12-activated CXCR4 associated with Janus kinase 2 and 3 (JAK2 and JAK3) [93,94]. Activated JAK2 and JAK3 can recruit and phosphorylate members of the STAT family of transcription factors. The phospho-STATs subsequently dimerize and translocate to the nucleus to mediate their transcriptional activity. STAT3 has been shown to mediate chemoresistance and also promote breast cancer stemness. At this juncture, more research is needed to dissect the precise role of JAK-STAT pathway in breast cancer.

Cross-talk of CXCR4 with Other Receptor and Non-receptor Tyrosine Kinases and its Interaction with Specific Adaptors

CXCR4 has been demonstrated to cross-talk with signaling pathways involving receptor tyrosine kinases such as epidermal growth factor receptor (EGFR), human epidermal growth factor receptor2 (HER2) [95], and insulin-like growth factor1 receptor (IGF-1R) [96]. This cross-talk of CXCR4 with various tyrosine kinases promotes cell motility, local invasion, and metastasis. HER2 in turn can enhance the expression of CXCR4 at the protein level. CXCR4 has been shown to be required for HER2-mediated breast cancer cell invasion *in vitro* and for metastasis to the lungs *in vivo* [95]. CXCR4 can also transactivate HER2 through activation of c-*Src* [97]. Cross-talk and transactivation of these various proteins could thereby reduce the efficacy of targeting a single receptor. Aside from interaction of CXCR4 with other receptors, it can also directly interact with the adaptor protein LIM and SH3 protein 1 (LASP1). Stable knock down of LASP1 abrogated the CXCR4-mediated invasion of the Matrigel by the TNBC cells *in vitro* [98]. Furthermore, LASP1 linked CXCR4 signaling to eIF4A pathway which is involved in translation of oncogenic proteins [55].

Stromal Cell Recruitment to the TME

The chemokine CXCL12 is primarily secreted into the breast cancer microenvironment by the carcinoma-associated fibroblasts (CAFs) [99]. CAF-derived CXCL12 recruits endothelial progenitor cells from the bone marrow and promotes neoangiogenesis in the TME [100]. CXCL12 also facilitates infiltration of mesenchymal stem cells, retention of the hypersegmented, aged N2 neutrophils expressing CXCR4 (tumor- associated neutrophils), and development and maintenance of CXCR4$^+$-breast cancer stem cells in the TME. These cells through the extensive autocrine and paracrine signaling events orchestrate and promote tumor progression and metastasis [101 - 103]. Breast cancer is maintained by a subset of tumor cells with properties of stemness which can drive tumor progression and metastasis and are called breast cancer stem-like cells (BCSCs). BCSCs are regulated by TME and are intrinsically chemoresistant and responsible for the minimal residual disease, tumor relapse and therapy failure. BCSCs with the expression cell surface CD44$^+$/CD24$^{-/low}$ are more migratory and invasive and often display a higher expression of CXCR4 than pure aldehyde dehydrogenase positive (ALDH$^+$)-subset of BCSCs [104]. CD44 is a receptor the extracellular matrix protein, hyaluronan or hyaluronic acid. Interestingly, there are 2 isoforms of CD44 with opposite functions. The standard isoform of CD44 (CD44s) promotes BCSC stemness whereas the CD44 variant form (CD44v) opposes it [105]. CD44 is generally involved in cell-cell and cell-matrix adhesions as well as cell migration [106 - 107]. A subset of BCSCs co-expresses both CD44 and ALDH markers and is considered highly aggressive and metastatic [108 - 110]. ALDHs are enzymes that are involved in detoxifying the chemotherapeutic drugs to less harmful or harmless end products. This process provides intrinsic chemoresistance to BCSCs in addition to other ways through which they can gain drug resistance. Previous work had demonstrated that the non-migratory, intrinsic ALDH$^+$ pool of BCSC can generate or get converted to CXCR4$^+$ migratory BCSCs and enable metastasis [111]. Interestingly, a phosphoproteomics study on CXCR4$^+$-BCSCs outlined an unidentified pathway that may operate upon stimulation with CXCL12. It is mediated by protein kinase A culminating in ERK signaling node – CXCL12/CXCR4-protein kinase A- Mitogen-Activated Protein Kinase Kinase 2-ERK pathway (CXCL12/CXCR4-PKA-MAP2K2-ERK) [112]. It was further demonstrated that in CXCL12-perturbed BCSCs, there was a feedback regulation of proteins such as MEK, ERK1/2, p120-catenin and PPP1Cα. These proteins can be potential targets for BCSC-directed therapy.

Therapeutic Implications

CXCR4 plays a role in almost all of the solid tumors and hematological malignancies [113]. The bicyclam compound AMD3100 (Plerixafor) is a CXCR4 antagonist that was FDA-approved and has been successfully used to mobilize hematopoietic cells in congenital WHIM (Warts, Hypogammaglobulinemia, Infections, Myelokathexis) syndrome due to the presence of the constitutively active CXCR4 from germline truncations at the C-terminus of the receptor [114,115]. Though it is employed for hematological malignancies, concerns exist over the action of AMD3100 as a partial agonist for atypical chemokine receptor 3 (ACKR3) or CXCR7. AMD3465 has been employed to block CXCR4 signaling in murine model to regulate primary tumor growth and metastasis [116]. LY2510924 is a novel cyclic peptide antagonist to CXCR4 and was demonstrated to be a potent and selective inhibitor of CXCR4. This compound also inhibited lung metastasis in a murine model [117]. Balixafortide (Polyphor, Allschwil, Switzerland) is a potent, highly selective CXCR4 antagonist that was recently fast-track approved by FDA for stage IV breast cancer along with the non-taxane microtubule targeting agent Eribulin. The drug has been observed to be tolerated well in the clinical trial [118]. Despite concerns against AMD3100, blocking of CXCR4 with AMD3100 decreased desmoplasia, improved the infiltration of cytotoxic CD8$^+$-T-cells and immunotherapy in a metastatic mammary carcinoma murine model [119]. Furthermore, genetic deletion of CXCR4 in α-smooth muscle actin positive cells (CAFs and pericytes), enhanced the infiltration of CD8$^+$-T-cells. This led to synergy with immune check point blockers [119].

In breast cancer patients, the PI3K-AKT-mTOR pathway is one of the highly dysregulated pathways [120]. Aberrant activation of this pathway by oncogenic mutations in *PI3CA*, *PTEN*, *AKT*, *TSC1*, *TSC2*, *LKB1* and *MTOR* leads to increase in severity and grade of the breast tumors. 30% of the breast cancer patients have constitutively active mutant forms of p110α (*PIK3CA* gene) [121]. The hot spot mutations that occur in *PIK3CA* gene were E542K, E545K, and H1407R and are correlated with an adverse clinical outcome. Aberrant activation of PI3K through these mutations can activate downstream signaling independent of AKT activation such as the activation of serum/glucocorticoid regulated kinase 3 (SGK3). Expression of Inositol polyphosphate-4-phosphatases type II (INPP4B) enhanced the activation of SGK3 kinase that supported proliferation in three-dimensional matrices, invasive migration, and tumorigenesis *in vivo* [122]. Amplification of the *PDK1* copy number is shown to correlate with low survival rates. 20% of breast tumors exhibit *PDK1* amplification with a concomitant increase of the phospho-PDK1 (pS241-PDK1) levels [123]. The use of FDA-approved inhibitors of PI3K (Idelalisib and Copanlisib) and mTOR (Temsirolimus and Everolimus) have seen limited clinical efficacy. This is due to toxicity and development of chemoresistance associated with these drugs. Selective inhibitors against p110α catalytic subunit of the PI3K such as BYL719 (Alpelisib) and GDC0032 (Taselisib) are showing promising clinical activity in solid tumors including breast cancer [124]. New compounds with selectivity and improved therapeutic indices are needed and predictive biomarkers of therapy response would be of immense value to the clinicians [125].

Application of statins like simvastatin (that functions to reduce cholesterol and triglyceride levels) was demonstrated to modulate the Ets-1 transcription factor and DUSP4 through the MAPK pathway. Interestingly, the simvastatin treatment of triple-negative breast cancer (TNBC) cells restored the expression of DUSP4. DUSP4 would thereby inhibit the functionality of MAPK pathway [126]. Significantly increased expression of spliced isoform of MNK1 (MNK1b) was observed in tumors and predicted poor prognosis in TNBC [63]. Expression of MNK1b promoted cellular growth and expression of the anti-apoptotic protein MCL1 was observed *in vitro* [63]. Tomivosertib (eFT-508) is a potent, selective anti-MNK1/2 inhibitor and is in phase 2 clinical trials in combination with PD-1/PD-L1 inhibitors. The mRNA helicase eIF4A is downstream of both PI3K and ERK pathway. eFT226 is a highly potent and selective small molecule inhibitor against eIF4A and is slated for a phase I-II clinical trial.

CONCLUSION

CXCR4 is a chemokine GPCR that is $G_{\alpha i}$-coupled. Stimulation of CXCR4 by CXCL12 activates a variety of signaling pathways such as PI3K, MAPK, c-*Src*, and JAK-STAT. The tumor microenvironment plays a pivotal role in sustaining tumorigenesis, metastatic, and chemoresistance related to CXCR4 signaling [113]. Finally, a judicious choice of combination of targeted therapies is warranted for improving the clinical outcome of patients with metastatic breast cancer especially the TNBC type. Despite their refined mode of molecular action, targeted therapies are associated with diverse toxicities, which clinicians should be aware of and treat patients accordingly. Tumor-directed instead of a systemic therapy with nanotechnology may bring promising results in the near future.

CONSENT FOR PUBLICATION

Not applicable.

CONFLICT OF INTEREST

The author declares that there is no conflict of interest in this chapter.

ACKNOWLEDGEMENTS

This manuscript has been supported in part by National Institute of Health (NIH) / National Cancer Institute (NCI) grant R21CA202176, Ohio Cancer Research foundation (OCR) and University of Toledo startup grant (F110796) to DR; A competitive university fellowship from College of Graduate Studies (COGS) (to CMH).

REFERENCES

[1]   Mantovani A, Ponzetta A, Inforzato A, Jaillon S. Innate immunity, inflammation and tumour progression: double-edged swords. J Intern Med 2019; 285(5): 524-32.
[http://dx.doi.org/10.1111/joim.12886] [PMID: 30873708]

[2]   Robinson SC, Coussens LM. Soluble mediators of inflammation during tumor development. Adv Cancer Res 2005; 93: 159-87.
[http://dx.doi.org/10.1016/S0065-230X(05)93005-4] [PMID: 15797447]

[3]   Aggarwal BB, Shishodia S, Sandur SK, Pandey MK, Sethi G. Inflammation and cancer: how hot is the link? Biochem Pharmacol 2006; 72(11): 1605-21.
[http://dx.doi.org/10.1016/j.bcp.2006.06.029] [PMID: 16889756]

[4]   Szlosarek P, Charles KA, Balkwill FR. Tumour necrosis factor-alpha as a tumour promoter. Eur J Cancer 2006; 42(6): 745-50.
[http://dx.doi.org/10.1016/j.ejca.2006.01.012] [PMID: 16517151]

[5]   Martins D, Schmitt F. Microenvironment in breast tumorigenesis: Friend or foe? Histol Histopathol 2019; 34(1): 13-24.

[PMID: 29978449]

[6]   Eiro N, Gonzalez LO, Fraile M, Cid S, Schneider J, Vizoso FJ. Breast cancer tumor stroma: Cellular components, phenotypic heterogeneity, intercellular communication, prognostic implications and therapeutic opportunities. Cancers (Basel) 2019; 11(5): 6562436.
        [http://dx.doi.org/10.3390/cancers11050664] [PMID: 31086100]

[7]   Galdiero MR, Marone G, Mantovani A. Cancer Inflammation and Cytokines. Cold Spring Harb Perspect Biol 2018; 10(8): 10.
        [http://dx.doi.org/10.1101/cshperspect.a028662] [PMID: 28778871]

[8]   Patel S, Fu S, Mastio J, *et al.* Unique pattern of neutrophil migration and function during tumor progression. Nat Immunol 2018; 19(11): 1236-47.
        [http://dx.doi.org/10.1038/s41590-018-0229-5] [PMID: 30323345]

[9]   Zhou J, Nefedova Y, Lei A, Gabrilovich D. Neutrophils and PMN-MDSC: Their biological role and interaction with stromal cells. Semin Immunol 2018; 35: 19-28.
        [http://dx.doi.org/10.1016/j.smim.2017.12.004] [PMID: 29254756]

[10]   Galdiero MR, Varricchi G, Loffredo S, Mantovani A, Marone G. Roles of neutrophils in cancer growth and progression. J Leukoc Biol 2018; 103(3): 457-64.
        [http://dx.doi.org/10.1002/JLB.3MR0717-292R] [PMID: 29345348]

[11]   Tcyganov E, Mastio J, Chen E, Gabrilovich DI. Plasticity of myeloid-derived suppressor cells in cancer. Curr Opin Immunol 2018; 51: 76-82, 5943174.
        [http://dx.doi.org/10.1016/j.coi.2018.03.009] [PMID: 29547768]

[12]   Veglia F, Perego M, Gabrilovich D. Myeloid-derived suppressor cells coming of age. Nat Immunol 2018; 19(2): 108-19.
        [http://dx.doi.org/10.1038/s41590-017-0022-x] [PMID: 29348500]

[13]   Richter-Ehrenstein C, Rentzsch J, Runkel S, Schneider A, Schönfelder G. Endothelial progenitor cells in breast cancer patients. Breast Cancer Res Treat 2007; 106(3): 343-9.
        [http://dx.doi.org/10.1007/s10549-007-9505-z] [PMID: 17972175]

[14]   Bussard KM, Mutkus L, Stumpf K, Gomez-Manzano C, Marini FC. Tumor-associated stromal cells as key contributors to the tumor microenvironment. Breast Cancer Res 2016; 18(1): 84.
        [http://dx.doi.org/10.1186/s13058-016-0740-2] [PMID: 27515302]

[15]   Alba-Castellón L, Olivera-Salguero R, Mestre-Farrera A, *et al.* Snail1-dependent activation of cancer-associated fibroblast controls epithelial tumor cell invasion and metastasis. Cancer Res 2016; 76(21): 6205-17.
        [http://dx.doi.org/10.1158/0008-5472.CAN-16-0176] [PMID: 27503928]

[16]   Su S, Chen J, Yao H, *et al.* CD10(+)GPR77(+) cancer493 associated fibroblasts promote cancer formation and chemoresistance by sustaining cancer 494 stemness. Cell 172 2018; 841-56.

[17]   Ren Y, Jia HH, Xu YQ, *et al.* Paracrine and epigenetic control of CAF-induced metastasis: the role of HOTAIR stimulated by TGF-ß1 secretion. Mol Cancer 2018; 17(1): 5.
        [http://dx.doi.org/10.1186/s12943-018-0758-4] [PMID: 29325547]

[18]   Janssens R, Struyf S, Proost P. The unique structural and functional features of CXCL12. Cell Mol Immunol 2018; 15(4): 299-311.
        [http://dx.doi.org/10.1038/cmi.2017.107] [PMID: 29082918]

[19]   Shirozu M, Nakano T, Inazawa J, *et al.* Structure and chromosomal localization of the human stromal cell-derived factor 1 (SDF1) gene. Genomics 1995; 28(3): 495-500.
        [http://dx.doi.org/10.1006/geno.1995.1180] [PMID: 7490086]

[20]   Hesselgesser J, Liang M, Hoxie J, *et al.* Identification and characterization of the CXCR4 chemokine receptor in human T cell lines: ligand binding, biological activity, and HIV-1 infectivity. J Immunol 1998; 160(2): 877-83.
        [PMID: 9551924]

[21]   Yu L, Cecil J, Peng SB, *et al*. Identification and expression of novel isoforms of human stromal cell-derived factor 1. Gene 2006; 374: 174-9.
[http://dx.doi.org/10.1016/j.gene.2006.02.001] [PMID: 16626895]

[22]   Cavnar SP, Ray P, Moudgil P, *et al*. Microfluidic source-sink model reveals effects of biophysically distinct CXCL12 isoforms in breast cancer chemotaxis. Integr Biol 2014; 6(5): 564-76.
[http://dx.doi.org/10.1039/C4IB00015C] [PMID: 24675873]

[23]   Müller A, Homey B, Soto H, *et al*. Involvement of chemokine receptors in breast cancer metastasis. Nature 2001; 410(6824): 50-6.
[http://dx.doi.org/10.1038/35065016] [PMID: 11242036]

[24]   Zlotnik A, Burkhardt AM, Homey B. Homeostatic chemokine receptors and organ-specific metastasis. Nat Rev Immunol 2011; 11(9): 597-606.
[http://dx.doi.org/10.1038/nri3049] [PMID: 21866172]

[25]   Smith MC, Luker KE, Garbow JR, *et al*. CXCR4 regulates growth of both primary and metastatic breast cancer. Cancer Res 2004; 64(23): 8604-12.
[http://dx.doi.org/10.1158/0008-5472.CAN-04-1844] [PMID: 15574767]

[26]   Kirui JK, Xie Y, Wolff DW, Jiang H, Abel PW, Tu Y. Gβγ signaling promotes breast cancer cell migration and invasion. J Pharmacol Exp Ther 2010; 333(2): 393-403, 2872950.
[http://dx.doi.org/10.1124/jpet.109.164814] [PMID: 20110378]

[27]   Dillenburg-Pilla P, Patel V, Mikelis CM, *et al*. SDF-1/CXCL12 induces directional cell migration and spontaneous metastasis *via* a CXCR4/Gαi/mTORC1 axis. FASEB J 2015; 29(3): 1056-68.
[http://dx.doi.org/10.1096/fj.14-260083] [PMID: 25466898]

[28]   Teicher BA, Fricker SP. CXCL12 (SDF-1)/CXCR4 pathway in cancer. Clin Cancer Res 2010; 16(11): 2927-31.
[http://dx.doi.org/10.1158/1078-0432.CCR-09-2329] [PMID: 20484021]

[29]   Holland JD, Kochetkova M, Akekawatchai C, Dottore M, Lopez A, McColl SR. Differential functional activation of chemokine receptor CXCR4 is mediated by G proteins in breast cancer cells. Cancer Res 2006; 66(8): 4117-24.
[http://dx.doi.org/10.1158/0008-5472.CAN-05-1631] [PMID: 16618732]

[30]   Kang H, Watkins G, Parr C, Douglas-Jones A, Mansel R E, Jiang W G. Stromal cell derived factor-1: its influence on invasiveness and migration of breast cancer cells *in vitro*, and its association with prognosis and survival in human breast cancer. Breast Cancer Res 2005; 7(4): R402-10.
[http://dx.doi.org/10.1186/bcr1022]

[31]   Yagi H, Tan W, Dillenburg-Pilla P, *et al*. A synthetic biology approach reveals a CXCR4-G13-Rho signaling axis driving transendothelial migration of metastatic breast cancer cells. Sci Signal 2011; 4(191): ra60.
[http://dx.doi.org/10.1126/scisignal.2002221] [PMID: 21934106]

[32]   Tan W, Martin D, Gutkind JS. The Galpha13-Rho signaling axis is required for SDF-1-induced migration through CXCR4. J Biol Chem 2006; 281(51): 39542-9.
[http://dx.doi.org/10.1074/jbc.M609062200] [PMID: 17056591]

[33]   Heuninck J, Perpina Viciano C, Isbilir A, *et al*. Context-dependent signalling of CXC chemokine receptor 4 (CXCR4) and atypical chemokine receptor 3 (ACKR3) Mol Pharmacol 2019; 96(6): 778-93.

[34]   Bilanges B, Posor Y, Vanhaesebroeck B. PI3K isoforms in cell signalling and vesicle trafficking. Nat Rev Mol Cell Biol 2019; 20(9): 515-34.
[http://dx.doi.org/10.1038/s41580-019-0129-z] [PMID: 31110302]

[35]   Choi S, Anderson RA. IQGAP1 is a phosphoinositide effector and kinase scaffold. Adv Biol Regul 2016; 60: 29-35.
[http://dx.doi.org/10.1016/j.jbior.2015.10.004] [PMID: 26554303]

[36] Chen M, Choi S, Jung O, *et al.* The Specificity of EGF-Stimulated IQGAP1 Scaffold Towards the PI3K-Akt Pathway is Defined by the IQ3 motif. Sci Rep 2019; 9(1): 9126.
[http://dx.doi.org/10.1038/s41598-019-45671-5] [PMID: 31235839]

[37] Choi S, Anderson RA. And Akt-ion! IQGAP1 in control of signaling pathways. EMBO J 2017; 36(8): 967-9.
[http://dx.doi.org/10.15252/embj.201796827] [PMID: 28320738]

[38] Choi S, Thapa N, Hedman AC, Li Z, Sacks DB, Anderson RA. IQGAP1 is a novel phosphatidylinositol 4,5 bisphosphate effector in regulation of directional cell migration. EMBO J 2013; 32(19): 2617-30.
[http://dx.doi.org/10.1038/emboj.2013.191] [PMID: 23982733]

[39] Vlahakis SR, Villasis-Keever A, Gomez T, Vanegas M, Vlahakis N, Paya CV. G protein-coupled chemokine receptors induce both survival and apoptotic signaling pathways. J Immunol 2002; 169(10): 5546-54.
[http://dx.doi.org/10.4049/jimmunol.169.10.5546] [PMID: 12421931]

[40] Kayali AG, Van Gunst K, Campbell IL, *et al.* The stromal cell-derived factor-1alpha/CXCR4 ligand-receptor axis is critical for progenitor survival and migration in the pancreas. J Cell Biol 2003; 163(4): 859-69.
[http://dx.doi.org/10.1083/jcb.200304153] [PMID: 14638861]

[41] Rubin JB, Kung AL, Klein RS, *et al.* A small-molecule antagonist of CXCR4 inhibits intracranial growth of primary brain tumors. Proc Natl Acad Sci USA 2003; 100(23): 13513-8.
[http://dx.doi.org/10.1073/pnas.2235846100] [PMID: 14595012]

[42] Prasad A, Fernandis AZ, Rao Y, Ganju RK. Slit protein-mediated inhibition of CXCR4-induced chemotactic and chemoinvasive signaling pathways in breast cancer cells. J Biol Chem 2004; 279(10): 9115-24.
[http://dx.doi.org/10.1074/jbc.M308083200] [PMID: 14645233]

[43] Alessi DR, James SR, Downes CP, *et al.* Characterization of a 3-phosphoinositide-dependent protein kinase which phosphorylates and activates protein kinase Balpha. Curr Biol 1997; 7(4): 261-9.
[http://dx.doi.org/10.1016/S0960-9822(06)00122-9] [PMID: 9094314]

[44] Sarbassov DD, Guertin DA, Ali SM, Sabatini DM. Phosphorylation and regulation of Akt/PKB by the rictor-mTOR complex. Science 2005; 307(5712): 1098-101.
[http://dx.doi.org/10.1126/science.1106148] [PMID: 15718470]

[45] Stephens L, Anderson K, Stokoe D, *et al.* Protein kinase B kinases that mediate phosphatidylinositol 3,4,5-trisphosphate-dependent activation of protein kinase B. Science 1998; 279(5351): 710-4.
[http://dx.doi.org/10.1126/science.279.5351.710] [PMID: 9445477]

[46] Luker KE, Luker GD. Functions of CXCL12 and CXCR4 in breast cancer. Cancer Lett 2006; 238(1): 30-41.
[http://dx.doi.org/10.1016/j.canlet.2005.06.021] [PMID: 16046252]

[47] Luo J, Manning BD, Cantley LC. Targeting the PI3K-Akt pathway in human cancer: rationale and promise. Cancer Cell 2003; 4(4): 257-62.
[http://dx.doi.org/10.1016/S1535-6108(03)00248-4] [PMID: 14585353]

[48] Lee BC, Lee TH, Avraham S, Avraham HK. Involvement of the chemokine receptor CXCR4 and its ligand stromal cell-derived factor 1alpha in breast cancer cell migration through human brain microvascular endothelial cells. Mol Cancer Res 2004; 2(6): 327-38.
[PMID: 15235108]

[49] Vivanco I, Sawyers CL. The phosphatidylinositol 3-Kinase AKT pathway in human cancer. Nat Rev Cancer 2002; 2(7): 489-501.
[http://dx.doi.org/10.1038/nrc839] [PMID: 12094235]

[50] Helbig G, Christopherson KW II, Bhat-Nakshatri P, *et al.* NF-kappaB promotes breast cancer cell

migration and metastasis by inducing the expression of the chemokine receptor CXCR4. J Biol Chem 2003; 278(24): 21631-8.
[http://dx.doi.org/10.1074/jbc.M300609200] [PMID: 12690099]

[51]   Jiang XH, Sun JW, Xu M, Jiang XF, Liu CF, Lu Y. Frequent hyperphosphorylation of AS160 in breast cancer. Cancer Biol Ther 2010; 10(4): 362-7.
[http://dx.doi.org/10.4161/cbt.10.4.12426] [PMID: 20574165]

[52]   Bartrons R, Simon-Molas H, Rodríguez-García A, *et al.* Fructose 2,6-Bisphosphate in Cancer Cell Metabolism. Front Oncol 2018; 8(331): 331.
[http://dx.doi.org/10.3389/fonc.2018.00331] [PMID: 30234009]

[53]   Yang H, Jiang X, Li B, *et al.* Mechanisms of mTORC1 activation by RHEB and inhibition by PRAS40. Nature 2017; 552(7685): 368-73.
[http://dx.doi.org/10.1038/nature25023] [PMID: 29236692]

[54]   Gingras AC, Raught B, Gygi SP, *et al.* Hierarchical phosphorylation of the translation inhibitor 4E-BP1. Genes Dev 2001; 15(21): 2852-64.
[PMID: 11691836]

[55]   Howard CM, Bearss N, Subramaniyan B, *et al.* The CXCR4-LASP1-eIF4F axis promotes translation of oncogenic proteins in triple-negative breast cancer cells. Front Oncol 2019; 9(284): 284.
[http://dx.doi.org/10.3389/fonc.2019.00284] [PMID: 31106142]

[56]   Ziegler ME, Hatch MM, Wu N, Muawad SA, Hughes CC. mTORC2 mediates CXCL12-induced angiogenesis. Angiogenesis 2016; 19(3): 359-71.
[http://dx.doi.org/10.1007/s10456-016-9509-6] [PMID: 27106789]

[57]   Roberts PJ, Der CJ. Targeting the Raf-MEK-ERK mitogen-activated protein kinase cascade for the treatment of cancer. Oncogene 2007; 26(22): 3291-310.
[http://dx.doi.org/10.1038/sj.onc.1210422] [PMID: 17496923]

[58]   Johnson GL, Lapadat R. Mitogen-activated protein kinase pathways mediated by ERK, JNK, and p38 protein kinases. Science 2002; 298(5600): 1911-2.
[http://dx.doi.org/10.1126/science.1072682] [PMID: 12471242]

[59]   Wilsbacher JL, Goldsmith EJ, Cobb MH. Phosphorylation of MAP kinases by MAP/ERK involves multiple regions of MAP kinases. J Biol Chem 1999; 274(24): 16988-94.
[http://dx.doi.org/10.1074/jbc.274.24.16988] [PMID: 10358048]

[60]   Pearson G, Robinson F, Beers Gibson T, *et al.* Mitogen-activated protein (MAP) kinase pathways: regulation and physiological functions. Endocr Rev 2001; 22(2): 153-83.
[PMID: 11294822]

[61]   Ueda Y, Neel NF, Schutyser E, Raman D, Richmond A. Deletion of the COOH-terminal domain of CXC chemokine receptor 4 leads to the down-regulation of cell-to-cell contact, enhanced motility and proliferation in breast carcinoma cells. Cancer Res 2006; 66(11): 5665-75.
[http://dx.doi.org/10.1158/0008-5472.CAN-05-3579] [PMID: 16740704]

[62]   Yoon S, Seger R. The extracellular signal-regulated kinase: multiple substrates regulate diverse cellular functions. Growth Factors 2006; 24(1): 21-44.
[http://dx.doi.org/10.1080/02699050500284218] [PMID: 16393692]

[63]   Pinto-Díez C, García-Recio EM, Pérez-Morgado MI, *et al.* Increased expression of MNK1b, the spliced isoform of MNK1, predicts poor prognosis and is associated with triple-negative breast cancer. Oncotarget 2018; 9(17): 13501-16.
[http://dx.doi.org/10.18632/oncotarget.24417] [PMID: 29568373]

[64]   Chrestensen CA, Shuman JK, Eschenroeder A, Worthington M, Gram H, Sturgill TW. MNK1 and MNK2 regulation in HER2-overexpressing breast cancer lines. J Biol Chem 2007; 282(7): 4243-52.
[http://dx.doi.org/10.1074/jbc.M607368200] [PMID: 17130135]

[65]   Pyronnet S, Imataka H, Gingras AC, Fukunaga R, Hunter T, Sonenberg N. Human eukaryotic

translation initiation factor 4G (eIF4G) recruits mnk1 to phosphorylate eIF4E. EMBO J 1999; 18(1): 270-9.
[http://dx.doi.org/10.1093/emboj/18.1.270] [PMID: 9878069]

[66]   Siddiqui N, Sonenberg N. Signalling to eIF4E in cancer. Biochem Soc Trans 2015; 43(5): 763-72.
[http://dx.doi.org/10.1042/BST20150126] [PMID: 26517881]

[67]   Robichaud N, del Rincon SV, Huor B, *et al.* Phosphorylation of eIF4E promotes EMT and metastasis *via* translational control of SNAIL and MMP-3. Oncogene 2015; 34(16): 2032-42.
[http://dx.doi.org/10.1038/onc.2014.146] [PMID: 24909168]

[68]   Robichaud N, Hsu B E, Istomine R, *et al.* Translational control in the tumor microenvironment promotes lung metastasis phosphorylation of eIF4E in neutrophils. Proc Natl Acad Sci 2018; 115: E2202-9.

[69]   Raught B, Peiretti F, Gingras A C, *et al.* Phosphorylation of eucaryotic translation initiation factor 4B Ser422 is modulated by S6 kinases The EMBO journal 23 2004. 1761-1769

[70]   Shahbazian D, Roux PP, Mieulet V, *et al.* The mTOR/PI3K and MAPK pathways converge on eIF4B to control its phosphorylation and activity. EMBO J 2006; 25(12): 2781-91.
[http://dx.doi.org/10.1038/sj.emboj.7601166] [PMID: 16763566]

[71]   Marais R, Wynne J, Treisman R. The SRF accessory protein Elk-1 contains a growth factor-regulated transcriptional activation domain. Cell 1993; 73(2): 381-93.
[http://dx.doi.org/10.1016/0092-8674(93)90237-K] [PMID: 8386592]

[72]   Zhang K, Corsa CA, Ponik SM, *et al.* The collagen receptor discoidin domain receptor 2 stabilizes SNAIL1 to facilitate breast cancer metastasis. Nat Cell Biol 2013; 15(6): 677-87.
[http://dx.doi.org/10.1038/ncb2743] [PMID: 23644467]

[73]   Zhou X, Liu Y, You J, Zhang H, Zhang X, Ye L. Myosin light-chain kinase contributes to the proliferation and migration of breast cancer cells through cross-talk with activated ERK1/2. Cancer Lett 2008; 270(2): 312-27.
[http://dx.doi.org/10.1016/j.canlet.2008.05.028] [PMID: 18710790]

[74]   Khuon S, Liang L, Dettman RW, Sporn PH, Wysolmerski RB, Chew TL. Myosin light chain kinase mediates transcellular intravasation of breast cancer cells through the underlying endothelial cells: a three-dimensional FRET study. J Cell Sci 2010; 123(Pt 3): 431-40.
[http://dx.doi.org/10.1242/jcs.053793] [PMID: 20067998]

[75]   Nguyen DH, Catling AD, Webb DJ, *et al.* Myosin light chain kinase functions downstream of Ras/ERK to promote migration of urokinase-type plasminogen activator-stimulated cells in an integrin-selective manner. J Cell Biol 1999; 146(1): 149-64.
[http://dx.doi.org/10.1083/jcb.146.1.149] [PMID: 10402467]

[76]   Talotta F, Mega T, Bossis G, *et al.* Heterodimerization with Fra-1 cooperates with the ERK pathway to stabilize c-Jun in response to the RAS oncoprotein. Oncogene 2010; 29(33): 4732-40.
[http://dx.doi.org/10.1038/onc.2010.211] [PMID: 20543861]

[77]   Owens DM, Keyse SM. Differential regulation of MAP kinase signalling by dual-specificity protein phosphatases. Oncogene 2007; 26(22): 3203-13.
[http://dx.doi.org/10.1038/sj.onc.1210412] [PMID: 17496916]

[78]   Balko JM, Schwarz LJ, Bhola NE, *et al.* Activation of MAPK pathways due to DUSP4 loss promotes cancer stem cell-like phenotypes in basal-like breast cancer. Cancer Res 2013; 73(20): 6346-58.
[http://dx.doi.org/10.1158/0008-5472.CAN-13-1385] [PMID: 23966295]

[79]   Balko JM, Cook RS, Vaught DB, *et al.* Profiling of residual breast cancers after neoadjuvant chemotherapy identifies DUSP4 deficiency as a mechanism of drug resistance. Nat Med 2012; 18(7): 1052-9.
[http://dx.doi.org/10.1038/nm.2795] [PMID: 22683778]

[80]   Mazumdar A, Poage GM, Shepherd J, *et al.* Analysis of phosphatases in ER-negative breast cancers

identifies DUSP4 as a critical regulator of growth and invasion. Breast Cancer Res Treat 2016; 158(3): 441-54.
[http://dx.doi.org/10.1007/s10549-016-3892-y] [PMID: 27393618]

[81]   Gaggianesi M, Turdo A, Chinnici A, *et al.* IL4 Primes the dynamics of breast cancer progression *via* DUSP4 inhibition. Cancer Res 2017; 77(12): 3268-79.
[http://dx.doi.org/10.1158/0008-5472.CAN-16-3126] [PMID: 28400477]

[82]   Rottenberg S, Jonkers J. MEK inhibition as a strategy for targeting residual breast cancer cells with low DUSP4 expression. Breast Cancer Res 2012; 14(6): 324.
[http://dx.doi.org/10.1186/bcr3327] [PMID: 23127286]

[83]   Fernandis AZ, Prasad A, Band H, Klösel R, Ganju RK. Regulation of CXCR4-mediated chemotaxis and chemoinvasion of breast cancer cells. Oncogene 2004; 23(1): 157-67.
[http://dx.doi.org/10.1038/sj.onc.1206910] [PMID: 14712221]

[84]   Fernandis AZ, Cherla RP, Ganju RK. Differential regulation of CXCR4-mediated T-cell chemotaxis and mitogen-activated protein kinase activation by the membrane tyrosine phosphatase, CD45. J Biol Chem 2003; 278(11): 9536-43.
[http://dx.doi.org/10.1074/jbc.M211803200] [PMID: 12519755]

[85]   Luo C, Pan H, Mines M, Watson K, Zhang J, Fan GH. CXCL12 induces tyrosine phosphorylation of cortactin, which plays a role in CXC chemokine receptor 4-mediated extracellular signal-regulated kinase activation and chemotaxis. J Biol Chem 2006; 281(40): 30081-93.
[http://dx.doi.org/10.1074/jbc.M605837200] [PMID: 16905744]

[86]   Bowden ET, Onikoyi E, Slack R, *et al.* Co-localization of cortactin and phosphotyrosine identifies active invadopodia in human breast cancer cells. Exp Cell Res 2006; 312(8): 1240-53.
[http://dx.doi.org/10.1016/j.yexcr.2005.12.012] [PMID: 16442522]

[87]   Buday L, Downward J. Roles of cortactin in tumor pathogenesis. Biochim Biophys Acta 2007; 1775(2): 263-73.
[PMID: 17292556]

[88]   Weaver AM. Cortactin in tumor invasiveness. Cancer Lett 2008; 265(2): 157-66.
[http://dx.doi.org/10.1016/j.canlet.2008.02.066] [PMID: 18406052]

[89]   Kirkbride KC, Sung BH, Sinha S, Weaver AM. Cortactin: a multifunctional regulator of cellular invasiveness. Cell Adhes Migr 2011; 5(2): 187-98.
[http://dx.doi.org/10.4161/cam.5.2.14773] [PMID: 21258212]

[90]   Rosenberg BJ, Gil-Henn H, Mader CC, *et al.* Phosphorylated cortactin recruits Vav2 guanine nucleotide exchange factor to activate Rac3 and promote invadopodial function in invasive breast cancer cells. Mol Biol Cell 2017; 28(10): 1347-60.
[http://dx.doi.org/10.1091/mbc.e16-12-0885] [PMID: 28356423]

[91]   Li Y, Tondravi M, Liu J, *et al.* Cortactin potentiates bone metastasis of breast cancer cells. Cancer Res 2001; 61(18): 6906-11.
[PMID: 11559568]

[92]   Fan Y, Si W, Ji W, *et al.* Rack1 mediates tyrosine phosphorylation of Anxa2 by Src and promotes invasion and metastasis in drug-resistant breast cancer cells. Breast Cancer Res 2019; 21(1): 66.
[http://dx.doi.org/10.1186/s13058-019-1147-7] [PMID: 31113450]

[93]   Vila-Coro AJ, Rodríguez-Frade JM, Martín De Ana A, Moreno-Ortíz MC, Martínez-A C, Mellado M. The chemokine SDF-1alpha triggers CXCR4 receptor dimerization and activates the JAK/STAT pathway. FASEB J 1999; 13(13): 1699-710.
[http://dx.doi.org/10.1096/fasebj.13.13.1699] [PMID: 10506573]

[94]   Ahr B, Denizot M, Robert-Hebmann V, Brelot A, Biard-Piechaczyk M. Identification of the cytoplasmic domains of CXCR4 involved in Jak2 and STAT3 phosphorylation. J Biol Chem 2005; 280(8): 6692-700.

[http://dx.doi.org/10.1074/jbc.M408481200] [PMID: 15615703]

[95] Li YM, Pan Y, Wei Y, *et al.* Upregulation of CXCR4 is essential for HER2-mediated tumor metastasis. Cancer Cell 2004; 6(5): 459-69.
[http://dx.doi.org/10.1016/j.ccr.2004.09.027] [PMID: 15542430]

[96] Akekawatchai C, Holland JD, Kochetkova M, Wallace JC, McColl SR. Transactivation of CXCR4 by the insulin-like growth factor-1 receptor (IGF-1R) in human MDA-MB-231 breast cancer epithelial cells. J Biol Chem 2005; 280(48): 39701-8.
[http://dx.doi.org/10.1074/jbc.M509829200] [PMID: 16172123]

[97] Cabioglu N, Summy J, Miller C, *et al.* CXCL-12/stromal cell-derived factor-1alpha transactivates HER2-neu in breast cancer cells by a novel pathway involving Src kinase activation. Cancer Res 2005; 65(15): 6493-7.
[http://dx.doi.org/10.1158/0008-5472.CAN-04-1303] [PMID: 16061624]

[98] Duvall-Noelle N, Karwandyar A, Richmond A, Raman D. LASP-1: a nuclear hub for the UHRF1-DNMT1-G9a-Snail1 complex. Oncogene 2016; 35(9): 1122-33.
[http://dx.doi.org/10.1038/onc.2015.166] [PMID: 25982273]

[99] Orimo A, Gupta PB, Sgroi DC, *et al.* Stromal fibroblasts present in invasive human breast carcinomas promote tumor growth and angiogenesis through elevated SDF-1/CXCL12 secretion. Cell 2005; 121(3): 335-48.
[http://dx.doi.org/10.1016/j.cell.2005.02.034] [PMID: 15882617]

[100] Orimo A, Weinberg RA. Stromal fibroblasts in cancer: a novel tumor-promoting cell type. Cell Cycle 2006; 5(15): 1597-601.
[http://dx.doi.org/10.4161/cc.5.15.3112] [PMID: 16880743]

[101] Lazennec G, Richmond A. Chemokines and chemokine receptors: new insights into cancer-related inflammation. Trends Mol Med 2010; 16(3): 133-44.
[http://dx.doi.org/10.1016/j.molmed.2010.01.003] [PMID: 20163989]

[102] Raman D, Baugher PJ, Thu YM, Richmond A. Role of chemokines in tumor growth. Cancer Lett 2007; 256(2): 137-65.
[http://dx.doi.org/10.1016/j.canlet.2007.05.013] [PMID: 17629396]

[103] Raman D, Sobolik-Delmaire T, Richmond A. Chemokines in health and disease. Exp Cell Res 2011; 317(5): 575-89.
[http://dx.doi.org/10.1016/j.yexcr.2011.01.005] [PMID: 21223965]

[104] Sheridan C, Kishimoto H, Fuchs RK, *et al.* CD44+/CD24- breast cancer cells exhibit enhanced invasive properties: an early step necessary for metastasis. Breast Cancer Res 2006; 8(5): R59.
[http://dx.doi.org/10.1186/bcr1610] [PMID: 17062128]

[105] Zhang H, Brown RL, Wei Y, *et al.* CD44 splice isoform switching determines breast cancer stem cell state. Genes Dev 2019; 33(3-4): 166-79.
[http://dx.doi.org/10.1101/gad.319889.118] [PMID: 30692202]

[106] Liu X, Taftaf R, Kawaguchi M, *et al.* Homophilic CD44 interactions mediate tumor cell aggregation and polyclonal metastasis in patient-derived breast cancer models. Cancer Discov 2019; 9(1): 96-113.
[http://dx.doi.org/10.1158/2159-8290.CD-18-0065] [PMID: 30361447]

[107] Senbanjo LT, Chellaiah MA. CD44: A multifunctional cell surface adhesion receptor is a regulator of progression and metastasis of cancer cells. Front Cell Dev Biol 2017; 5(18): 18.
[http://dx.doi.org/10.3389/fcell.2017.00018] [PMID: 28326306]

[108] Işman FK, Kucukgergin C, Daşdemir S, Cakmakoglu B, Sanli O, Seckin S. Association between SDF1-3'A or CXCR4 gene polymorphisms with predisposition to and clinicopathological characteristics of prostate cancer with or without metastases. Mol Biol Rep 2012; 39(12): 11073-9.
[http://dx.doi.org/10.1007/s11033-012-2010-4] [PMID: 23053994]

[109] Al-Hajj M, Wicha MS, Benito-Hernandez A, Morrison SJ, Clarke MF. Prospective identification of tumorigenic breast cancer cells. Proc Natl Acad Sci USA 2003; 100(7): 3983-8.
[http://dx.doi.org/10.1073/pnas.0530291100] [PMID: 12629218]

[110] Qiu Y, Pu T, Guo P, *et al.* ALDH(+)/CD44(+) cells in breast cancer are associated with worse prognosis and poor clinical outcome. Exp Mol Pathol 2016; 100(1): 145-50.
[http://dx.doi.org/10.1016/j.yexmp.2015.11.032] [PMID: 26687806]

[111] Mukherjee S, Manna A, Bhattacharjee P, *et al.* Non-migratory tumorigenic intrinsic cancer stem cells ensure breast cancer metastasis by generation of CXCR4(+) migrating cancer stem cells. Oncogene 2016; 35(37): 4937-48.
[http://dx.doi.org/10.1038/onc.2016.26] [PMID: 26923331]

[112] Yi T, Zhai B, Yu Y, *et al.* Quantitative phosphoproteomic analysis reveals system-wide signaling pathways downstream of SDF-1/CXCR4 in breast cancer stem cells. Proc Natl Acad Sci 2014; 111: E2182-2190.

[113] Scala S. Molecular Pathways: Targeting the CXCR4-CXCL12 Axis--Untapped Potential in the Tumor Microenvironment. Clin Cancer Res 2015; 21(19): 4278-85.
[http://dx.doi.org/10.1158/1078-0432.CCR-14-0914] [PMID: 26199389]

[114] Xu L, Hunter ZR, Tsakmaklis N, *et al.* Clonal architecture of CXCR4 WHIM-like mutations in Waldenström Macroglobulinaemia. Br J Haematol 2016; 172(5): 735-744, 5409813.
[http://dx.doi.org/10.1111/bjh.13897] [PMID: 26659815]

[115] McDermott DH, Liu Q, Ulrick J, *et al.* The CXCR4 antagonist plerixafor corrects panleukopenia in patients with WHIM syndrome. Blood 2011; 118(18): 4957-4962, 3208300.
[http://dx.doi.org/10.1182/blood-2011-07-368084] [PMID: 21890643]

[116] Ling X, Spaeth E, Chen Y, *et al.* The CXCR4 antagonist AMD3465 regulates oncogenic signaling and invasiveness *in vitro* and prevents breast cancer growth and metastasis *in vivo.* PLoS One 2013; 8(3): e58426.
[http://dx.doi.org/10.1371/journal.pone.0058426] [PMID: 23484027]

[117] Peng SB, Zhang X, Paul D, *et al.* Identification of LY2510924, a novel cyclic peptide CXCR4 antagonist that exhibits antitumor activities in solid tumor and breast cancer metastatic models. Mol Cancer Ther 2015; 14(2): 480-90.
[http://dx.doi.org/10.1158/1535-7163.MCT-14-0850] [PMID: 25504752]

[118] Pernas S, Martin M, Kaufman PA, *et al.* Balixafortide plus eribulin in HER2-negative metastatic breast cancer: a phase 1, single-arm, dose-escalation trial. Lancet Oncol 2018; 19(6): 812-24.
[http://dx.doi.org/10.1016/S1470-2045(18)30147-5] [PMID: 29706375]

[119] Chen IX, Chauhan VP, Posada J, *et al.* Blocking CXCR4 alleviates desmoplasia, increases T-lymphocyte infiltration, and improves immunotherapy in metastatic breast cancer. Proc Natl Acad Sci USA 2019; 116(10): 4558-4566, 6410779.
[http://dx.doi.org/10.1073/pnas.1815515116] [PMID: 30700545]

[120] Jin W, Wu L, Liang K, Liu B, Lu Y, Fan Z. Roles of the PI-3K and MEK pathways in Ras-mediated chemoresistance in breast cancer cells. Br J Cancer 2003; 89(1): 185-191, 2394213.
[http://dx.doi.org/10.1038/sj.bjc.6601048] [PMID: 12838322]

[121] Zhang Y, Kwok-Shing Ng P, Kucherlapati M, *et al.* A Pan-Cancer Proteogenomic Atlas of PI3K/AKT/mTOR Pathway Alterations. Cancer Cell 2017; 31(6): 820-32.

[122] Gasser JA, Inuzuka H, Lau AW, Wei W, Beroukhim R, Toker A. SGK3 mediates INPP4B-dependent PI3K signaling in breast cancer. Mol Cell 2014; 56(4): 595-607.
[http://dx.doi.org/10.1016/j.molcel.2014.09.023] [PMID: 25458846]

[123] Maurer M, Su T, Saal LH, *et al.* 3-Phosphoinositide-dependent kinase 1 potentiates upstream lesions on the phosphatidylinositol 3-kinase pathway in breast carcinoma. Cancer Res 2009; 69(15): 6299-306.
[http://dx.doi.org/10.1158/0008-5472.CAN-09-0820] [PMID: 19602588]

[124]   Arafeh R, Samuels Y. PIK3CA in cancer: The past 30 years. Semin Cancer Biol 2019; 59: 36-49.
[http://dx.doi.org/10.1016/j.semcancer.2019.02.002] [PMID: 30742905]

[125]   Janku F, Yap TA, Meric-Bernstam F. Targeting the PI3K pathway in cancer: are we making headway?
Nat Rev Clin Oncol 2018; 15(5): 273-91.
[http://dx.doi.org/10.1038/nrclinonc.2018.28] [PMID: 29508857]

[126]   Jung HH, Lee SH, Kim JY, Ahn JS, Park YH, Im YH. Statins affect ETS1-overexpressing triple-
negative breast cancer cells by restoring DUSP4 deficiency. Sci Rep 2016; 6(33035): 33035.
[http://dx.doi.org/10.1038/srep33035] [PMID: 27604655]

CHAPTER 3

Epidermal Growth Factor Receptor Signaling in Colon Cancer

Avtar S. Meena[1,*] and **Pradeep K. Shukla**[2,*]

¹ CSIR-Centre for Cellular and Molecular Biology (CCMB) Habsiguda, Uppal Road Hyderabad - 500 007 Telangana, India

² Department of Physiology, College of Medicine, University of Tennessee Health Science Center, Memphis, TN, USA

Abstract: Epidermal growth factor receptor (EGFR) expression regulates cancer cell proliferation, survival, and metastatic potential and is associated with the majority of human carcinomas, including colorectal carcinoma. The relationship between EGFR expression and its prognosis in cancer patients, however, has not been proven in clinical settings. Various preclinical studies suggest that the oncogenic potential of EGFR is associated with levels of EGFR ligands. Mutations in EGFR family ligands and their receptors are characteristic of many different kinds of tumors. Therefore, this signaling axis is an attractive target for the development of targeted therapies. Various small molecule inhibitors and antibodies are in clinical trials that specifically target EGFR.

Here, we will discuss the current literature's attempts to identify markers, which contribute resistance and sensitivity to small molecule EGFR inhibitors. Moreover, we will summarize the role of EGFR in the development of colon cancer. We will discuss the mechanistic basis for EGFR interaction with various molecules, its consequences for biology, and its prospective importance as a target for colon cancer therapy.

Keywords: Cancer therapy, Cancer cell proliferation, Colon cancer, EGFR ligands, Epidermal growth factor receptor (EGFR), Targeted therapies.

COLORECTAL CANCER AND RISK FACTORS

Colorectal cancer (CRC) is the second most prevalent human malignant disease. It is one of the prominent causes of cancer-related mortalities globally [1]. The development of CRC comprises a complex multistage process in which sequential

*** Corresponding authors Pradeep K. Shukla and Avtar S. Meena:** Department of Physiology, College of Medicine, University of Tennessee Health Science Center, Memphis, TN, USA; Tel: 38163-2113; (901) 448-3019 and CSIR-Centre for Cellular and Molecular Biology (CCMB), Habsiguda, Uppal Road, Hyderabad-500007 Telangana, India; Tel: +91-40-27160222; E-mails: pshukla2@uthsc.edu and avtarsingh@ccmb.res.in, respectively

Manoj K. Pandey & Vijay P. Kale (Eds.)

mutational events occur along with the progression of cancer. The 5 -year survival of patients diagnosed with metastatic colorectal cancer (mCRC) is approximately 13-18%. Early detection and treatments are essential for the prevention of colon cancer-related death. Approximately 60-80% of CRC patients exhibit overexpression of EGFR, which is associated with poor prognosis [2]. Various treatment agents have recently been established to demonstrate prominent efficacy in the treatment of mCRC.

For this reason, EGFR has been the central target for treatment with small-molecule inhibitor and monoclonal antibodies, cetuximab and panitumumab, which have been useful for patients with RAS wild type in randomized clinical trials [3 - 5]. There are multiple significant risk factors for the development of CRC, which are crucial for an increase in the rate of genetic mutation occurring in tumor suppressor genes and various oncogenes as well. These factors generally include environmental exposure, personal or family history of CRC, genetic mutation, location, and associated disease(s). Environmental exposures such as smoking, alcohol use, sedentary lifestyle, diet, and abdominal radiation are associated with an increased risk of CRC [6 - 12]. Supplementation of a high-fat Western diet promotes the development of colon cancer *via* an EGFR mediated mechanism [13]. Various habits or personal behaviors are major risk factors for the development of colorectal cancer (CRC). As with many cancers, the risk of CRC increases with age without gender differences [14]. Other than the age, people who have diabetes, obesity, and inflammatory bowel disease (IBD) are at higher risk of developing CRC, respectively [15 - 17]. We will discuss EGFR signaling, the development of anti-EGFR therapies, and mechanisms of resistance to EGFR therapies in CRC.

EGFR SIGNALING IN CRC

EGFR is one of the crucial targets to be exploited in cancer treatment, including CRC. The receptor, which belongs to the receptor tyrosine kinase (RTK) family, also known as HER1 (human EGFR receptor), is a 170-kDa transmembrane protein that acts as a receptor for the EGF family. In addition to EGFR, the receptors belonging to the RTK superfamily are ErbB- 2 (HER/c-neu), ErbB-3 (Her 3), and ErbB-4 (Her 4). All of these receptors are composed of an extracellular ligand-binding domain (cysteine-rich domain), a hydrophobic transmembrane region, a short juxta-membrane section, and an intracytoplasmic tyrosine kinase C-terminal domain (Fig. **1A**). EGFR and ErbB4 receptor exhibit a similar structure and are involved in ligand-dependent homo- or heterodi-merization. In contrast, erbB2 lacks a ligand-binding domain and has been shown to elicit both ligand-dependent and independent dimerization [18, 19]. ErbB3 also undergoes ligand-dependent dimerization; however, these receptors have been shown defective in their intrinsic tyrosine kinase activities. Therefore, they require heterodimerization with another member of the erbB family for the activation of signaling cascade [20]. Autophosphorylation of one intracellular kinase domain by the others promotes downstream signaling cascades. In general, there are seven combinations of receptor dimers and ten ligands binding partners that play a crucial role in the activation of downstream signaling cascade [21]. Various combinations of receptors and their ligands involved in signaling pathways summarized in Fig. (**1B**) and (**1C**). EGFR is expressed on all stromal and epithelial cells and is presented on various glial and smooth muscle cells as well [22]. Because of its involvement in cancers, EGFR has been a focus for the development of drug targets. Multiple studies suggest the role of EGFR in neoplastic progression. Three crucial mechanisms have been documented so far. First, a mutation in the EGFR gene, which leads to its constitutive activation even in the absence of ligand [23, 24]. Second, increased EGFR expression in breast, non-small cell lung, and colon cancer [25, 26]. However, it has remained unclear whether increased expression correlated with oncogenic activity. Third, EGFR signaling involves the binding of specific soluble ligands (*e.g.*, EGF, amphiregulin, epiregulin, betacellulin, or neuregulin), and mediate downstream signaling. Downstream signaling regulates cellular activities, including cell growth, survival, proliferation, inhibition of apoptosis, and differentiation in mammalian cells [27]. Binding of ligand to EGFR induces conformational changes in the receptor that promotes homo- or heterodimer formation between receptors. Receptor dimerization is crucial for the activation of intracellular tyrosine kinase and phosphorylation of the C-terminal domains, which provide a docking site for cytoplasmic proteins harboring phosphotyrosine-binding and Src homology-2 domains [28]. EGFR family activates Ras/Raf/MEK/MAPK, PLCγ-1/PKC, phosphatidylinositol-3 kinase/Akt, and STAT pathways (Fig. **2**). In the next section, we will discuss the role of the EGF-like growth factors, MAPK, and PI3K/ Akt signaling pathways, which have pivotal roles in CRC development and progression (Fig. **2**). Moreover, various signaling molecules and their mutation status involved in CRC progression are summarized in Table **1**.

Table 1. Summary of Signaling pathways altered in CRC.

Gene	Protein Function	Observed Alteration	Mutation	Ref.
EGFR	Transmembrane tyrosine kinase receptor	Mutation	Very Rare	[42]
		Protein Expression	30-90%	[148]
		Increased Copy Number	0-50%	[149]
KRAS	GDP/GTP binding protein facilitates EGFR downstream signaling	Activating Mutation	35-40%	[112, 113, 150]

(Table 1) cont.....

Gene	Protein Function	Observed Alteration	Mutation	Ref.
NRAS	GDP/GTP binding protein facilitates EGFR downstream signaling	Mutation	3-5%	[112, 113, 151]
HRAS	GDP/GTP binding protein facilitates EGFR downstream signaling	Mutation	Negligible	[112, 113]
BRAF	Serine/ Threonine kinase protein, act downstream of Ras protein	Activating Mutation (V600E)	10%	[120, 121, 152]
PIK3CA	Involved in PI3K/ Akt signaling cascade	Activating Mutation (exon 9 and 20)	10-20%	[127, 153]
PTEN	Phosphatase enzyme act as a tumor suppressor gene and negatively regulate PI3K pathway	Loss of PTEN activity; Mutation, Loss of Heterozygosity	25-45%	[126]

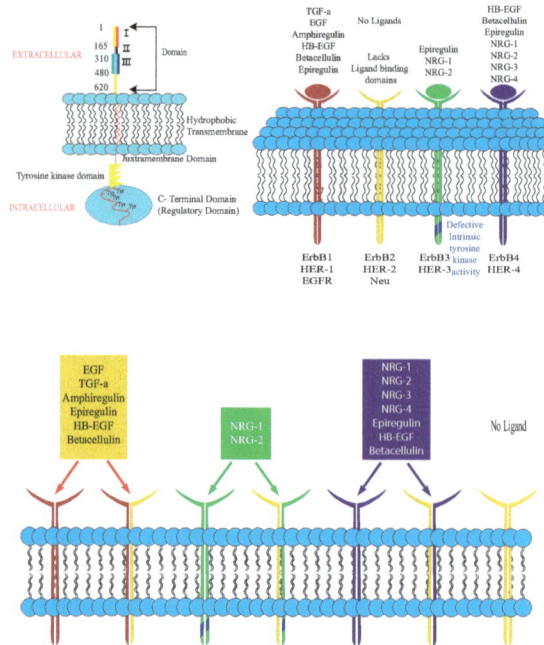

Fig. (1). The ErbB receptors and their ligands.

The ErbB family of receptor consists of extracellular domains (domain I to IV; I and II are leucine-rich domains, and III & IV are cysteine-rich domains), transmembrane domain, a short juxta-membrane segment and c-terminal intracellular domain. C- terminal contains regulatory sites and phosphorylation sites, acts as a docking site, and involved in the activation of the downstream signaling cascade. Ligands that bind to specific receptor are depicted on the top in Fig. (**1B**). The different EGFR dimers and their interacting ligands are shown in Fig. (**1C**). Note that erbB2 dimers work even without presence of ligands and ErbB3 lacks intrinsic tyrosine kinase activity. Abbreviation: TGF-α, transforming growth factor- α; EGF, epidermal growth factor; NRG, neuregulin; HB-EGF, heparin-binding EGF.

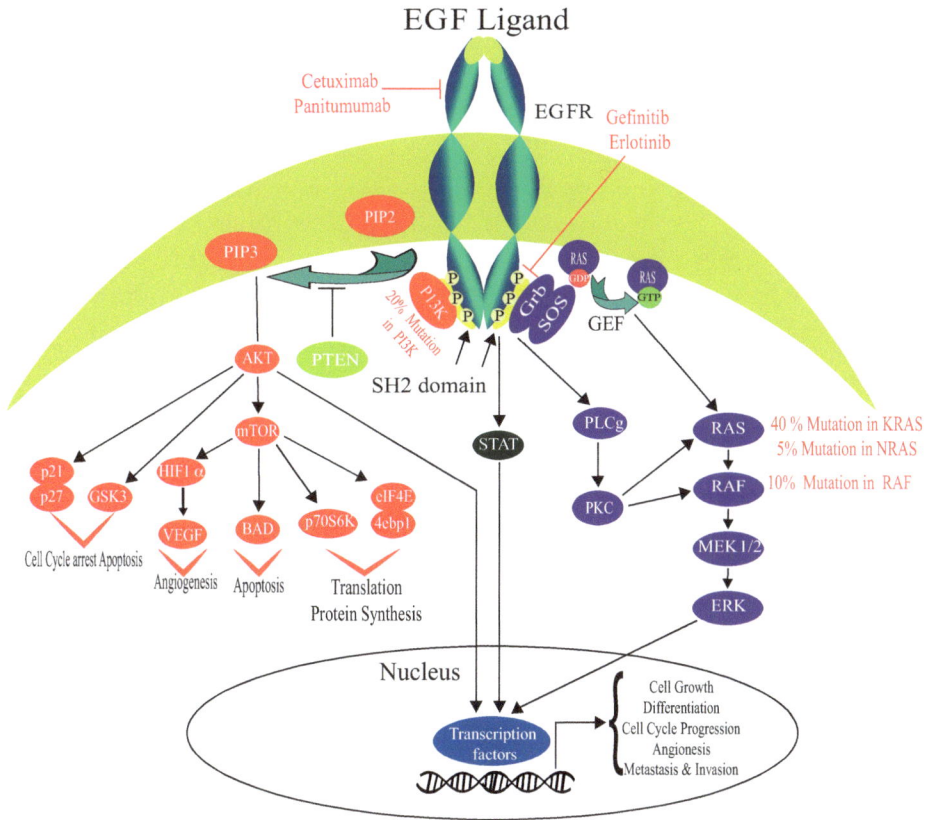

Fig. (2). Schematic diagram of the EGFR signaling pathway.
Growth factor binding induces dimerization, autophosphorylation of the c-terminal intracellular tyrosine kinase domain and leads to the activation of EGFR signaling pathways including PI3K/AKT, RAS/MAPK and other signaling pathways, promoting the processes of cell growth, proliferation, survival, angiogenesis, metastasis/ invasion, and inhibition of apoptosis. EGFR moAbs, cetuximab and panitumumab, prevent the binding of ligands to EGFR. Erlotinib and gefitinib inhibit the TK activity of the EGFR TK domain. Both agents block signaling pathways critical in the survival and proliferation of cancer cells. *PTEN* inhibits the PI3K/Akt signaling by dephosphorylating PIP3. *Regular arrow: activates, Arrow ending with a straight line: inhibits.*

EGF-like Growth Factors

The majority of human carcinomas including breast, lung, colon, ovary, and head and neck cancers express different levels of their specific EGF-like growth factors (Table **2**). TGF-α expression has been found in colon adenomas, suggesting a potential role in early tumorigenesis and resistance to cetuximab through the EGFR-MET axis [29]. However, various studies failed to establish a correlation between TGF- α expression and patient outcome. It may be due to the co-expression of other EGF-like peptides in most human carcinomas [30, 31]. In colon carcinomas, expression of amphiregulin correlates with more differentiated phenotypes [32 - 34]. The expression of amphiregulin frequently occurs in healthy tissues. In contrast, its loss has been demonstrated in the tissues surrounding both breast and colon carcinomas [32, 34, 35]. The expression of heparin-binding EGF (HB-EGF) is negatively regulated by the aggressiveness of the tumors. Its transcripts or protein levels detected in colon, hepatocellular, and gastric carcinomas [36 - 39]. The occurrence of HB-EGF is higher in colon adenomas as compared with other carcinomas, suggesting its involvement in early tumorigenesis. Expressions of TGF- α, amphiregulin, and HB-EGF proteins were detected by immunohistochemistry in 50-90%, 50-77%, and 28% colon carcinomas, respectively.

Table 2. Expression of EGFR ligands in human cancer.

EGFR Ligand	Colon	Breast	Lung	Ovary	Ref.
TGF-α	55-90%	42-75%	70-100%	60-100%	[30, 31, 154, 155]
Amphiregulin	55-80%	40-85%	15-80%	20-75%	[32, 34, 35, 155]
Heparin-binding EGFR	Not assessed	25-30%	Not assessed	80-92%	[37, 38, 157, 158]
Heregulin/Neuregulin	30%	75%	0%	55%	[156, 159-162]

MAPK Signaling

EGFR signaling pathways have an adaptor protein complex that comprises the son of sevenless (SOS) and the growth factor receptor-bound protein 2 (Grb2). This complex binds to phosphorylated residues on the cytoplasmic domain of the EGFR, which further activates Ras-GTP and promotes a signaling cascade of Ras-Raf-MEK and ERK through phosphorylation. The Ras-Raf-ERK signaling cascade plays a crucial role in the regulation of cell survival, differentiation, and growth. Dysregulation of this cascade promotes malignant transformation and tumor progression through increased cell survival, invasion, angiogenesis, proliferation, and anti-apoptosis. The EGFR/MAPK signaling pathway is correlated with oncogenic potential and, therefore, crucial in the development of tumor growth and the progression of CRC [40, 41]. Aberrant expression of these pathways is a documented target for CRC treatment [42, 43]. Ras and Raf proteins are essential signaling molecules located downstream of EGFR pathways, and these often mutate in the development of CRC.

PI3K/ Akt Signaling

PI3Ks are heterodimeric lipid/protein kinases that differ in their structure, tissue distribution, activation, specificity, and regulation. PI3K activation increases various downstream pathways responsible for cellular transformation, adhesion, cell growth, apoptosis, motility, and survival [44]. PI3K is one of the essential pathways, which is stimulated by EGFR signaling. Subunits of PI3K such as p110a (catalytic subunit) and p85 (regulatory subunit), play a crucial role in tumorigenesis, as p110a subunit frequently found to be mutated in several tumors including CRC [45]. Akt, a serine/threonine-protein kinase (Ser/Thr kinase) located in downstream of PI3K signaling cascade, confers tumor growth, development, cell proliferation, and inhibition of apoptosis in human CRCs. Many molecules have developed to inhibit the PI3K/Akt pathway for CRC treatment [46]. Stimulation of receptor tyrosine kinase (RTK) or activation of Ras, leads to the activation of PI3K signaling in which p85 subunit binds to phosphor-tyrosine residues of RTK, and displaces p110 (inhibitor effect). Activated PI3K generates phosphatidylinositol 3,4,5 triphosphate (PIP3) through phosphorylation of phosphatidylinositol 4,5 biphosphate (PIP2). PIP3 then activates AKT, which plays a pivotal role in cell proliferation and cell survival. The mammalian target of rapamycin (mTOR) is activated downstream of Akt, and it promotes protein translation, metabolism, angiogenesis, and growth. Phosphatase and tensin homolog protein (*PTEN*) acts as a tumor suppressor molecule and downregulates the PI3K/Akt pathway through dephosphorylation of PIP3. It suggests that PI3K signaling cascade serves as an oncogenic potential in the initiation and progression of CRC [47]. Multiple reports demonstrate that targeted inhibition of PI3K causes an increase in apoptosis and a decrease in CRC growth [46].

Emerging Role of EGFR in the Development of Colon Cancer

Homeobox A3 (HOXA3) is a transcription factor that regulates gene expression during embryonic development. HOXA3 expression has reported to be associated with several cancers, including colon cancer. *In vitro* and *in vivo* studies suggest that HOXA3 expression increases in colon tumor tissues and cell lines, which is associated with a low survival rate. Downregulation of HOXA3 suppresses the activation of the EGFR downstream signaling pathway, suggesting that HOXA3 acts as a promoter for colon cancer development by regulating EGFR signaling. HOXA3 might be a potential therapeutic target in the treatment of colon cancer [48]. A recent study suggests the involvement of microRNA in colon cancer and demonstrates that targeting microRNA 375 (MIR375) possesses a therapeutic value in the treatment of colon cancer. In this study, the author showed that the connective tissue growth factor is a direct gene of MIR375, a ligand of EGFR, and significantly increases in CRC tissues in comparison to normal colon tissues. Using xenograft of MIR375-overexpressing colorectal cells in mice, the author showed that MIR375 regulates cell growth and proliferation, migration, cell cycle in colon cells. Also, overexpression of MIR375, along with cetuximab treatment-induced apoptosis and necrosis, suggests that MIR372 may have therapeutic value in the treatment of CRC [49]. EGF plays a crucial role in the regulation of EGFR expression and affecting migration, invasion, and proliferative abilities of cancer cells. Besides these, it regulates MEK1/2-ERK, JAK/STT, and PI3K-Akt pathways. Distinct involvements of these signaling and targeting pathways will help to design a novel agent to treat colon cancer [50]. C-terminal tensin-like (CTEN; TNS4) is a focal adhesion molecule that belongs to the tensin family. CTEN expression increased by EGF, and induced EGF- mediated metastasis. In the presence of CTEN, EGF binding elevated EGFR protein expression and extended half-life of EGFR. CTEN reduced degradation of EGFR by binding to c-Cbl and decreasing EGFR ubiquitination. These data demonstrate that CTEN enhanced cancer cell migration through elevated EGFR signaling by reducing degradation [51]. Direct visualization of endogenous expression of EGFR is not possible. Therefore, Yang *et al.* developed a system using CRISPR/Cas9, in which a fluorescent reporter gene helps to detect EGFR by binding to its C-terminus. Upon stimulation with EGF or amphiregulin, a very distinct pattern of EGFR internalization and trafficking was observed. Moreover, EGFR localizes mostly to the crypt rather than the villus compartment, and its expression is seen more frequently in epithelial tumors that other intestinal tumors. This report will permit *in vivo* monitoring of the dynamics of EGFR localization and trafficking in normal and disease conditions [52]. Expression of EGFR in myeloid cells from the stroma of human CRC is associated with tumor metastasis and shorter life span. Deletion of EGFR in myeloid cells, but not intestinal epithelial cells, protects mice from colitis-induced colon cancer. EGFR signaling in myeloid cells resulted in severe colitis after DSS administration, increased intestinal inflammation, barrier dysfunction, and promoted activation of STAT3. These data demonstrate that expression of EGFR in myeloid cells, rather than cancer cells, contributes to tumor progression [53]. Deoxycholic acid (DCA) treatment increased intracellular calcium level and CAM-kinase II, which leads to MAPK activation through recruitment of c-Src. The combination of DCA and EGF, synergistically activates MAPK signaling in a non-canonical manner. This mechanism prevents EGFR degradation, and allows constitutive activation, which is crucial for tumor-promoting effects in colon cancer [54]. Expressions of ephrinA5 and EGFR expression were analyzed in both colon and normal tissues, and revealed that ephrinA5 mRNA and protein levels downregulated in colon cancer compared to normal counterparts. The expression of ephrinA5 was negatively associated with tumor aggressiveness. EphrinA5 inhibited colon cancer progression by promoting c-Cbl mediated ubiquitination and degradation of EGFR, thus suppressing resistance, cell growth, and migration ability of cancer cells [55]. Fibroblast growth factor (FGF) expression is strongly associated with cancer progression. FGF9 overexpression in the CRC cell line induces resistance to anti-EGFR therapy, which is blocked by the FGFR9 inhibitor, suggests that combined treatment of anti-EGFR and FGFR inhibitor would be a better treatment in CRC patients where FGFR9 is upregulated [56]. Several studies suggest that sialyation has crucial involvement in the progression of cancer. NEU3 is a plasma membrane-associated sialidase whose deregulation frequently observed in various cancers including cervical, and CRC. The report suggests that NEU3 has interacted with EGFR, and overexpression of wild type NEU3 increased receptor without affecting mRNA and protein expression [57].

EGFR THERAPIES

The EGFR signaling cascade plays a crucial involvement in tumor development and the advancement of numerous cancers, including CRC. EGFR is highly regulated by its inhibitory mechanisms, which involve *de novo* expression of EGFR inhibitors, and dephosphorylation by protein tyrosine phosphatases [58]. Dysregulation of feedback mechanisms contributes to the development of cancer through hyperactivation of RTK, and the constitutive activation of downstream effector molecules [59]. EGFR protein or mRNA expression has shown a prominent factor in the majority of the cancer studies. The frequency of EGFR expression in human cancer is high, and detected by immunohistochemistry, which is associated with poor survival and tumor progression. An elevated level of EGFR expression has been reported in 26% to 80% of colon cancer, with an average of approximately 51%. However, the clinical significance of EGFR protein expression is uncertain in CRC. One research group demonstrated an association of EGFR overexpression and reduced CRC survival rates, while another group found no association between them. Other studies exhibit an association of EGFR expression with tumor grade in CRC, while some do not show this association [60 - 63]. Observations from preclinical and clinical studies demonstrate that cancer with low expression of EGFR may respond to anti-EGFR agents [64]. Therefore, it is crucial to define a standardized and unique technique for evaluating EGFR expression in tumors that reflect the existence of tools such as anti-EGFR agents currently used to treat patients.

Anti-EGFR Receptor Therapy

The first-line treatment for patients with metastatic colorectal cancer (mCRC), is based on patient history, tumor-related factors, and molecular evidence to evaluate the individualized treatment. This receptor has become a promising candidate for anticancer therapies due to the significant involvement of EGFR and its downstream signaling in tumor growth and disease progression. Preclinical and clinical studies evaluated that blocking EGFR and downstream pathways may lead to cancer cell growth inhibition, resulting in significant benefits for cancer patients. Several therapies targeting EGFR have been investigated, and most of them have been tested in clinical trials. Two classes of agents are developed and used in cancer treatment that targets EGFR explicitly: 1) tyrosine kinase inhibitors (TKI), are small molecules that bind to the tyrosine kinase domain in EGFR and block its activity. TKIs are erlotinib and gefitinib. 2) monoclonal antibodies (mAbs) bind to the extracellular complex of EGFR and prevent ligands binding to the receptor. Cetuximab and Panitumumab are mAbs used for the treatment of CRC. Both approaches lead to the inhibition of EGFR autophosphorylation [65]. Multiple studies have demonstrated that TKI application is restricted to the cases where the EGFR mutation occurs in the kinase domain of exons 18-21 (except for exon 20 variations, which appear to be blocked only by irreversible TKIs). Therefore, CRC patients whose mutation is rarely detected, cannot benefit from TKI administration [42, 66]. Anti-EGFR mAbs cetuximab or panitumumab are prominent and effective treatment regimen for EGFR expressing CRC. Several clinical trials have been performed to evaluate the effectiveness of anti-EGFR mAbs or TKIs alone and in combination with chemotherapeutic drugs in treating mCRC patients, too (Table **3**).

Table 3. Anti-EGFR therapies (mAbs and TKI).

Treatment Regimen	Number of Patients Recruited	Population	Response Rate (RR, in %)	Overall Survival (OS, in months)	Progression-Free Survival (PFS, in months)	Ref.
CETUXIMAB						
Cetuximab+ FOLFIRI *vs.* FOLFIRI	1198	Intent to treat	46.9 *vs.* 38.7	19.9 *vs.* 18.6	8.9 *vs.* 8.0	[5]
	666	*KRAS wild type*	57.3 *vs.* 39.7	23.5 *vs.* 20.0	9.9 *vs.* 8.4	
	397	*KRAS mutant*	31.3 *vs.* 36.1	16.2 *vs.* 16.7	7.4 *vs.* 7.7	
Cetuximab+ FOLFOX *vs.* FOLFOX	337	Intent to treat	46.0 *vs.* 36.0	18.3 *vs.* 18.0	7.2 *vs.* 7.2	[76]
	179	*KRAS wild type*	57.0 *vs.* 34.0	22.8 *vs.* 18.5	8.3 *vs.* 7.2	
	136	*KRAS mutant*	34.0 *vs.* 53.0	13.4 *vs.* 17.5	5.5 *vs.* 8.6	
Cetuximab + FLOFOX/XELOX *vs.* FLOFOX/XELOX	729	*KRAS wild type*	64.0 *vs.* 57.0	17.0 *vs.* 17.9	8.6 *vs.* 8.6	[4]

Treatment Regimen	Number of Patients Recruited	Population	Response Rate (RR, in %)	Overall Survival (OS, in months)	Progression-Free Survival (PFS, in months)	Ref.
Cetuximab+ FLOX *vs.* Intermittent Cetuximab+ FLOX *vs.* FLOX	566	Intent to treat	49.0 *vs.* 47.0 *vs.* 41.0	19.7 *vs.* 20.3 *vs.* 20.4	8.3 *vs.* 7.3 *vs.* 7.9	[77]
	303	*KRAS wild type*	46.0 *vs.* 51.0 *vs.* 47.0	20.1 *vs.* 21.4 *vs.* 22.0	7.9 *vs.* 7.5 *vs.* 8.7	
	137	*KRAS mutant*	49.0 *vs.* 42.0 *vs.* 40.0	21.1 *vs.* 20.5 *vs.* 20.4	9.2 *vs.* 7.2 *vs.* 7.8	
PANITUMUMAB						
Panitumumab+ FOLFOX *vs.* FOLFOX	512	*KRAS wild type*	NR	25.8 *vs.* 202	10.1 *vs.* 7.9	[3, 80]
	656	*KRAS wild type*	55.0 *vs.* 48.0	23.9 *vs.* 19.7	9.6 *vs.* 8.0	
	548	*KRAS mutant*	NR	15.5 *vs.* 18.7	7.3 *vs.* 8.7	
	440	*KRAS mutant*	40.0 *vs.* 40.0	15.5 *vs.* 19.3	7.3 *vs.* 8.8	
ERLOTINIB						
Erlotinib+ XELOX	32	Phase II trial	25%	14.7	5.4	[86, 87, 163]
Erlotinib+FOLFOX4+B evacizumab	30	Phase II trial	57%	12.4	10.9	[88]
Erlotinib+FOLFIRI	6	Phase I trial	1%	--	5	
GEFITINIB						
Gefitinib	115	Phase II trial	< 1	6.3	--	[92]
Gefitinib+ FOLFOX4	27	Phase II trial	78	--	--	[95]
Gefitinib+ FOLFOX4	27	Phase II trial	33	12	5.4	[96]
Gefitinib+ Irinotecan	39	Phase I/II trial	11.1	9.3	--	[97]
Gefitinib+FOLFIRI	16	Phase I trial	25	--	--	[164]

FOLFIRI: fluoropyrimidine + irinotecan ; FOLFOX: fluoropyrimidine + oxaliplatin, FLOX, fluoropyrimidine + folinic acid + oxaliplatin; XELOX: Capecitabine + oxaliplatin

Anti-EGFR Monoclonal Antibodies

Cetuximab

Cetuximab is a recombinant human/mouse IgG1 mAb used for the treatment of metastatic CRC, metastatic non-small cell lung cancer (NSCLC), and head and neck cancer. Cetuximab binds to the extracellular endogenous binding domain of EGFR with high affinity, and subsequently, inhibits the binding of EGFR with their ligands. Consequently, it inhibits the activation of receptor tyrosine kinase and downstream signaling pathways that are related to cell proliferation, survival, angiogenesis, and metastasis [66 - 68]. Cetuximab inhibits cancer growth with parallel inhibition of STAT3 activity in tumor xenograft animal studies. Knockdown of protein tyrosine phosphatase receptor delta, enhanced STAT3 activity, and promoted resistance to cetuximab treatment. HN5 cells exhibit acquired drug resistance to AG1478 and display increased STAT3 activity. These cells sensitized to AG1478, cetuximab, and erlotinib. When combined with the STAT3 inhibitor, they may provide therapeutic benefits for CRC patients [69]. Cetuximab treatment increases HER3 and its phosphorylation through AKT inhibition. Lapatinib, EGFR, and HER tyrosine kinase inhibitors, are shown to exert their effects by preventing cetuximab-induced-HER2/HER3 dimerization and HER3 phosphorylation [70]. In CRC, anti-EGFR antibodies routinely used as a therapy. Various studies suggest that mutation in EGFR kinase domains such as G719S and G724S, plays a role in oncogenic function. Studies performed *in vitro* suggest that cetuximab is very effective against colon cancer-derived G719S and G724S mutants and may benefit as first-line therapy [71]. Celecoxib is a nonsteroidal anti-inflammatory drug (NSAID), specifically a COX-2 inhibitor, which reduces inflammation. Celecoxib is shown to induce phosphorylation of ERk1/2, and increased EGFR mRNA and protein expression in colon tumor-associated fibroblasts, promoting EGFR binding and internalization, increasing responsiveness to anti- EGFR therapy [72]. Zhang *et al.*, showed that cetuximab, effectively inhibited AOM/DSS-induced colitis-associated tumorigenesis, downregulated M2-related markers, and decreased F4/80+/CD206+ macrophage populations *in vivo* [73]. These data suggest that knockdown of EGFR signaling in colon cancer cells regulates the secretion of cytokines, and prevents M1-to-M2 macrophage polarization, hence reduces cancer cell proliferation. Mechanism of blocking EGFR pathway by cetuximab supported at both preclinical and clinical settings, where it demonstrated cytostatic activity alone, and in combination with chemotherapeutic drugs potentiated antitumor activities. In the BOND1 study, cetuximab was used as a single agent or in combination with irinotecan in 329 CRC patients refracting to irinotecan-based chemotherapy. Response rate (RR), time to progression (TTP) and, stable disease (SD) were significantly higher in cetuximab/ irinotecan arm in comparison to cetuximab alone [74, 75]. The

BOND1 trials led to the approval of cetuximab for CRC patients were refractory to irinotecan therapy. In the CRYSTAL study, 1,198 untreated patients with mCRC were randomized to assess fluoropyrimidine plus irinotecan (FOLFIRI) alone or in combination with cetuximab. In the intent-to-treat (ITT) population, progression free-survival (PFS) significantly improved in the combination arm compared to FOLFIRI alone (8.9 *vs.* 8.0 months), but not overall survival (OS). Interestingly, patients with wild type *KRAS*, combination arm significantly improved PFS (9.9 v/s 8.4 months) and OS (23.5 *vs.* 20 months) [75]. In OPUS trial, cetuximab used in combination with fluoropyrimidine plus oxaliplatin (FOLFOX) or FOLFOX alone. In patients with wild type *KRAS*, the combination arm showed statistically significant benefit in terms of PFS (8.3 v/s 7.2 months) and OS (22.8 *vs.* 18.5 months) [76]. In the COIN trial, cetuximab combined with FOLFOX/ capecitabine plus oxaliplatin (XELOX) or FOLFOX/ XELOX. Cetuximab plus FOLFOX/ XELOX was superior to FOLFOX/ XELOX alone in response rate (RR) (64% *vs.* 57%; p = 0.0049), neither PFS (8.6 *vs.* 8.6 months) nor OS (17.0 *vs.* 17.9 months) was improved by adding cetuximab to FOLFOX/ XELOX [4]. Similarly, in the NORDIC trial, patients with wt *KRAS* showed no benefit by adding cetuximab to fluoropyrimidine plus folinic acid plus oxaliplatin (FLOX) in terms of OS (20.1 *vs.* 22 months) or PFS 7.9 *vs.* 8.7 months) [77].

Panitumumab

Panitumumab, fully humanized IgG2 mAb, and has approved in the US and Europe as a third-line treatment of CRC patients. Panitumumab binds to extracellular domains of EGFR and prevents its binding with transforming growth factor-α and inhibits downstream signaling, which is involved in the proliferation of cancer cells [78]. Interestingly, panitumumab also showed similar promising outcomes in a group of mCRC chemotherapy-refractory patients as compared to cetuximab treated patients and also requires wt *KRAS* for efficacy [3]. In a randomized phase III clinical trial, the effect of panitumumab plus best supportive care (BSC) evaluated with BSC alone in mCRC patients (n=463, with 184 are *KRAS* mutation). Patients with panitumumab plus BSC showed a significant improvement in PFS compared to BSC alone. Besides it, RR got improved in combination *vs.* BSC alone (28% *vs.* 8%). However, there were no significant differences observed in median OS [79]. In the first-line treatment, the panitumumab's effect evaluated in combination with FOLFLOX. PRIME study demonstrated that 512 CRC patients exhibited wild type Ras genes, and, confers significant improvement in OS (25.8 *vs.* 20.2 months), and PFS (10.1 *vs.* 7.9 months). In another study of 548 patients with RAS mutation, the addition of panitumumab to FOLFLOX has a detrimental effect on OS (15.5 *vs.* 18.7 months) and PFS 7.3 *vs.* 8.7 months) [80]. These suggest that wt RAS gene is a predictor for the effectiveness of monoclonal antibodies. Overall, except in the COIN study, these studies demonstrated improved outcomes in the patients of wt RAS gene with a combination of either cetuximab or panitumumab to chemotherapeutic drugs. The reasons for the contradictory findings of the COIN study, and the shorter median survival compared with other recent trials, are still unclear. EGFR mAbs have evaluated as first-, second-, or third-line therapy, either as a single agent or in combination with chemotherapeutic drugs. Both antibodies showed a reduction in the tumor burden, and improved quality of life of patients with refractory CRC [42, 67, 81].

Anti-EGFR Tyrosine Kinase Inhibitors

Small molecule EGFR RTK inhibitors, such as erlotinib and gefitinib, are investigated vastly in mCRC.

Erlotinib

Erlotinib (Tarceva) is a potent inhibitor of EGFR-TK used in the treatment of non-small cell lung cancer (NSCLC), pancreatic cancer, and CRC. It binds reversibly to the adenosine triphosphate (ATP) binding site of EGFR-tyrosine kinase domains and inhibits intracellular phosphorylation. The mechanism of clinical antitumor action of erlotinib is not fully understood yet. However, erlotinib effect is evaluated in a phase II study to assess its activity in patients with mCRC. Continuous administration of erlotinib (150 mg/day) alone does not show any beneficial effect in the advanced CRC patients [82, 83]. A combination of capecitabine plus erlotinib was also not effective in terms of RR, time to progression (TTP), and overall survival (OS) compared to capecitabine alone. However, combination treatment regime increases cytotoxicity in comparison to alone treated with capecitabine [84]. A combination of erlotinib and FOLFOX treatment therapy showed an RR of 40%. However, it was associated with adverse effects such as nausea, rash, diarrhea, and stomatitis [85, 86]. In another phase II trial, a combination of erlotinib and XELOX evaluated; patients pretreated with therapy experience a 25% RR, 14.7-month OS, and 44% had stable disease (SD) [87]. In another phase II trial, erlotinib added with FOLFOX/ bevacizumab was used to treat 30 CRC patients. The combination regimen overall increased 57% RR, 12.4 month- OS, and 38% SD. However, the phase II trial was closed prematurely due to associated toxicity of grade 3, including nausea, dehydration, anorexia, diarrhea, rash, and fatigue [88]. The combined effect of erlotinib and FOLFIRI evaluated in another phase II clinical trial in 6 CRS patients; however, it was stopped early due to unexpected severe toxicity [89].

Gefitinib

Gefitinib is an oral, reversible, selective inhibitor of EGFR TKI domains, and acts similar to erlotinib. Gefitinib showed promising effects when combined with chemotherapeutic agents in preclinical models of CRC [90]. In a significant phase II trial, 115 patients previously treated with irinotecan and 5-fluorouracil (5-FU) were randomized to receive gefitinib at a dose of 250 mg/day or 500 mg/day. Only one patient showed 1% RR, although 18% had SD. In another study, the gefitinib dose increased to 750mg/day; however, it did not exhibit better outcomes [91, 92]. In another phase I/ II trial, a combination of gefitinib with capecitabine or oxaliplatin showed no promising result; however, toxicity associated with the combination regimen [93, 94]. A combination of gefitinib and FOLFOX4 exhibited 78% RR in CRC patients with no history of chemotherapy and 33% RR along with 12-month OS in CRC patients who were treated previously with irinotecan and 5-FU. In this study, there was no evidence of mutation status; it emerges that gefitinib enhances the effect of FOLFLOX independent of mutational status [95, 96]. In another phase I/ II trial, 39 patients with advanced fluoropyrimidine-refractory CRC were treated with 250mg/day gefitinib and showed an 11.1% RR and 9.3-month OS. In this study, gefitinib did not increase the efficacy of irinotecan [97]. A combination of irinotecan, gefitinib, and capecitabine examined in 13 patients, but the study stopped due to severe toxicity [98]. In another phase II trial, 13 patients recruited and treated with gefitinib and FOLFIRI, seven patients required hospitalization due to toxicity [99]. In phase I clinical trial, gefitinib with either 250 mg/day or 500 mg/day along with FOLFIRI, showed 25% RR with no effect in OS.

MECHANISM OF RESISTANCE TO ANTI-EGFR THERAPY

Cetuximab and panitumumab are anti-EGFR monoclonal antibodies used to treat metastatic CRC. However, its effectiveness often compromised because of intrinsic or acquired resistance. Preclinical and clinical models demonstrated alterations in the pathways which are involved in the resistance towards anti-EGFR. Multiple factors may act synergistically or individually, and contribute towards major failure, eventually leading to par below expected outcome in cancer therapy. Clinical specimens confirmed that genetic alteration in the EGFR signaling pathways, HER2 amplification, MET amplification, and receptor tyrosine kinase (RTK) are significant players in developing the anti-EGFR therapy which eventually leads in the reactivation of AKT signaling. Besides, EGFR mutation at S492R appears to play a crucial role in acquired resistance to these therapies [100]. EGFR is considered as a potential candidate for therapies in cancer, ever since FDA approved kinase inhibitors such as Gefitinib and Osimertinib. Due to the development of resistance to current therapies, studies are now underway to find the most efficient inhibitors. Cancer cells resist EGFR kinase inhibitors through multiple mechanisms, including T790M mutations and amplification of the HER2 gene. Therefore, multi-targeted medicine to treat TKI-resistant cancer cells, along with an inhibitor of EGFR/HER2, will help overcome drug resistance [101]. In one study, an experiment designed to transfer condition media from resistant cells to sensitive parental cells. Cancer cells exhibit drug resistance to cetuximab therapy, secrete inflammatory cytokines such as IL8, IL1A, and 1B following EGFR pathway activation, promoting resistance in healthy cells to anti-EGFR therapy. This data demonstrates that inhibition of these cytokines in combination with cetuximab, may bear promise as a treatment therapy for CRC patients [102]. The activation of EGFR maintained by a balance of kinases and phosphatases activity in cancers. Protein tyrosine phosphatase receptor type O (PTPRO) is downregulated in CRC patients and is associated with poor prognosis. PTPRO acts as a phosphatase that negatively regulates SRC by dephosphorylating Y416, followed by phosphorylation of EGFR (Y845) and c-CBL ubiquitin ligase (Y731). Phosphorylation of EGFR and c-CBL enhanced EGFR receptor activity, and stability. Loss of PTPRO leads to activation of SRC/EGFR conferring resistance to EGFR inhibitors and hence, suggests that anti-SRC therapy will be beneficial where expression of PTPRO is reduced [103].

Low Expression of Amphiregulin, Epiregulin, and EGFR Gene Copy Number

Early clinical studies demonstrated that anti-EGFR therapies were ineffective in almost 80% of unselected mCRC cases, suggesting that the inherent mechanism is crucial in the development of resistance to CRC [104]. Alteration in EGFR, including EGFR-specific ligand and low EGFR gene copy numbers, have been associated with responses to EGFR- therapies in retrospective clinical studies [105, 106]. In clinical studies of 110 mCRC patients treated with cetuximab; gene expression data show that tumors expressing a high level of amphiregulin and epiregulin are more likely to respond to cetuximab in comparison to patients with low expression of these ligands. Also, low expression of amphiregulin and epiregulin were associated with inadequate response and reduced progression free survival and overall survival after treatment with cetuximab or a combination of cetuximab and irinotecan. Reduced expression of amphiregulin and epiregulin in tumors are less dependent on EGFR and, therefore, develop intrinsic resistance to EGFR inhibitors [106, 107].

Mutations in EGFR correlated with clinical responsiveness to EGFR TKI in non-small cell lung cancer patients [108]. Similarly, the response observed in breast cancer patients treated with trastuzumab [109]. Therefore, most of the studies are focused on an altered gene copy number of EGFR [110]. Results from clinical studies showed that a low EGFR gene copy number is associated with less or no response to panitumumab or cetuximab (with or without irinotecan) treatment, and with reduced OS and PFS [111]. Mechanisms behind nonresponse to anti-

EGFR therapy in cases of low EGFR gene copy number remains unknown and requires more exploration. Overall, both findings demonstrate that anti-EGFR treatment is likely to work effectively against overexpressed targets.

EGFR Downstream Effectors

RAS

Activation of RAS has commonly occurred in CRC. It is detected in about 50% of CRC patients (40% in *KRAS*, 3-5% *NRAS* and negligible in *HRAS*) [112, 113]. Mutations in the RAS gene lead to constitutive activation of RAS protein and downstream cascade, which in turn activate molecular pathways involved in metastasis and cancer cell proliferation without the influence of EGFR and RTKs. In CRC, the most common RAS mutations in the codons of 12, 13, and 61 maintain RAS in its active, GTP-bound state. are resistant to GAPs. This resistance prevents hydrolysis of GTP into GDP [114, 115]. Mutations in the *KRAS* are also found in approximately 41% of colorectal adenomas, and 74% of CRC [116]. *KRAS* is frequently mutated and induces resistance to anti-EGFR antibody. *KRAS* siRNA with anti- EGFR was targeted and internalized by the EGFR receptor. This internalized complex suppressed proliferation, viability, and apoptosis *in vitro* and reduced tumor growth shown in the xenograft model [117]. Besides, *KRAS* mutations were also found to be associated with the resistance to cetuximab in CRC [80, 118]. These results suggest that RAS is a crucial downstream of EGFR, and its mutation correlated with resistance to EGFR inhibitors in carcinomas.

RAF

RAF is a serine/threonine kinase that acts downstream of *KRAS* in the MAPK signaling pathway, and is the only *RAF* protein mutated in cancer [119]. *BRAF* activates mitogen- activated protein kinase (MAPKK/ MEK), which leads to cell proliferation. Mutation in the *BRAF* gene (V600E) causes a constitutive activation and is associated with poor prognosis, and a higher risk of recurrence compared with *KRAS* mutation in CRC patients [120]. A recent study suggests that *BRAF*^{V600E} confers aggressive cancer phenotype compared to wild- type *BRAF* [121]. *BRAF* mutation believed to be a predictor for resistance to EGFR moAbs in the chemotherapy-refractory settings. In retrospective clinical trials with 1022 mCRC patients, result shown that *BRAF*^{V600E} mutation is associated with poor RR than wild-type tumors (8.3% *vs.* 38%) when treated with cetuximab and chemotherapeutic drug. These data indicated that *BRAF*^{V600E} contributes to resistance to anti-EGFR therapy in chemotherapy- refractory wild type tumors [114]. In another study, *BRAF* mutations were associated with reduced OS and PFS after treatment with panitumumab or cetuximab (with or without chemotherapeutic drugs) [122]. Colon cancer patients who harbor $BRAF^{V600E}$ oncogenic lesions demonstrate poor prognosis and show limited response to PLX4032 (vemurafenib only). In another study, inhibition of EGFR and $BRAF^{V600E}$ by cetuximab or the small- molecule drugs gefitinib or erlotinib, shows synergism, both *in vitro* and *in vivo*. These data demonstrate that $BRAF^{V600E}$ colon cancer, with no targeted therapies available, might benefit from combination therapy and utilizing EGFR and *BRAF* inhibitors [123]. These studies indicate the association of *BRAF* mutation with resistance to anti-EGFR therapy in mCRC. Moreover, *BRAF* mutations are limited to tumors that do not carry the RAS mutation. Therefore, while treating mCRC patients with anti-EGFR, we should consider the mutational status of both RAS and RAF.

PIK3CA

Very few studies have been performed to evaluate the predictive effects of PI3KCA mutation in CRC patients treated with anti-EGFR therapy. Cancer cell lines harboring PI3KCA mutations (or that are *PTEN*-negative), exhibit resistance to cetuximab compared to healthy cells because of variation at exon 20 in PI3KCA [124 - 126]. In a more extensive retrospective study with *KRAS* wild type background, *PIK3CA* exon 20 mutations were evaluated in response to cetuximab-based therapy. They showed lower RR than wild type *PIK3CA* (0% *vs.* 36.8). Studies from a meta-analysis of 13 cohort studies suggested that mutation in exon 20 of *PIK3CA* genes is associated with less or no response to anti-EGFR therapy [127]. These dates show that variation at exon 20 may play a crucial role in the development of resistance to EGFR therapy. Also, *KRAS* and *BRAF* mutations coexist with PI3KCA mutation; it will be challenging to ascertain EGFR target therapy and its clinical significance.

PTEN

PTEN is a tumor suppressor gene and negatively regulates PI3K/Akt signaling through its lipid phosphatase activity. Loss of *PTEN* activity observed in about 25-45% of mCRC patients, which is associated with constitutive activation of PI3K/Akt signaling, leading to cancer cell survival and proliferation. Several studies have performed to evaluate the role of *PTEN* in CRC; however, they showed conflicting and inconsistent observations of anti-EGFR resistance. One group demonstrated that loss of *PTEN* is associated with a reduction in OS, PFS, and RR of mCRC patients treated with cetuximab or panitumumab in chemotherapy-refractory mCRC [126, 128]. However, other groups reported no significant differences in OS, PFS, and RR in association with the expression of *PTEN* in larger patients' series [129]. Further, randomized clinical trials and examinations are essential to confirm the *PTEN* expression role in mCRC patients to anti-EGFR therapy.

ROLE OF EGFR IN OTHER DISEASE MODELS

EGFR and Probiotics

Probiotics bacteria are live entities and secrete soluble factors, which have beneficial effects on various intestinal disorders. *Lactobacillus rhamnosus* GG produces a soluble protein, p40, which blocks apoptosis in intestinal cells. Recombinant 40 proteins activated EGFR, leads to Akt activation, and inhibition of cytokine-induced apoptosis, in *ex-vivo* and *in vitro*. Activation of EGFR by p40 required for the prevention of oxazolone-induced colitis, inflammation, and cell apoptosis [130]. Studies performed by Wang *et al.* demonstrate that the p40 soluble factor produces mucin production in the colonic epithelium, thereby thickening the mucus layer in wild type but not in EGFR-Tg mice (dominant-negative mutation in the EGFR kinase domain). Inhibition of mucin-type-O-linked glycosylation suppressed the effect on p40 in the protection of epithelial layers from TNF-induced apoptosis. These data suggest that p40-induced activation of EGFR mediated up-regulation of mucin production is crucial for the protection against epithelial injury [131]. Chronic alcohol consumption is known to cause alcoholic liver disease involving gut barrier dysfunction, endotoxemia, and toxin-mediated cellular injury. Our recent study showed that *Lactobacillus plantarum* not only blocks but also mitigates ethanol (EtOH) induced gut and liver damage in mice. *Lactobacillus plantarum* prevents EtOH-induced gut mucosal permeability, TJ disruption, inflammation, and protein thiol oxidation in wild type mice, but not in mice expressing dominant-negative form of EGFR. Additionally, *Lactobacillus plantarum* treatment after damage, accelerated the recovery from EtOH-induced tissue injury in the colon and liver [132].

EGFR and Inflammation

Enhanced EGFR signaling in myofibroblasts contributes to inflammation. TNF-α exposure to cancer cells increased EGFR with lysophosphatidic acid (LPA), induced phosphorylation at Y1068. Besides, a combination of LPA and TNF-α increased p42/p44 MAPK phosphorylation, and cyclooxygenase-2 (COX-2) expression blocked by MMP inhibitor, suggests that MMP releases EGFR ligand from the cell surface, and hence, activates EGFR signaling. Src inhibitor blocks LPA and TNF-α-induced COX-2, p42/p44 MAPK phosphorylation, GPCR, and phosphorylation of EGFR at Y1068, demonstrates that src is upstream in the transactivation of EGFR [133]. Recent studies showed that EGFR signaling in myeloid cells, specifically macrophages, plays an important role in colitis-induced CRC. In this study, the author showed that mice with myeloid-specific deletion of EGFR exhibit decreased tumor burden, reduced colitis, decreased macrophage, neutrophil, T-cell infiltration, and protection from dysplasia. These effects were absent in mice with gastrointestinal epithelial cell-specific EGFR deletion. These data suggest that EGFR signaling in macrophages acts as a biomarker for colitis-induced CRC or bears a therapeutic target in the treatment of inflammatory bowel disease [134]. A recent study suggests that the involvement of the EGFR-ER--MYC signaling pathway acts as a repressor of human β- defensin-1 (HBD1) expression. HBD1 is an antimicrobial peptide that constitutively and ubiquitously produces epithelial cells at the mucosal surface. HBD1 mechanisms are to kill gram-negative bacteria, candida genus, and viruses such as HIV-1. Decreased expression of HBD1 in various cancers, including prostate, renal oral squamous, and liver, suggests its role as a tumor suppressor gene. EGFR expression is hyperactivated in most of the cancers. These EGFR aberrations over-activate their downstream target and transcription factor, including MAPK and MYC gene. Bonamy *et al.* demonstrate that blocking EGFR by inhibitors (AG1478, Gefitinib and Erlotinib, *etc.*), or their downstream signaling molecule MEKK1/2 or MYC, mediated the EGFR- dependent regulation of HBD1 [135]. In ulcerative colitis, regeneration of epithelia is a crucial step in terms of recovery. Metalloproteinase-17 (ADAM17) predominantly expressed by regenerating epithelia as well as loss or inhibition of ADAM17 attenuated EGFR activation, barrier function, mucus production, and epithelial proliferation. It is crucial to maintain ADAM17 and EGFR axis signaling for the recovery from colitis and would target against TNF-α shedding [136]. Methyl-2-cyano-3, 12 dioxoolean-1, 9 diene-28-oate (CDDO-Me) acts as an antioxidant and anti-inflammatory that activates antioxidant response element (ARE) and nuclear factor-erythroid 2-related factor 2 (Nrf2) signaling cascade. In a recent study, CDDO-Me mitigates radiation-induced cellular damage *via* activating EGFR related DNA repair responses where EGFR is phosphorylated and translocated into the nucleus and interacts with DNA-PKcs. These data demonstrate that targeting EGFR using CDDO-Me may bear a promising radiation mitigator [137].

EGFR and Glutamine

Glutamine is a free amino acid and mostly utilized by intestinal cells. Reports suggest that alcohol consumption inhibits L-glutamine synthesis at the cellular level. Our studies demonstrate that L-Glutamine blocks acetaldehyde-induced decrease in transepithelial electrical resistance, and an increase in permeability to inulin and lipopolysaccharide in a time- and dose-dependent manner. L-Glutamine prevents acetaldehyde-induced redistribution of TJs, AJs, and actin cytoskeleton. The protective effect of L-Glutamine blocked by AG1478 treatment, indicates its protective effect by an EGF receptor-dependent mechanism. Our recent study showed that glutamine prevents EtOH-induced tissue injury in the large intestine. Doxycycline-induced expression of EGFR-Tg (a dominant-negative form of EGFR) blocked glutamine-mediated protection of epithelial tight junction disruption, gut permeability, and endotoxemia. Ethanol disrupted the actin cytoskeleton through cofilin activation, which was blocked by glutamine in an EGFR- dependent mechanism. Ethanol up-regulated chemokine and cytokine gene expression were blocked by glutamine in EGFR wild type mice. Glutamine promotes secretion of metalloproteinases into the medium, and metalloproteinase inhibitors blocked the glutamine-mediated prevention of barrier dysfunction. Results demonstrate that EGFR plays an essential role in glutamine-mediated prevention of alcoholic gut permeability and endotoxemia [138].

FUTURE DIRECTION

It is clear from present literature that various forms of alteration such as RAS mutation, *BRAF* mutation, *PIK3CA* mutation, inactivation of *PTEN*, HER-2 amplification, low EGFR copy number, and ligands results in the resistance to anti-EGFR therapy through constitutive activation of EGFR downstream cascade regardless of EGFR blockade. Therefore, it is entirely reasonable to anticipate that the blocking resistance pathway may sensitize CRC to anti-EGFR treatment. As a result, novel agents that target resistance signaling pathways along with anti-EGFR therapy may enhance the treatment efficacy. Although various biomarkers correlated with a lack of sensitivity, there is already a promising targeted strategy proposed in clinical and preclinical trials. For example, sorafenib, a potent inhibitor of $BRAF^{V600E}$, showed a promising effect in combination with cetuximab. Cetuximab was ineffective in $BRAF^{V600E}$ mutant cells compared to wild type *BRAF*. A combination of cetuximab and sorafenib enhanced sensitivity in the $BRAF^{V600E}$ mutant cells as compared to cetuximab treatment alone. In the clinical setting, the combination treatment of cetuximab and sorafenib resulted in SD for more than seven months in patients with $BRAF^{V600E}$ mutant mCRC, whose disease previously exhibited resistance to cetuximab [7]. Also, other inhibitors such as vemurafenib and dabrafenib have been approved for the treatment of advanced melanomas harboring $BRAF^{V600E}$; however, these drugs are less effective when used as monotherapy. Vemurafenib is more effective than sorafenib in treating *BRAF* mutant cell lines, and it showed the ability to inhibit MAPK signaling cascade [139]. In a phase II study, 21 mCRC patients when treated with vemurafenib exhibited RR (5%), median PFS (2.1 months), and OS (7.7 months). The combination with *BRAF* and MEK inhibitors significantly decreases MAPK signaling in $BRAF^{V600E}$ mutant cell lines [140, 141]. A combination of dabrafenib and trametinib in 43 mCRC patients showed that combination therapy is more effective than monotherapy. Combination of dabrafenib and trametinib demonstrated a decrease in downstream activation of the MAPK pathway as compared to either agent alone in melanoma [142]. In the VE-BASKET trial, a combination of vemurafenib and cetuximab tested in 27 mCRC patients in comparison to 10 mCRC patients treated with vemurafenib. The overall RR in combination was 4% (69% had SD), with a median PFS of 3.7 months and OS of 7.1 months [143]. Vemurafenib was also tested with panitumumab in 12 *BRAF* mutant CRC patients, and showed a RR of 13% (while 53% achieved SD) [144]. Overall, combined treatment regimen of *BRAF* inhibitor, and EGFR or MEK inhibitors, suggest an improvement in efficacy over *BRAF* inhibitor alone. Similar outcomes were observed in other clinical trials while combining anti-EGFR with inhibitors of different signaling pathways [145 - 147]. Another potential mechanism to counteract resistance pathways would be to target EGFR downstream signaling pathways such as MAPK and mTOR, which are downstream effectors of RAF and PI3K. Studies have demonstrated that dual EGFR and MAPK/ mTOR show improved outcomes in tumors harboring aberrant expression of markers such as *KRAS, BRAF*, and *PIK3CA*. Our current understanding of the mechanism of resistance to anti-EGFR therapies is poorly understood; an additional resistance mechanism may be involved, which has not been discovered yet. A more elaborate scheme of resistance mechanisms will be discovered, which will help us develop novel strategies to overcome both intrinsic and acquired resistance. Therefore, a rational combination treatment regimen that targets multiple signaling pathways are optimum approaches to block the anti-EGFR resistance pathway. Due to tumor heterogeneity, every individual responds differently to anti-EGFR therapy. Therefore, to overcome resistance and to enhance its drug efficacy, it is crucial to develop a formulation based on the mechanism of resistance in individual CRC patients. We envisage the emergence of additional therapeutic schemes to counteract resistance, and further progress in developing personalized medicine for CRC.

CONCLUSION

EGFR signaling plays a crucial role in the development of CRC and its management. Therefore, EGFR-targeted therapy has been developed, and has entered clinical practice. Various studies and data from preclinical and clinical studies with anti-EGFR mAb demonstrate that CRC with a low level of EGFR expression might respond to these agents. Due to the periodic development of resistance, it is mandatory to assess *NRAS* and *KRAS* mutations before introducing anti-EGFR agents. It is essential to develop and standardize highly sensitive techniques to detect EGFR expression that may help in the treatment of patients with anti-EGFR agents. Concise and precise information, based on the literature provided in this chapter, will help pharmaceutical companies as they develop new compounds designed to be used in conjunction with cetuximab and panitumumab that target EGFR and its downstream signaling axis (such as ErbB receptors) . Our understanding of the EGFR signaling network and its crosstalk with other oncogenic signaling is also leading to the foundation of therapeutic modalities involving combinational therapies. This research will lead to greater hope of survival for many more CRC patients, as well as the rational expectation of a cure in the not-too-distant future.

CONSENT FOR PUBLICATION

Not applicable.

CONFLICT OF INTEREST

The author declares that there is no conflict of interest in this chapter.

ACKNOWLEDGEMENTS

We thank Renu Sharma for her expertise and assistance in illustrating figures in this chapter.

REFERENCES

[1]   Siegel RL, Miller KD, Fedewa SA, *et al.* Colorectal cancer statistics, 2017. CA Cancer J Clin 2017; 67(3): 177-93.
        [http://dx.doi.org/10.3322/caac.21395] [PMID: 28248415]

[2]   Cohen RB. Epidermal growth factor receptor as a therapeutic target in colorectal cancer. Clin Colorectal Cancer 2003; 2(4): 246-51.
        [http://dx.doi.org/10.3816/CCC.2003.n.006] [PMID: 12620146]

[3]   Douillard JY, Siena S, Cassidy J, *et al.* Randomized, phase III trial of panitumumab with infusional fluorouracil, leucovorin, and oxaliplatin (FOLFOX4) *versus* FOLFOX4 alone as first-line treatment in patients with previously untreated metastatic colorectal cancer: the PRIME study. J Clin Oncol 2010; 28(31): 4697-705.
        [http://dx.doi.org/10.1200/JCO.2009.27.4860] [PMID: 20921465]

[4]   Maughan TS, Adams RA, Smith CG, *et al.* Addition of cetuximab to oxaliplatin-based first-line combination chemotherapy for treatment of advanced colorectal cancer: results of the randomised phase 3 MRC COIN trial. Lancet 2011; 377(9783): 2103-14.
        [http://dx.doi.org/10.1016/S0140-6736(11)60613-2] [PMID: 21641636]

[5]   Van Cutsem E, Köhne CH, Hitre E, *et al.* Cetuximab and chemotherapy as initial treatment for metastatic colorectal cancer. N Engl J Med 2009; 360(14): 1408-17.
        [http://dx.doi.org/10.1056/NEJMoa0805019] [PMID: 19339720]

[6]   Dinicola S, Masiello MG, Proietti S, *et al.* Nicotine increases colon cancer cell migration and invasion through epithelial to mesenchymal transition (EMT): COX-2 involvement. J Cell Physiol 2018; 233(6): 4935-48.
        [http://dx.doi.org/10.1002/jcp.26323] [PMID: 29215713]

[7]   Al-Marrawi MY, Saroya BS, Brennan MC, Yang Z, Dykes TM, El-Deiry WS. Off-label use of cetuximab plus sorafenib and panitumumab plus regorafenib to personalize therapy for a patient with V600E BRAF-mutant metastatic colon cancer. Cancer Biol Ther 2013; 14(8): 703-10.
        [http://dx.doi.org/10.4161/cbt.25191] [PMID: 23792568]

[8]   Fedirko V, Tramacere I, Bagnardi V, *et al.* Alcohol drinking and colorectal cancer risk: an overall and dose-response meta-analysis of published studies. Ann Oncol 2011; 22(9): 1958-72.
        [http://dx.doi.org/10.1093/annonc/mdq653] [PMID: 21307158]

[9] Mahmood S, MacInnis RJ, English DR, Karahalios A, Lynch BM. Domain-specific physical activity and sedentary behaviour in relation to colon and rectal cancer risk: a systematic review and meta-analysis. Int J Epidemiol 2017; 46(6): 1797-813.
[http://dx.doi.org/10.1093/ije/dyx137] [PMID: 29025130]

[10] Moskal A, Norat T, Ferrari P, Riboli E. Alcohol intake and colorectal cancer risk: a dose-response meta-analysis of published cohort studies. Int J Cancer 2007; 120(3): 664-71.
[http://dx.doi.org/10.1002/ijc.22299] [PMID: 17096321]

[11] Park SY, Boushey CJ, Wilkens LR, Haiman CA, Le Marchand L. High-quality diets associate with reduced risk of colorectal cancer: Analyses of diet quality indexes in the multiethnic cohort. Gastroenterology 2017; 153(2): 386-94.
[http://dx.doi.org/10.1053/j.gastro.2017.04.004] [PMID: 28428143]

[12] Sasaki K, Ishihara S, Hata K, et al. Radiation-associated colon cancer: A case report. Mol Clin Oncol 2017; 6(6): 817-20.
[http://dx.doi.org/10.3892/mco.2017.1252] [PMID: 28588770]

[13] Dougherty U, Cerasi D, Taylor I, et al. Epidermal growth factor receptor is required for colonic tumor promotion by dietary fat in the azoxymethane/dextran sulfate sodium model: roles of transforming growth factor-alpha and PTGS2. Clin Cancer Res 2009; 15(22): 6780-9.
[http://dx.doi.org/10.1158/1078-0432.CCR-09-1678] [PMID: 19903783]

[14] Patel SS, Nelson R, Sanchez J, et al. Elderly patients with colon cancer have unique tumor characteristics and poor survival. Cancer 2013; 119(4): 739-47.
[http://dx.doi.org/10.1002/cncr.27753] [PMID: 23011893]

[15] Ashraf I, Choudhary A, Arif M, et al. Ursodeoxycholic acid in patients with ulcerative colitis and primary sclerosing cholangitis for prevention of colon cancer: a meta-analysis. Indian J Gastroenterol 2012; 31(2): 69-74.
[http://dx.doi.org/10.1007/s12664-012-0175-3] [PMID: 22528343]

[16] Hale LP, Greer PK. A novel murine model of inflammatory bowel disease and inflammation-associated colon cancer with ulcerative colitis-like features. PLoS One 2012; 7(7): e41797.
[http://dx.doi.org/10.1371/journal.pone.0041797] [PMID: 22848611]

[17] Ryan BM, Wolff RK, Valeri N, et al. An analysis of genetic factors related to risk of inflammatory bowel disease and colon cancer. Cancer Epidemiol 2014; 38(5): 583-90.
[http://dx.doi.org/10.1016/j.canep.2014.07.003] [PMID: 25132422]

[18] Graus-Porta D, Beerli RR, Daly JM, Hynes NE. ErbB-2, the preferred heterodimerization partner of all ErbB receptors, is a mediator of lateral signaling. EMBO J 1997; 16(7): 1647-55.
[http://dx.doi.org/10.1093/emboj/16.7.1647] [PMID: 9130710]

[19] Brennan PJ, Kumagai T, Berezov A, Murali R, Greene MI. HER2/Neu: mechanisms of dimerization/oligomerization. Oncogene 2002; 21(2): 328.
[http://dx.doi.org/10.1038/sj.onc.1205119] [PMID: 11840330]

[20] Citri A, Skaria KB, Yarden Y. The deaf and the dumb: the biology of ErbB-2 and ErbB-3. Exp Cell Res 2003; 284(1): 54-65.
[http://dx.doi.org/10.1016/S0014-4827(02)00101-5] [PMID: 12648465]

[21] Seshacharyulu P, Ponnusamy MP, Haridas D, Jain M, Ganti AK, Batra SK. Targeting the EGFR signaling pathway in cancer therapy. Expert Opin Ther Targets 2012; 16(1): 15-31.
[http://dx.doi.org/10.1517/14728222.2011.648617] [PMID: 22239438]

[22] Wells A. EGF receptor. Int J Biochem Cell Biol 1999; 31(6): 637-43.
[http://dx.doi.org/10.1016/S1357-2725(99)00015-1] [PMID: 10404636]

[23] Pines G, Köstler WJ, Yarden Y. Oncogenic mutant forms of EGFR: lessons in signal transduction and targets for cancer therapy. FEBS Lett 2010; 584(12): 2699-706.
[http://dx.doi.org/10.1016/j.febslet.2010.04.019] [PMID: 20388509]

[24]   Endres NF, Das R, Smith AW, *et al.* Conformational coupling across the plasma membrane in activation of the EGF receptor. Cell 2013; 152(3): 543-56.
[http://dx.doi.org/10.1016/j.cell.2012.12.032] [PMID: 23374349]

[25]   Spano JP, Lagorce C, Atlan D, *et al.* Impact of EGFR expression on colorectal cancer patient prognosis and survival. Ann Oncol 2005; 16(1): 102-8.
[http://dx.doi.org/10.1093/annonc/mdi006] [PMID: 15598946]

[26]   Brabender J, Danenberg KD, Metzger R, *et al.* Epidermal growth factor receptor and HER2-neu mRNA expression in non-small cell lung cancer Is correlated with survival. Clin Cancer Res 2001; 7(7): 1850-5.
[PMID: 11448895]

[27]   Wee P, Wang Z. Epidermal growth factor receptor cell proliferation signaling pathways. Cancers (Basel) 2017; 9(5): E52.
[PMID: 28513565]

[28]   Pawson T. Specificity in signal transduction: from phosphotyrosine-SH2 domain interactions to complex cellular systems. Cell 2004; 116(2): 191-203.
[http://dx.doi.org/10.1016/S0092-8674(03)01077-8] [PMID: 14744431]

[29]   Troiani T, Martinelli E, Napolitano S, *et al.* Increased TGF-α as a mechanism of acquired resistance to the anti-EGFR inhibitor cetuximab through EGFR-MET interaction and activation of MET signaling in colon cancer cells. Clin Cancer Res 2013; 19(24): 6751-65.
[http://dx.doi.org/10.1158/1078-0432.CCR-13-0423] [PMID: 24122793]

[30]   Normanno N, Bianco C, De Luca A, Salomon DS. The role of EGF-related peptides in tumor growth. Front Biosci 2001; 6: D685-707.
[http://dx.doi.org/10.2741/A635] [PMID: 11333208]

[31]   Salomon DS, Kim N, Saeki T, Ciardiello F. Transforming growth factor-alpha: An oncodevelopmental growth factor. Cancer Cells 1990; 2(12): 389-97.
[PMID: 2088454]

[32]   De Angelis E, Grassi M, Gullick WJ, *et al.* Expression of cripto and amphiregulin in colon mucosa from high risk colon cancer families. Int J Oncol 1999; 14(3): 437-40.
[http://dx.doi.org/10.3892/ijo.14.3.437] [PMID: 10024674]

[33]   Kuramochi H, Nakajima GO, Hayashi K, Araida T, Yamamoto M. *Amphiregulin/epiregulin* mRNA Expression and Primary Tumor Location in Colorectal Cancer. Anticancer Res 2019; 39(9): 4729-36.
[http://dx.doi.org/10.21873/anticanres.13655] [PMID: 31519572]

[34]   Saeki T, Stromberg K, Qi CF, *et al.* Differential immunohistochemical detection of amphiregulin and cripto in human normal colon and colorectal tumors. Cancer Res 1992; 52(12): 3467-73.
[PMID: 1596904]

[35]   Qi CF, Liscia DS, Normanno N, *et al.* Expression of transforming growth factor alpha, amphiregulin and cripto-1 in human breast carcinomas. Br J Cancer 1994; 69(5): 903-10.
[http://dx.doi.org/10.1038/bjc.1994.174] [PMID: 8180021]

[36]   Inui Y, Higashiyama S, Kawata S, *et al.* Expression of heparin-binding epidermal growth factor in human hepatocellular carcinoma. Gastroenterology 1994; 107(6): 1799-804.
[http://dx.doi.org/10.1016/0016-5085(94)90823-0] [PMID: 7958694]

[37]   Ito Y, Higashiyama S, Takeda T, Okada M, Matsuura N. Bimodal expression of heparin-binding EGF-like growth factor in colonic neoplasms. Anticancer Res 2001; 21(2B): 1391-4.
[PMID: 11396220]

[38]   Miyamoto S, Hirata M, Yamazaki A, *et al.* Heparin-binding EGF-like growth factor is a promising target for ovarian cancer therapy. Cancer Res 2004; 64(16): 5720-7.
[http://dx.doi.org/10.1158/0008-5472.CAN-04-0811] [PMID: 15313912]

[39]   Naef M, Yokoyama M, Friess H, Büchler MW, Korc M. Co-expression of heparin-binding EGF-like growth factor and related peptides in human gastric carcinoma. Int J Cancer 1996; 66(3): 315-21.
[http://dx.doi.org/10.1002/(SICI)1097-0215(19960503)66:3<315::AID-IJC8>3.0.CO;2-1]   [PMID: 8621250]

[40]   Jeong WJ, Ro EJ, Choi KY. Interaction between Wnt/β-catenin and RAS-ERK pathways and an anti-cancer strategy via degradations of β-catenin and RAS by targeting the Wnt/β-catenin pathway. NPJ Precis Oncol 2018; 2(1): 5.
[http://dx.doi.org/10.1038/s41698-018-0049-y] [PMID: 29872723]

[41]   Tabana YM. D.S., Shah AM, Majid A, Major signaling pathways of colorectal carcinogenesis. Recent Adv Colon Cancer 2016; 1: 1-2.

[42]   Saletti P. M.F., Dosso S, Frattini M, EGFR signaling in colorectal cancer: a clinical perspective. Gastrointest Cancer 2015; 5: 21-38.

[43]   Hutchinson RA, Adams RA, McArt DG, Salto-Tellez M, Jasani B, Hamilton PW. Epidermal growth factor receptor immunohistochemistry: new opportunities in metastatic colorectal cancer. J Transl Med 2015; 13: 217.
[http://dx.doi.org/10.1186/s12967-015-0531-z] [PMID: 26149458]

[44]   Kirouac DC, Du J, Lahdenranta J, et al. HER²⁺ cancer cell dependence on PI3K vs. MAPK signaling axes is determined by expression of EGFR, ERBB3 and CDKN1B. PLOS Comput Biol 2016; 12(4): e1004827.
[http://dx.doi.org/10.1371/journal.pcbi.1004827] [PMID: 27035903]

[45]   Papadatos-Pastos D, Rabbie R, Ross P, Sarker D. The role of the PI3K pathway in colorectal cancer. Crit Rev Oncol Hematol 2015; 94(1): 18-30.
[http://dx.doi.org/10.1016/j.critrevonc.2014.12.006] [PMID: 25591826]

[46]   Temiz TK. A.A., Turgut N, Balcı E, Investigation of the effects of drugs effective on PI3K–AKT signaling pathway in colorectal cancer alone and in combination. Cumhuriyet Med J 2014; 36(2): 167-77.
[http://dx.doi.org/10.7197/cmj.v36i2.5000033144]

[47]   McDonald GT, Sullivan R, Paré GC, Graham CH. Inhibition of phosphatidylinositol 3-kinase promotes tumor cell resistance to chemotherapeutic agents via a mechanism involving delay in cell cycle progression. Exp Cell Res 2010; 316(19): 3197-206.
[http://dx.doi.org/10.1016/j.yexcr.2010.08.007] [PMID: 20736003]

[48]   Zhang X, Liu G, Ding L, et al. HOXA3 promotes tumor growth of human colon cancer through activating EGFR/Ras/Raf/MEK/ERK signaling pathway. J Cell Biochem 2018; 119(3): 2864-74.
[http://dx.doi.org/10.1002/jcb.26461] [PMID: 29073728]

[49]   Alam KJ, Mo JS, Han SH, et al. MicroRNA 375 regulates proliferation and migration of colon cancer cells by suppressing the CTGF-EGFR signaling pathway. Int J Cancer 2017; 141(8): 1614-29.
[http://dx.doi.org/10.1002/ijc.30861] [PMID: 28670764]

[50]   Ellina MI, Bouris P, Aletras AJ, Theocharis AD, Kletsas D, Karamanos NK. EGFR and HER2 exert distinct roles on colon cancer cell functional properties and expression of matrix macromolecules. Biochim Biophys Acta 2014; 1840(8): 2651-61.
[http://dx.doi.org/10.1016/j.bbagen.2014.04.019] [PMID: 24792576]

[51]   Hong SY, Shih YP, Li T, Carraway KL III, Lo SH. CTEN prolongs signaling by EGFR through reducing its ligand-induced degradation. Cancer Res 2013; 73(16): 5266-76.
[http://dx.doi.org/10.1158/0008-5472.CAN-12-4441] [PMID: 23774213]

[52]   Yang YP, Ma H, Starchenko A, et al. A chimeric egfr protein reporter mouse reveals egfr localization and trafficking In Vivo. Cell Rep 2017; 19(6): 1257-67.
[http://dx.doi.org/10.1016/j.celrep.2017.04.048] [PMID: 28494873]

[53]   Srivatsa S, Paul MC, Cardone C, et al. EGFR in tumor-associated myeloid cells promotes

development of colorectal cancer in mice and associates with outcomes of patients. Gastroenterology 2017; 153(1): 178-90.
[http://dx.doi.org/10.1053/j.gastro.2017.03.053] [PMID: 28400195]

[54] Centuori SM, Gomes CJ, Trujillo J, *et al.* Deoxycholic acid mediates non-canonical EGFR-MAPK activation through the induction of calcium signaling in colon cancer cells. Biochim Biophys Acta 2016; 1861(7): 663-70.
[http://dx.doi.org/10.1016/j.bbalip.2016.04.006] [PMID: 27086143]

[55] Wang TH, Chang JL, Ho JY, Wu HC, Chen TC. EphrinA5 suppresses colon cancer development by negatively regulating epidermal growth factor receptor stability. FEBS J 2012; 279(2): 251-63.
[http://dx.doi.org/10.1111/j.1742-4658.2011.08419.x] [PMID: 22074469]

[56] Mizukami T, Togashi Y, Naruki S, *et al.* Significance of FGF9 gene in resistance to anti-EGFR therapies targeting colorectal cancer: A subset of colorectal cancer patients with FGF9 upregulation may be resistant to anti-EGFR therapies. Mol Carcinog 2017; 56(1): 106-17.
[http://dx.doi.org/10.1002/mc.22476] [PMID: 26916220]

[57] Mozzi A, Forcella M, Riva A, *et al.* NEU3 activity enhances EGFR activation without affecting EGFR expression and acts on its sialylation levels. Glycobiology 2015; 25(8): 855-68.
[http://dx.doi.org/10.1093/glycob/cwv026] [PMID: 25922362]

[58] Tarcic G, Boguslavsky SK, Wakim J, *et al.* An unbiased screen identifies DEP-1 tumor suppressor as a phosphatase controlling EGFR endocytosis. Curr Biol 2009; 19(21): 1788-98.
[http://dx.doi.org/10.1016/j.cub.2009.09.048] [PMID: 19836242]

[59] McKay JA, Murray LJ, Curran S, *et al.* Evaluation of the epidermal growth factor receptor (EGFR) in colorectal tumours and lymph node metastases. Eur J Cancer 2002; 38(17): 2258-64.
[http://dx.doi.org/10.1016/S0959-8049(02)00234-4] [PMID: 12441262]

[60] Koskensalo S, Louhimo J, Hagström J, Lundin M, Stenman UH, Haglund C. Concomitant tumor expression of EGFR and TATI/SPINK1 associates with better prognosis in colorectal cancer. PLoS One 2013; 8(10): e76906.
[http://dx.doi.org/10.1371/journal.pone.0076906] [PMID: 24204699]

[61] Mouzakiti A, Nastos C, Vlachodimitropoulos D, Gennatas C, Kondi-Pafiti A, Voros D. Prognostic significance of EGFR and COX-2 expression in colorectal cancer and their association. A study in Greek population. J BUON 2018; 23(1): 23-8.
[PMID: 29552755]

[62] Piyush T, Chacko AR, Sindrewicz P, Hilkens J, Rhodes JM, Yu LG. Interaction of galectin-3 with MUC1 on cell surface promotes EGFR dimerization and activation in human epithelial cancer cells. Cell Death Differ 2017; 24(11): 1937-47.
[http://dx.doi.org/10.1038/cdd.2017.119] [PMID: 28731466]

[63] Shimamoto Y, Nukatsuka M, Takechi T, Fukushima M. Association between mRNA expression of chemotherapy-related genes and clinicopathological features in colorectal cancer: A large-scale population analysis. Int J Mol Med 2016; 37(2): 319-28.
[http://dx.doi.org/10.3892/ijmm.2015.2427] [PMID: 26676887]

[64] Campiglio M, Locatelli A, Olgiati C, *et al.* Inhibition of proliferation and induction of apoptosis in breast cancer cells by the epidermal growth factor receptor (EGFR) tyrosine kinase inhibitor ZD1839 ('Iressa') is independent of EGFR expression level. J Cell Physiol 2004; 198(2): 259-68.
[http://dx.doi.org/10.1002/jcp.10411] [PMID: 14603528]

[65] Grünwald V, Hidalgo M. Developing inhibitors of the epidermal growth factor receptor for cancer treatment. J Natl Cancer Inst 2003; 95(12): 851-67.
[http://dx.doi.org/10.1093/jnci/95.12.851] [PMID: 12813169]

[66] Ciardiello F, Tortora G. EGFR antagonists in cancer treatment. N Engl J Med 2008; 358(11): 1160-74.
[http://dx.doi.org/10.1056/NEJMra0707704] [PMID: 18337605]

[67] Jonker DJ, O'Callaghan CJ, Karapetis CS, *et al.* Cetuximab for the treatment of colorectal cancer. N Engl J Med 2007; 357(20): 2040-8.
[http://dx.doi.org/10.1056/NEJMoa071834] [PMID: 18003960]

[68] Amado RG, Wolf M, Peeters M, *et al.* Wild-type KRAS is required for panitumumab efficacy in patients with metastatic colorectal cancer. J Clin Oncol 2008; 26(10): 1626-34.
[http://dx.doi.org/10.1200/JCO.2007.14.7116] [PMID: 18316791]

[69] Ung N, Putoczki TL, Stylli SS, *et al.* Anti-EGFR therapeutic efficacy correlates directly with inhibition of STAT3 activity. Cancer Biol Ther 2014; 15(5): 623-32.
[http://dx.doi.org/10.4161/cbt.28179] [PMID: 24556630]

[70] Bosch-Vilaró A, Jacobs B, Pomella V, *et al.* Feedback activation of HER3 attenuates response to EGFR inhibitors in colon cancer cells. Oncotarget 2017; 8(3): 4277-88.
[http://dx.doi.org/10.18632/oncotarget.13834] [PMID: 28032592]

[71] Cho J, Bass AJ, Lawrence MS, *et al.* Colon cancer-derived oncogenic EGFR G724S mutant identified by whole genome sequence analysis is dependent on asymmetric dimerization and sensitive to cetuximab. Mol Cancer 2014; 13: 141.
[http://dx.doi.org/10.1186/1476-4598-13-141] [PMID: 24894453]

[72] Venè R, Tosetti F, Minghelli S, Poggi A, Ferrari N, Benelli R. Celecoxib increases EGF signaling in colon tumor associated fibroblasts, modulating EGFR expression and degradation. Oncotarget 2015; 6(14): 12310-25.
[http://dx.doi.org/10.18632/oncotarget.3678] [PMID: 25987127]

[73] Zhang W, Chen L, Ma K, *et al.* Polarization of macrophages in the tumor microenvironment is influenced by EGFR signaling within colon cancer cells. Oncotarget 2016; 7(46): 75366-78.
[http://dx.doi.org/10.18632/oncotarget.12207] [PMID: 27683110]

[74] Cunningham D, Humblet Y, Siena S, *et al.* Cetuximab monotherapy and cetuximab plus irinotecan in irinotecan-refractory metastatic colorectal cancer. N Engl J Med 2004; 351(4): 337-45.
[http://dx.doi.org/10.1056/NEJMoa033025] [PMID: 15269313]

[75] Tejpar S, Stintzing S, Ciardiello F, *et al.* Prognostic and predictive relevance of primary tumor location in patients with ras wild-type metastatic colorectal cancer: Retrospective analyses of the crystal and fire-3 trials. JAMA Oncol 2017; 3(2): 194-201.
[http://dx.doi.org/10.1001/jamaoncol.2016.3797] [PMID: 27722750]

[76] Bokemeyer C, Bondarenko I, Makhson A, *et al.* Fluorouracil, leucovorin, and oxaliplatin with and without cetuximab in the first-line treatment of metastatic colorectal cancer. J Clin Oncol 2009; 27(5): 663-71.
[http://dx.doi.org/10.1200/JCO.2008.20.8397] [PMID: 19114683]

[77] Tveit KM, Guren T, Glimelius B, *et al.* Phase III trial of cetuximab with continuous or intermittent fluorouracil, leucovorin, and oxaliplatin (Nordic FLOX) *versus* FLOX alone in first-line treatment of metastatic colorectal cancer: the NORDIC-VII study. J Clin Oncol 2012; 30(15): 1755-62.
[http://dx.doi.org/10.1200/JCO.2011.38.0915] [PMID: 22473155]

[78] Lynch DH, Yang XD. Therapeutic potential of ABX-EGF: a fully human anti-epidermal growth factor receptor monoclonal antibody for cancer treatment. Semin Oncol 2002; 29(1) (Suppl. 4): 47-50.
[http://dx.doi.org/10.1053/sonc.2002.31522] [PMID: 11894013]

[79] Peeters M, Siena S, Van Cutsem E, *et al.* Association of progression-free survival, overall survival, and patient-reported outcomes by skin toxicity and KRAS status in patients receiving panitumumab monotherapy. Cancer 2009; 115(7): 1544-54.
[http://dx.doi.org/10.1002/cncr.24088] [PMID: 19189371]

[80] Douillard JY, Oliner KS, Siena S, *et al.* Panitumumab-FOLFOX4 treatment and RAS mutations in colorectal cancer. N Engl J Med 2013; 369(11): 1023-34.
[http://dx.doi.org/10.1056/NEJMoa1305275] [PMID: 24024839]

[81]   Saltz LB, Meropol NJ, Loehrer PJ Sr, Needle MN, Kopit J, Mayer RJ. Phase II trial of cetuximab in patients with refractory colorectal cancer that expresses the epidermal growth factor receptor. J Clin Oncol 2004; 22(7): 1201-8.
[http://dx.doi.org/10.1200/JCO.2004.10.182] [PMID: 14993230]

[82]   Keilholz U, Arnold D, Niederle N, *et al.* Erlotinib as 2nd or 3rd line monotherapy in patients with metastatic colorectal cancer. Results of a multicenter two-cohort phase II trial. J Clin Oncol 2005; 23(16): 3575.

[83]   Townsley CA, Major P, Siu LL, *et al.* Phase II study of erlotinib (OSI-774) in patients with metastatic colorectal cancer. Br J Cancer 2006; 94(8): 1136-43.
[http://dx.doi.org/10.1038/sj.bjc.6603055] [PMID: 16570047]

[84]   Vincent MD, Breadner D, Soulieres D, *et al.* Phase II trial of capecitabine plus erlotinib *versus* capecitabine alone in patients with advanced colorectal cancer. Future Oncol 2017; 13(9): 777-86.
[http://dx.doi.org/10.2217/fon-2016-0444] [PMID: 28045335]

[85]   Hanauske AR, Cassidy J, Sastre J, *et al.* Phase 1b dose escalation study of erlotinib in combination with infusional 5-Fluorouracil, leucovorin, and oxaliplatin in patients with advanced solid tumors. Clin Cancer Res 2007; 13(2 Pt 1): 523-31.
[http://dx.doi.org/10.1158/1078-0432.CCR-06-1627] [PMID: 17255274]

[86]   Meyerhardt JA, Stuart K, Fuchs CS, *et al.* Phase II study of FOLFOX, bevacizumab and erlotinib as first-line therapy for patients with metastatic colorectal cancer. Ann Oncol 2007; 18(7): 1185-9.
[http://dx.doi.org/10.1093/annonc/mdm124] [PMID: 17483115]

[87]   Meyerhardt JA, Ancukiewicz M, Abrams TA, *et al.* Phase I study of cetuximab, irinotecan, and vandetanib (ZD6474) as therapy for patients with previously treated metastastic colorectal cancer. PLoS One 2012; 7(6): e38231.
[http://dx.doi.org/10.1371/journal.pone.0038231] [PMID: 22701615]

[88]   Spigel DR. H.J., Burris HA, *et al.*, Phase II study of FOLFOX4, bevacizumab and erlotinib as first-line therapy in patients with advanced colorectal cancer. Presented at the 2006 ASCO Gastrointestinal Cancers Symposium.

[89]   Messersmith WA, Laheru DA, Senzer NN, *et al.* Phase I trial of irinotecan, infusional 5-fluorouracil, and leucovorin (FOLFIRI) with erlotinib (OSI-774): early termination due to increased toxicities. Clin Cancer Res 2004; 10(19): 6522-7.
[http://dx.doi.org/10.1158/1078-0432.CCR-04-0746] [PMID: 15475439]

[90]   Blanke CD. Gefitinib in colorectal cancer: if wishes were horses. J Clin Oncol 2005; 23(24): 5446-9.
[http://dx.doi.org/10.1200/JCO.2005.05.904] [PMID: 16110007]

[91]   Mackenzie MJ, Hirte HW, Glenwood G, *et al.* A phase II trial of ZD1839 (Iressa) 750 mg per day, an oral epidermal growth factor receptor-tyrosine kinase inhibitor, in patients with metastatic colorectal cancer. Invest New Drugs 2005; 23(2): 165-70.
[http://dx.doi.org/10.1007/s10637-005-5862-9] [PMID: 15744593]

[92]   Rothenberg ML, LaFleur B, Levy DE, *et al.* Randomized phase II trial of the clinical and biological effects of two dose levels of gefitinib in patients with recurrent colorectal adenocarcinoma. J Clin Oncol 2005; 23(36): 9265-74.
[http://dx.doi.org/10.1200/JCO.2005.03.0536] [PMID: 16361624]

[93]   Kindler HL, Friberg G, Skoog L, Wade-Oliver K, Vokes EE. Phase I/II trial of gefitinib and oxaliplatin in patients with advanced colorectal cancer. Am J Clin Oncol 2005; 28(4): 340-4.
[http://dx.doi.org/10.1097/01.coc.0000159558.19631.d5] [PMID: 16062074]

[94]   Jimeno A, Grávalos C, Escudero P, *et al.* Phase I/II study of gefitinib and capecitabine in patients with colorectal cancer. Clin Transl Oncol 2008; 10(1): 52-7.
[http://dx.doi.org/10.1007/s12094-008-0153-5] [PMID: 18208793]

[95]   Fisher GA, Kuo T, Ramsey M, *et al.* A phase II study of gefitinib, 5-fluorouracil, leucovorin, and

oxaliplatin in previously untreated patients with metastatic colorectal cancer. Clin Cancer Res 2008; 14(21): 7074-9.
[http://dx.doi.org/10.1158/1078-0432.CCR-08-1014] [PMID: 18981005]

[96]   Kuo T, Cho CD, Halsey J, *et al.* Phase II study of gefitinib, fluorouracil, leucovorin, and oxaliplatin therapy in previously treated patients with metastatic colorectal cancer. J Clin Oncol 2005; 23(24): 5613-9.
[http://dx.doi.org/10.1200/JCO.2005.08.359] [PMID: 16110021]

[97]   Chau I, Cunningham D, Hickish T, *et al.* Gefitinib and irinotecan in patients with fluoropyrimidine-refractory, irinotecan-naive advanced colorectal cancer: a phase I-II study. Ann Oncol 2007; 18(4): 730-7.
[http://dx.doi.org/10.1093/annonc/mdl481] [PMID: 17237473]

[98]   Arnold DCC, Seufferlein T, *et al.* Phase I study of gefitinib in combination with capecitabine and irinotecan for 2nd and/or 3rd line treatment in patients with metastatic colorectal cancer. J Clin Oncol 2005; 23(16) (Suppl.): 293.
[http://dx.doi.org/10.1200/jco.2005.23.16_suppl.3691]

[99]   Veronese ML, Sun W, Giantonio B, *et al.* A phase II trial of gefitinib with 5-fluorouracil, leucovorin, and irinotecan in patients with colorectal cancer. Br J Cancer 2005; 92(10): 1846-9.
[http://dx.doi.org/10.1038/sj.bjc.6602569] [PMID: 15870719]

[100]   Van Emburgh BO, Sartore-Bianchi A, Di Nicolantonio F, Siena S, Bardelli A. Acquired resistance to EGFR-targeted therapies incolorectal cancer. Mol Oncol 2014; 8(6): 1084-94.
[http://dx.doi.org/10.1016/j.molonc.2014.05.003] [PMID: 24913799]

[101]   Milik SN, Lasheen DS, Serya RAT, Abouzid KAM. How to train your inhibitor: Design strategies to overcome resistance to Epidermal Growth Factor Receptor inhibitors. Eur J Med Chem 2017; 142: 131-51.
[http://dx.doi.org/10.1016/j.ejmech.2017.07.023] [PMID: 28754471]

[102]   Gelfo V, Rodia MT, Pucci M, *et al.* A module of inflammatory cytokines defines resistance of colorectal cancer to EGFR inhibitors. Oncotarget 2016; 7(44): 72167-83.
[http://dx.doi.org/10.18632/oncotarget.12354] [PMID: 27708224]

[103]   Asbagh LA, Vazquez I, Vecchione L, *et al.* The tyrosine phosphatase PTPRO sensitizes colon cancer cells to anti-EGFR therapy through activation of SRC-mediated EGFR signaling. Oncotarget 2014; 5(20): 10070-83.
[http://dx.doi.org/10.18632/oncotarget.2458] [PMID: 25301722]

[104]   Bardelli A, Siena S. Molecular mechanisms of resistance to cetuximab and panitumumab in colorectal cancer. J Clin Oncol 2010; 28(7): 1254-61.
[http://dx.doi.org/10.1200/JCO.2009.24.6116] [PMID: 20100961]

[105]   Moroni M, Veronese S, Benvenuti S, *et al.* Gene copy number for epidermal growth factor receptor (EGFR) and clinical response to antiEGFR treatment in colorectal cancer: a cohort study. Lancet Oncol 2005; 6(5): 279-86.
[http://dx.doi.org/10.1016/S1470-2045(05)70102-9] [PMID: 15863375]

[106]   Khambata-Ford S, Garrett CR, Meropol NJ, *et al.* Expression of epiregulin and amphiregulin and K-ras mutation status predict disease control in metastatic colorectal cancer patients treated with cetuximab. J Clin Oncol 2007; 25(22): 3230-7.
[http://dx.doi.org/10.1200/JCO.2006.10.5437] [PMID: 17664471]

[107]   Jacobs B, De Roock W, Piessevaux H, *et al.* Amphiregulin and epiregulin mRNA expression in primary tumors predicts outcome in metastatic colorectal cancer treated with cetuximab. J Clin Oncol 2009; 27(30): 5068-74.
[http://dx.doi.org/10.1200/JCO.2008.21.3744] [PMID: 19738126]

[108]   Lynch TJ, Bell DW, Sordella R, *et al.* Activating mutations in the epidermal growth factor receptor underlying responsiveness of non-small-cell lung cancer to gefitinib. N Engl J Med 2004; 350(21):

2129-39.
[http://dx.doi.org/10.1056/NEJMoa040938] [PMID: 15118073]

[109] Vogel CL, Cobleigh MA, Tripathy D, *et al.* Efficacy and safety of trastuzumab as a single agent in first-line treatment of HER2-overexpressing metastatic breast cancer. J Clin Oncol 2002; 20(3): 719-26.
[http://dx.doi.org/10.1200/JCO.2002.20.3.719] [PMID: 11821453]

[110] Barber TD, Vogelstein B, Kinzler KW, Velculescu VE. Somatic mutations of EGFR in colorectal cancers and glioblastomas. N Engl J Med 2004; 351(27): 2883.
[http://dx.doi.org/10.1056/NEJM200412303512724] [PMID: 15625347]

[111] Sartore-Bianchi A, Moroni M, Veronese S, *et al.* Epidermal growth factor receptor gene copy number and clinical outcome of metastatic colorectal cancer treated with panitumumab. J Clin Oncol 2007; 25(22): 3238-45.
[http://dx.doi.org/10.1200/JCO.2007.11.5956] [PMID: 17664472]

[112] Bos JL. ras oncogenes in human cancer: a review. Cancer Res 1989; 49(17): 4682-9.
[PMID: 2547513]

[113] Fernández-Medarde A, Santos E. Ras in cancer and developmental diseases. Genes Cancer 2011; 2(3): 344-58.
[http://dx.doi.org/10.1177/1947601911411084] [PMID: 21779504]

[114] De Roock W, Jonker DJ, Di Nicolantonio F, *et al.* Association of KRAS p.G13D mutation with outcome in patients with chemotherapy-refractory metastatic colorectal cancer treated with cetuximab. JAMA 2010; 304(16): 1812-20.
[http://dx.doi.org/10.1001/jama.2010.1535] [PMID: 20978259]

[115] De Roock W, Claes B, Bernasconi D, *et al.* Effects of KRAS, BRAF, NRAS, and PIK3CA mutations on the efficacy of cetuximab plus chemotherapy in chemotherapy-refractory metastatic colorectal cancer: a retrospective consortium analysis. Lancet Oncol 2010; 11(8): 753-62.
[http://dx.doi.org/10.1016/S1470-2045(10)70130-3] [PMID: 20619739]

[116] McDermott U, Longley DB, Johnston PG. Molecular and biochemical markers in colorectal cancer. Ann Oncol 2002; 13 (Suppl. 4): 235-45.
[http://dx.doi.org/10.1093/annonc/mdf665] [PMID: 12401696]

[117] Bäumer S, Bäumer N, Appel N, *et al.* Antibody-mediated delivery of anti-KRAS-siRNA *in vivo* overcomes therapy resistance in colon cancer. Clin Cancer Res 2015; 21(6): 1383-94.
[http://dx.doi.org/10.1158/1078-0432.CCR-13-2017] [PMID: 25589625]

[118] Peeters M, Oliner KS, Parker A, *et al.* Massively parallel tumor multigene sequencing to evaluate response to panitumumab in a randomized phase III study of metastatic colorectal cancer. Clin Cancer Res 2013; 19(7): 1902-12.
[http://dx.doi.org/10.1158/1078-0432.CCR-12-1913] [PMID: 23325582]

[119] Michaloglou C, Vredeveld LC, Mooi WJ, Peeper DS. BRAF(E600) in benign and malignant human tumours. Oncogene 2008; 27(7): 877-95.
[http://dx.doi.org/10.1038/sj.onc.1210704] [PMID: 17724477]

[120] Davies H, Bignell GR, Cox C, *et al.* Mutations of the BRAF gene in human cancer. Nature 2002; 417(6892): 949-54.
[http://dx.doi.org/10.1038/nature00766] [PMID: 12068308]

[121] Martínez JRW, Vargas-Salas S, Gamboa SU, *et al.* The combination of ret, braf and demographic data identifies subsets of patients with aggressive papillary thyroid cancer. Horm Cancer 2019; 10(2-3): 97-106.
[http://dx.doi.org/10.1007/s12672-019-0359-8] [PMID: 30903583]

[122] Rowland A, Dias MM, Wiese MD, *et al.* Meta-analysis of BRAF mutation as a predictive biomarker of benefit from anti-EGFR monoclonal antibody therapy for RAS wild-type metastatic colorectal

cancer. Br J Cancer 2015; 112(12): 1888-94.
[http://dx.doi.org/10.1038/bjc.2015.173] [PMID: 25989278]

[123] Prahallad A, Sun C, Huang S, *et al.* Unresponsiveness of colon cancer to BRAF(V600E) inhibition through feedback activation of EGFR. Nature 2012; 483(7387): 100-3.
[http://dx.doi.org/10.1038/nature10868] [PMID: 22281684]

[124] Jhawer M, Goel S, Wilson AJ, *et al.* PIK3CA mutation/PTEN expression status predicts response of colon cancer cells to the epidermal growth factor receptor inhibitor cetuximab. Cancer Res 2008; 68(6): 1953-61.
[http://dx.doi.org/10.1158/0008-5472.CAN-07-5659] [PMID: 18339877]

[125] Prenen H, De Schutter J, Jacobs B, *et al.* PIK3CA mutations are not a major determinant of resistance to the epidermal growth factor receptor inhibitor cetuximab in metastatic colorectal cancer. Clin Cancer Res 2009; 15(9): 3184-8.
[http://dx.doi.org/10.1158/1078-0432.CCR-08-2961] [PMID: 19366826]

[126] Sartore-Bianchi A, Martini M, Molinari F, *et al.* PIK3CA mutations in colorectal cancer are associated with clinical resistance to EGFR-targeted monoclonal antibodies. Cancer Res 2009; 69(5): 1851-7.
[http://dx.doi.org/10.1158/0008-5472.CAN-08-2466] [PMID: 19223544]

[127] Mao C, Yang ZY, Hu XF, Chen Q, Tang JL. PIK3CA exon 20 mutations as a potential biomarker for resistance to anti-EGFR monoclonal antibodies in KRAS wild-type metastatic colorectal cancer: a systematic review and meta-analysis. Ann Oncol 2012; 23(6): 1518-25.
[http://dx.doi.org/10.1093/annonc/mdr464] [PMID: 22039088]

[128] Razis E, Briasoulis E, Vrettou E, *et al.* Potential value of PTEN in predicting cetuximab response in colorectal cancer: an exploratory study. BMC Cancer 2008; 8: 234.
[http://dx.doi.org/10.1186/1471-2407-8-234] [PMID: 18700047]

[129] Laurent-Puig P, Cayre A, Manceau G, *et al.* Analysis of PTEN, BRAF, and EGFR status in determining benefit from cetuximab therapy in wild-type KRAS metastatic colon cancer. J Clin Oncol 2009; 27(35): 5924-30.
[http://dx.doi.org/10.1200/JCO.2008.21.6796] [PMID: 19884556]

[130] Yan F, Cao H, Cover TL, *et al.* Colon-specific delivery of a probiotic-derived soluble protein ameliorates intestinal inflammation in mice through an EGFR-dependent mechanism. J Clin Invest 2011; 121(6): 2242-53.
[http://dx.doi.org/10.1172/JCI44031] [PMID: 21606592]

[131] Wang L, Cao H, Liu L, *et al.* Activation of epidermal growth factor receptor mediates mucin production stimulated by p40, a Lactobacillus rhamnosus GG-derived protein. J Biol Chem 2014; 289(29): 20234-44.
[http://dx.doi.org/10.1074/jbc.M114.553800] [PMID: 24895124]

[132] Shukla PK, Meena AS, Manda B, *et al.* Lactobacillus plantarum prevents and mitigates alcohol-induced disruption of colonic epithelial tight junctions, endotoxemia, and liver damage by an EGF receptor-dependent mechanism. FASEB J 2018; 32(11): fj201800351R.
[http://dx.doi.org/10.1096/fj.201800351R] [PMID: 29912589]

[133] Yoo J, Rodriguez Perez CE, Nie W, Sinnett-Smith J, Rozengurt E. TNF-α and LPA promote synergistic expression of COX-2 in human colonic myofibroblasts: role of LPA-mediated transactivation of upregulated EGFR. BMC Gastroenterol 2013; 13: 90.
[http://dx.doi.org/10.1186/1471-230X-13-90] [PMID: 23688423]

[134] Hardbower DM, Coburn LA, Asim M, *et al.* EGFR-mediated macrophage activation promotes colitis-associated tumorigenesis. Oncogene 2017; 36(27): 3807-19.
[http://dx.doi.org/10.1038/onc.2017.23] [PMID: 28263971]

[135] Bonamy C, Sechet E, Amiot A, *et al.* Expression of the human antimicrobial peptide β-defensin-1 is repressed by the EGFR-ERK-MYC axis in colonic epithelial cells. Sci Rep 2018; 8(1): 18043.
[http://dx.doi.org/10.1038/s41598-018-36387-z] [PMID: 30575780]

[136] Shimoda M, Horiuchi K, Sasaki A, *et al.* Epithelial cell-derived a disintegrin and metalloproteinase-17 confers resistance to colonic inflammation through EGFR activation. EBioMedicine 2016; 5: 114-24.
[http://dx.doi.org/10.1016/j.ebiom.2016.02.007] [PMID: 27077118]

[137] Kim SB, Ly P, Kaisani A, Zhang L, Wright WE, Shay JW. Mitigation of radiation-induced damage by targeting EGFR in noncancerous human epithelial cells. Radiat Res 2013; 180(3): 259-67.
[http://dx.doi.org/10.1667/RR3371.1] [PMID: 23919312]

[138] Meena AS, Shukla PK, Sheth P, Rao R. EGF receptor plays a role in the mechanism of glutamine-mediated prevention of alcohol-induced gut barrier dysfunction and liver injury. J Nutr Biochem 2019; 64: 128-43.
[http://dx.doi.org/10.1016/j.jnutbio.2018.10.016] [PMID: 30502657]

[139] Yang H, Higgins B, Kolinsky K, *et al.* Antitumor activity of BRAF inhibitor vemurafenib in preclinical models of BRAF-mutant colorectal cancer. Cancer Res 2012; 72(3): 779-89.
[http://dx.doi.org/10.1158/0008-5472.CAN-11-2941] [PMID: 22180495]

[140] Johnson DB, Flaherty KT, Weber JS, *et al.* Combined BRAF (Dabrafenib) and MEK inhibition (Trametinib) in patients with BRAFV600-mutant melanoma experiencing progression with single-agent BRAF inhibitor. J Clin Oncol 2014; 32(33): 3697-704.
[http://dx.doi.org/10.1200/JCO.2014.57.3535] [PMID: 25287827]

[141] Montero-Conde C, Ruiz-Llorente S, Dominguez JM, *et al.* Relief of feedback inhibition of HER3 transcription by RAF and MEK inhibitors attenuates their antitumor effects in BRAF-mutant thyroid carcinomas. Cancer Discov 2013; 3(5): 520-33.
[http://dx.doi.org/10.1158/2159-8290.CD-12-0531] [PMID: 23365119]

[142] Corcoran RB, Atreya CE, Falchook GS, *et al.* Combined BRAF and MEK Inhibition With Dabrafenib and Trametinib in BRAF V600-Mutant Colorectal Cancer. J Clin Oncol 2015; 33(34): 4023-31.
[http://dx.doi.org/10.1200/JCO.2015.63.2471] [PMID: 26392102]

[143] Hyman DM, Puzanov I, Subbiah V, *et al.* Vemurafenib in multiple nonmelanoma cancers with BRAF V600 mutations. N Engl J Med 2015; 373(8): 726-36.
[http://dx.doi.org/10.1056/NEJMoa1502309] [PMID: 26287849]

[144] Yaeger R, Cercek A, O'Reilly EM, *et al.* Pilot trial of combined BRAF and EGFR inhibition in BRAF-mutant metastatic colorectal cancer patients. Clin Cancer Res 2015; 21(6): 1313-20.
[http://dx.doi.org/10.1158/1078-0432.CCR-14-2779] [PMID: 25589621]

[145] Zhang YJ, Tian XQ, Sun DF, Zhao SL, Xiong H, Fang JY. Combined inhibition of MEK and mTOR signaling inhibits initiation and progression of colorectal cancer. Cancer Invest 2009; 27(3): 273-85.
[http://dx.doi.org/10.1080/07357900802314893] [PMID: 19194827]

[146] Markman B, Atzori F, Pérez-García J, Tabernero J, Baselga J. Status of PI3K inhibition and biomarker development in cancer therapeutics. Ann Oncol 2010; 21(4): 683-91.
[http://dx.doi.org/10.1093/annonc/mdp347] [PMID: 19713247]

[147] Richman SD, Southward K, Chambers P, *et al.* HER2 overexpression and amplification as a potential therapeutic target in colorectal cancer: analysis of 3256 patients enrolled in the QUASAR, FOCUS and PICCOLO colorectal cancer trials. J Pathol 2016; 238(4): 562-70.
[http://dx.doi.org/10.1002/path.4679] [PMID: 26690310]

[148] Krasinskas AM. EGFR Signaling in Colorectal Carcinoma. Pathol Res Int 2011; 2011: 932932.
[http://dx.doi.org/10.4061/2011/932932] [PMID: 21403829]

[149] Wu WK, Wang XJ, Cheng AS, *et al.* Dysregulation and crosstalk of cellular signaling pathways in colon carcinogenesis. Crit Rev Oncol Hematol 2013; 86(3): 251-77.
[http://dx.doi.org/10.1016/j.critrevonc.2012.11.009] [PMID: 23287077]

[150] Inamura K. Colorectal cancers: An update on their molecular pathology. Cancers (Basel) 2018; 10(1): E26.
[http://dx.doi.org/10.3390/cancers10010026] [PMID: 29361689]

[151] Takane K, Akagi K, Fukuyo M, Yagi K, Takayama T, Kaneda A. DNA methylation epigenotype and clinical features of NRAS-mutation(+) colorectal cancer. Cancer Med 2017; 6(5): 1023-35.
[http://dx.doi.org/10.1002/cam4.1061] [PMID: 28378457]

[152] Summers MG, Smith CG, Maughan TS, Kaplan R, Escott-Price V, Cheadle JP. *BRAF* and *NRAS* Locus-Specific Variants Have Different Outcomes on Survival to Colorectal Cancer. Clin Cancer Res 2017; 23(11): 2742-9.
[http://dx.doi.org/10.1158/1078-0432.CCR-16-1541] [PMID: 27815357]

[153] Malapelle U, Pisapia P, Sgariglia R, *et al.* Less frequently mutated genes in colorectal cancer: evidences from next-generation sequencing of 653 routine cases. J Clin Pathol 2016; 69(9): 767-71.
[http://dx.doi.org/10.1136/jclinpath-2015-203403] [PMID: 26797410]

[154] Salomon DS, Brandt R, Ciardiello F, Normanno N. Epidermal growth factor-related peptides and their receptors in human malignancies. Crit Rev Oncol Hematol 1995; 19(3): 183-232.
[http://dx.doi.org/10.1016/1040-8428(94)00144-I] [PMID: 7612182]

[155] D'Antonio A, Losito S, Pignata S, *et al.* Transforming growth factor alpha, amphiregulin and cripto-1 are frequently expressed in advanced human ovarian carcinomas. Int J Oncol 2002; 21(5): 941-8.
[PMID: 12370739]

[156] Normanno N, Kim N, Wen D, *et al.* Expression of messenger RNA for amphiregulin, heregulin, and cripto-1, three new members of the epidermal growth factor family, in human breast carcinomas. Breast Cancer Res Treat 1995; 35(3): 293-7.
[http://dx.doi.org/10.1007/BF00665981] [PMID: 7579500]

[157] Ito Y, Takeda T, Higashiyama S, Noguchi S, Matsuura N. Expression of heparin-binding epidermal growth factor-like growth factor in breast carcinoma. Breast Cancer Res Treat 2001; 67(1): 81-5.
[http://dx.doi.org/10.1023/A:1010667108371] [PMID: 11518469]

[158] Chong IW, Lin SR, Lin MS, Huang MS, Tsai MS, Hwang JJ. Heparin-binding epidermal growth factor-like growth factor and transforming growth factor-alpha in human non-small cell lung cancers. J Formos Med Assoc 1997; 96(8): 579-85.
[PMID: 9290266]

[159] Bacus SS, Gudkov AV, Zelnick CR, *et al.* Neu differentiation factor (heregulin) induces expression of intercellular adhesion molecule 1: implications for mammary tumors. Cancer Res 1993; 53(21): 5251-61.
[PMID: 8106145]

[160] Gilmour LM, Macleod KG, McCaig A, *et al.* Neuregulin expression, function, and signaling in human ovarian cancer cells. Clin Cancer Res 2002; 8(12): 3933-42.
[PMID: 12473609]

[161] Ingold Heppner B, Behrens HM, Balschun K, *et al.* HER2/neu testing in primary colorectal carcinoma. Br J Cancer 2014; 111(10): 1977-84.
[http://dx.doi.org/10.1038/bjc.2014.483] [PMID: 25211663]

[162] Shabbir A, Mirza T, Khalid AB, Qureshi MA, Asim SA. Frequency of Her2/neu expression in colorectal adenocarcinoma: a study from developing South Asian Country. BMC Cancer 2016; 16(1): 855.
[http://dx.doi.org/10.1186/s12885-016-2912-y] [PMID: 27821098]

[163] Meyerhardt JA, Zhu AX, Enzinger PC, *et al.* Phase II study of capecitabine, oxaliplatin, and erlotinib in previously treated patients with metastatic colorectal cancer. J Clin Oncol 2006; 24(12): 1892-7.
[http://dx.doi.org/10.1200/JCO.2005.05.3728] [PMID: 16622264]

[164] Wolpin BM, Clark JW, Meyerhardt JA, *et al.* Phase I study of gefitinib plus FOLFIRI in previously untreated patients with metastatic colorectal cancer. Clin Colorectal Cancer 2006; 6(3): 208-13.
[http://dx.doi.org/10.3816/CCC.2006.n.037] [PMID: 17026790]

CHAPTER 4

Targeting the PI3K/AKT/mTOR Signaling Pathway in Hepatocellular Carcinoma: Current State and Future Trends

Neelam Yadav[*] and **Yoganchal Mishra**[1]

[1] *Department of Biochemistry, Dr. Rammanohar Lohia Avadh University, Faizabad-224001, India*

Abstract: Hepatocellular carcinoma (HCC) is the most common liver cancer and the leading cause of cancer-related deaths. Advanced HCC has a poor prognosis with limited treatment option. Chronic liver diseases and cirrhosis are the main risk factors for the development of HCC. Phosphoinositide 3-kinase PI3K/AKT/mTOR, intracellular mediators play a very important role in the development and progression of HCC. This signaling pathway is frequently activated in HCC patients. Therefore, signaling pathways have become the main source of targets for new treatments in HCC patients.

In our chapter, we will discuss the role of PI3K/AKT/mTOR signaling pathway in the pathology of HCC and provide an update on the preclinical and clinical approaches for the development of various molecular agents targeting this proliferation/survival pathway, which include various PI3K/Akt/mTOR inhibitors and other agents for the treatment of HCC.

Keywords: Hepatocellular carcinoma, Inhibitors, Signaling pathways, Sorafenib, Therapy.

INTRODUCTION

Hepatocellular carcinoma (HCC) is an aggressive tumor of the liver and the third most common cause of death in human beings [1, 2]. Its poor prognosis is due to relapse and metastasis [3 - 5]. In HCC patients, metastasis is an essential cause of high mortality [6 - 8]. Ji *et al.* [9], reported that the clinical diagnosis and treatment of HCC patients have made great progress in the last few years. HCC occurs mainly in patients suffering with chronic liver disease and cirrhosis. Most of the mortality in HCC patients results from liver cirrhosis related problems like ascites, hepatic encephalopathy, hepatorenal syndrome and variceal hemorrhage.

[*] **Corresponding author Neelam Yadav:** Department of Biochemistry, Dr. Rammanohar Lohia Avadh University, Faizabad-224001, India; Tel: +91 9453731722; neelam2k4@gmail.com

Several genes are responsible for the tumorigenesis and progression of HCC and many molecular changes play a crucial role in the development of this aggressive malignancy [10, 11].

Due to the activation of many signal transduction pathways that regulate cell proliferation and tumor progression and complex molecular alteration in hepatic tissue, treatment of HCC is not successful [12]. The phosphoinositide 3-kinase (PI3K)/AKT/mTOR signaling pathway is repeatedly activated in HCC.

Many patients with HCC are diagnosed at the advanced stage of the disease. Current treatment therapies for HCC are locoregional ablative approaches, surgical removal and interventional ablation techniques. Although these treatments could increase few year's survival rate in 70% patients of HCC, however, long-term survival remains low due to the high rate of recurrence and metastasis after surgical resection [13 - 15]. Therefore, novel evidence-based therapies for this aggressive malignancy is urgently needed.

Risk Factors for HCC

In HCC patients, no early noticeable symptoms appear during tumor development. Its occurrence is associated mainly with aflatoxin B1 contaminated food and endemic hepatitis C virus (HCV) and hepatitis B virus (HBV) infection, obesity and non-alcoholic steatohepatitis. Despite the food storage conditions and implementation of vaccinations to reduce the risk of aflatoxin B1 and contamination and hepatitis B infection respectively, the incidence of liver cancer is not decreasing. Early risk factors responsible for the development of HCC are immune-mediated chronic inflammation in hepatitis that results into progressive fibrosis and development of liver cirrhosis [16, 17].

Pathophysiology

The development of hepatocellular carcinoma is a complex process that involves many steps. It mainly occurs after liver cirrhosis and is associated with the diversity of aetiologies of the major chronic liver disease. In liver cirrhosis, HCC follows a sequence of events that involves pre-cancerous cirrhotic nodules development known as low-grade dysplastic nodules (LGDNs). High-grade dysplastic nodules (HGDNs) develop from LGDNs and convert into early-stage HCC and than more advanced HCC. Various cells, including mature hepatocytes and stem or progenitor cells, play an important role in malignant transformation into HCC [18]. The accumulation of somatic genomic alterations in driver and passenger cancer genes is responsible for HCC. However, genomic alterations are not accumulated, which suggests that many signaling pathways may involve in the promotion of carcinogenesis [19].

In HCC progression, several pathways and processes have been involved (Table 1). A number of epigenetic and genetic changes like rearrangements and deletions of chromosomes, mutations, aneuploidy, gene amplification, and DNA methylations have been observed in HCC.

Table 1. Major gene alterations reported in advanced hepatocellular carcinoma.

Name of Pathway(s)	Gene(s) Name	Type of Alteration	Frequency Percentage (%) in HCC
AKT–mTOR– MAPK signalling	PTEN RPS6KA3 TSC1 and TSC2 FGF3, FGF4 and FGF19 P13KCA	Mutation or deletion Mutation Mutation or deletion Amplification Mutation	1-3% 2-9% 3-8% 4-6% 0-2%
WNT-β– catenin signalling	AXIN1 CTNNB1	Mutation or deletion Mutation	5-15% 11-37%
Angiogenesis	VEGFA	Amplification	3-7%
Oxidative stress	KEAP1 NFE2L2	Mutation Mutation	2-8% 3-6%
Telomere maintenance	TERT	Amplification Promoter mutation	5-6% 54-60%
Cell cycle control	RB1 CCND1 TP53 CDKN2A	Deletion or Mutation Amplification Mutation or Deletion Mutation or Deletion	3-8% 7% 12-48% 2-12%

AXIN1, axin 1; *CCND1*, cyclin D1; *CDKN2A*, cyclin-dependent kinase inhibitor 2A; *CTNNB1*, β-catenin; *FGF*, fibroblast growth factor; *KEAP1*, kelch like ECH associated protein 1; *NFE2L2*, nuclear factor, *PI3K*, phosphoinositide 3-kinase; *PTEN*, phosphatase and tensin homologue; *RB1*, retinoblastoma 1; *RPS6KA3*, ribosomal protein S6 kinase, 90kDa *TSC*, tuberous sclerosis; *TERT*, telomerase reverse transcriptase; *TP53*, cellular tumor antigen p53; *VEGFA*, vascular endothelial growth factor A.

Basic Signaling Pathways

Llovet *et al.* [20], reported that the oxidative stress, chromatin remodeling, Wnt/ beta catenin and other signaling pathways including epidermal growth factor (EGF), insulin growth factor, vascular endothelial growth factor (VEGF), fibroblast-derived growth factor (FGF), platelet-derived growth factor (PDGF), and intracellular mediators RAS–RAF–MAPK (MAP kinase) and PI3/AKT are critical signaling pathways in HCC (Table 1).

Many growth factors signaling (IGF, EGF, PDGF, FGF, and HGF), angiogenesis (VEGF) and cell differentiation (*e.g.*, WNT, Hedgehog, Notch) modules are deregulated in hepatocellular carcinoma [21]. In HCC, PI3K/AKT/mTOR and the MAP kinase pathways are continuously activated. Approximately 5% of tumors are caused by amplification of *FGF3*, *FGF4* and *FGF19 region*, and 3–8% of cases by inactivating mutations in tuberous sclerosis 1 (*TSC1*) or *TSC2* or 1–3% of cases can be related to phosphates and tensin homologue (*PTEN*).

PI3K/AKT/MTOR SIGNALING PATHWAY

Phosphatidylinositide 3-kinases (PI3Ks) are important kinases and play an important role in cellular functions. In HCC, these enzymes are involved in cell survival growth, proliferation, differentiation and intracellular trafficking [22, 23]. These enzymes are divided into three classes. The Class IA has three (p110a, b and d) catalytic subunits and a regulatory subunit (p85) [23]. In response to cytokines or growth factors stimulation and the subsequent activation of G protein-coupled receptors and receptor tyrosine kinases (RTKs), PI3K is recruited to the membrane by direct or indirect interaction with the activated receptors. On the lipid membrane, the activated PI3K generates the second messenger phosphatidylinositol (3–5)-trisphosphate (PIP3) from phosphatidylinositol 4,5-bisphosphate (PIP2) by phosphorylating inositols. Then PI3K downstream target, serine-threonine kinase Akt is recruited to the membrane *via* conjugating with PIP3, resulting in its phosphorylation by phosphoinositide-dependent kinases [24]. Akt plays an important role in cell survival pathways by inhibiting cell death processes.

After activation, Akt regulates downstream signaling of cell survival, proliferation, migration, cell cycle progression, and angiogenesis. Akt then activates phosphorylation of mTORC1, a serine/threonine kinase. By phosphorylation, the mTOR protein regulates its downstream effectors, translational repressor protein 4E-BP1 and p70S6. Both of the proteins regulate the translation of several important proliferative and angiogenic factors (cyclinD1, c-myc, VEGF and HIF1a) [25, 26]. The PI3K/Akt/ mTOR signaling is activated by various growth factors and cytokines and down regulated by tumor suppressor, PTEN homolog, which dephosphorylates PIP3 (Fig. **1**). PI Tenins (PITs) and SH2-containing inositol phosphatase-1 (SHIP1) are negative regulators of this pathway [27 - 29].

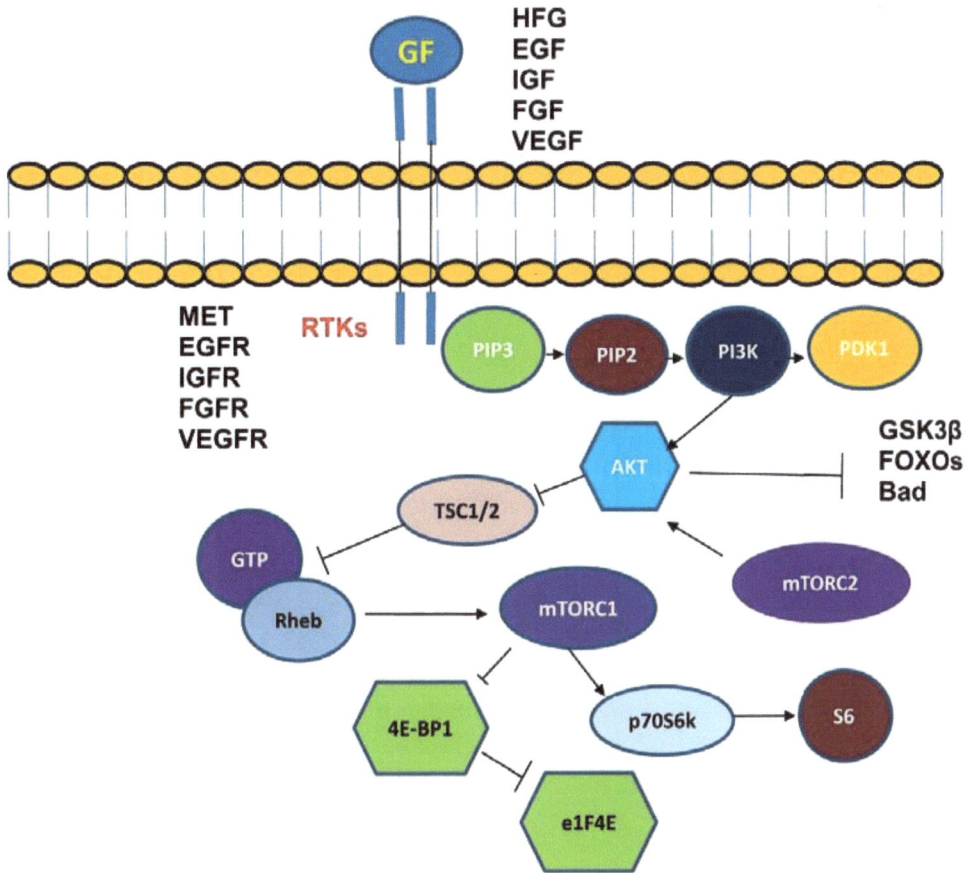

Fig. (1). The PI3K/Akt/mTOR signaling pathway in hepatocellular carcinoma.

After stimulation of growth factors (GFs), RTKs stimulate activity of class PI3K. From PIP2, PI3K generates PIP3. On the membrane, PIP3 recruits Akt and PDK1 and phosphorylation of AKT on Thr308 takes place by PDK1. Akt activated by phosphotrylation on Ser473 by mTORC2. After activation, Akt play important role in the inactivation of many substrates, including FOXOs, Bad and GSK3b. TSC1 associated TSC2 activity, also phoshorylated and inhibited by Akt. These inactivated TSC1/TSC2 complex allows to the Rheb (small G protein) for the accumulation into GTP. Then mTORC1 kinase activity upregulated by Rheb-GTP, although complete mechanism has not yet been examined. Two main downstream effectors, p70S6k and 4E-BP1 of translation are phosphorylated by mTORC1. A downstream effector of p70S6k is ribosomal S6 protein. mTORC2 is activated by complex of TSC1/TSC2.

Activated events indicated by arrows, however, inhibitory events showed by perpendicular lines. Abbreviation: *RTK,* Receptor tyrosine kinase; *GF,* Growth factor; *PIP2,* Phosphatidylinositol 4,5-bisphosphate; *GTP,* Guanosine triphosphate; *PIP3,* Phosphatidylinositol (3–5)-trisphosphate.

Adapted source: [63].

Activation of PI3K/Akt/mTOR Pathway

In HCC, many evidences exhibit that abnormal activation continuously occurs in PI3K/Akt/mTOR signaling pathway. In 45% of HCC, phosphorylation of mTOR and the expression of its downstream effectors (p70S6k) are unregulated [30]. Villanueva *et al.* [31] also reported that S6 was over activated in 50% of the HCC patients. In 40% of HCC cases, mTOR is found to be activated [32]. The PI3K/Akt/mTOR pathway is more significantly activated in high-grade HCC tumors. Akt and S6 phosphorylation is associated with poor prognosis and poor survival in HCC patients [33]. In HCC, the underlying cellular mechanism for the activation of the PI3K/Akt/mTOR pathway is not fully understood. However, one mechanism is activation by upstream receptor kinases. These may involve overexpression of EGFR, IGF1-R and c-Met. In 68% of HCC, EGFR was found to be overexpressed. Similarly, in 83% of HCC, c-Met has been found to be overexpressed [34, 35]. In HCC development, the carcinogenic role of c-Met signaling in transgenic mice model was reported by Sakata *et al.* [36].

Recently, genome sequencing studies in HCC also revealed the involvement of genomic alteration in the PI3K pathway. In 5% HCC, somatic loss of *PTEN* by gene mutation or deletion is found, which result to Akt activation. H1047R and E545K are two common PIK3CA mutations in HCC. The increase in PIP3 levels activates Akt and results into cellular transformation [22, 37 - 39]. The above evidence suggests that many events are responsible for the activation of the PI3K/Akt/mTOR pathway in the development of HCC.

Targeting PI3K/Akt/mTOR Signaling Pathway

In HCC, the activated PI3K signaling pathway contributes to the cell proliferation, survival and angiogenesis of tumor. Therefore, for targeting PI3K and other important molecules of the signaling pathway many inhibitory agents have been developed (Fig. **2**).

Targeting PI3K

Three classes of PI3Ks have been reported. First-class IA has three catalytic subunits. Wortmannin and LY294002 are first-generation pan-PI3K inhibitors. A specific and irreversible inhibitor of PI3K is Wortmannin (a furanosteroid metabolite of the fungi *Talaromyces (Penicillium) wortmannii*). *In vitro* condition, it exhibits same potency for the inhibition of all three PI3K class member's activities. LY294002 was the first synthetic molecule, which reversibly inhibits the class members of PI3K. Unfortunately, IC50 of both of the above preclinical compounds was very less, and no preferential selectivity was observed for individual isoforms of PI3K. Furthermore, an unfavorable pharmacokinetic and significant toxicities have been observed in LY294002 or Wortmannin administered animals [40 - 42]. Dry skin, bodyweight loss, and mortality were reported in treated animals; therefore, both compounds are not useful for clinical applications. Many PI3K inhibitors targeting PI3K are in clinical trials.

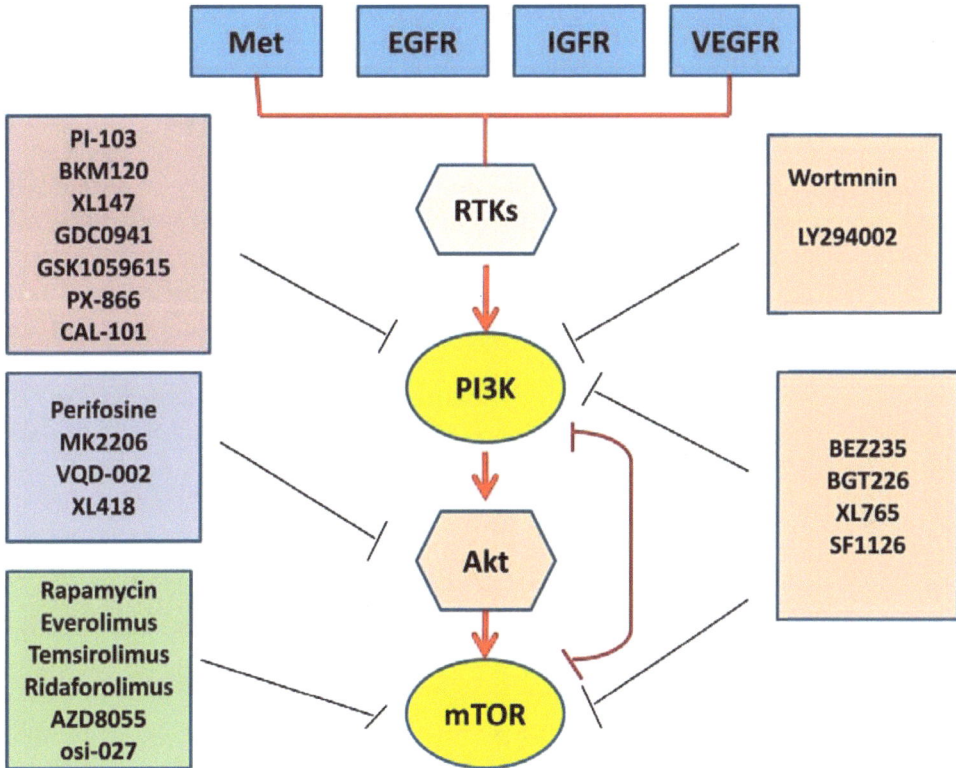

Fig. (2). Inhibitors involved for targeting the PI3K/Akt/mTOR signaling pathway.
Abbreviation: *IGFR*: Insulin-like growth factor; RTK: Receptor tyrosine kinase; *VEGFR*: Vascular endothelial growth factor; *EGFR*: Epidermal growth factor.

Targeting Akt

The potential downstream effector of the PI3K pathway is Akt; therefore, it is the most important therapeutic target for HCC. Akt1, Akt2 and Akt3 are three isoforms of Akt. Many pan-Akt inhibitors have been reported. A lipid-based phosphatidylinositol analog, Perifosine binds to the pleckstrin homology domain of Akt. It prevents binding of Akt to PIP3 and consequential membrane translocation [43]. In HCC patients, Phase II trial of Perifosine has been examined [44]. In this trial, 3% HCC treated patients showed a partial response and 47%

achieved a stable condition for three months [44]. Furthermore, sorafenib and MK2206 combination was also effective in HCC [45], suggesting the practicable use of PI3K/Akt/mTOR inhibitors for the treatment of HCC patients.

Targeting mTOR

mTORC1 and mTORC2 are two different forms of mTOR. The mTOR inhibitors were specific for targeting mTORC1. Rapamycin, or sirolimus (Rapamune®; Wyeth, NJ, USA), is a bacterially derived natural compound with antifungal [46], immunosuppressive [47] and antitumor activity [48 - 51]. It is a prototype inhibitor of mTORC1. It is associated with FK506-binding protein 12 (FKBP12), an intracellular receptor, which then binds to mTORC1 and suppresses the phosphorylation of p70S6k and 4E-BP1 (downstream substrates) [49, 51]. Due to insoluble nature of rapamycin in aqueous solution, it was not very useful for clinical applications. Recently, temsirolimus (CCI-779/Torisel®; Wyeth), and everolimus (RAD001/Afinitor®; Novartis, Basel, Switzerland), analogs of rapamycin have been reported. For the inhibition of mTORC1, these analogs follow the common mechanism of rapamycin, but have superior medical properties for cancer treatment. In various cancer patients, clinical trials of mTOR inhibitors have been evaluated [49].

Clinical Perspectives of the Current State

Hepatocellular carcinoma is diagnosed in an advanced stage, with a poor survival rate from 6 to 20 months [52]. HCC has limited treatment options. During last ten years, sorafenib, a multi-tyrosine kinase inhibitor (TKI), has been used as a systemic agent for first-line treatment of HCC [53]. Recently, another multi-TKI, lenvatinib, was also reported after III RREFLECT trial. For second-line treatment, two multi- TKIs, regorafenib (2016) and cabozantinib (2018) were approved. An anti-PD-1 antibody, nivolumab and Ramucirumab, will soon be available as other targeted therapies for HCC treatment. Masuda [54] reported that these agents generally lead to stabilization of disease rather than shrinkage of tumor. With above systemic compounds treatment of HCC still remains rare; however curative breakthroughs for this disease are urgently required.

Recently, Hindupur *et al.* [55] reported that phospholysine phosphohistidine inorganic pyrophosphate, LHPP acts as a tumor suppressor in HCC. They demonstrated that histidine phosphorylation play an important role in HCC development. In 50% of HCC patients, mTOR pathway is upregulated and associated with the resistance to sorafenib as well as poor prognosis [19, 56, 57]. For their study, they used liver-specific double-knockout (L-dKO) mice lacking PTEN and TSC1 (tumor suppressors) of the mTOR pathway, thereby causing constitutive activation of PI3K/AKT/ mTOR signaling. LHPP was specifically down-regulated in the hepatic tumors. Furthermore, decreased expression of LHPP was observed in clinical tissue samples of HCC, and low expressions of LHPP mRNA were correlated with poor prognosis. Finally, Hindupur *et al.* [55], concluded that LHHP is a tumor suppressor and histidine phosphorylation play an important role in the development of HCC.

Challenges in Targeting PI3K/Akt/mTOR Pathway

There are many challenges in targeting PI3K/Akt/mTOR pathway in HCC. The PI3K target specificity is the first challenge. The complex of both isoforms of Class IA PI3Ks (p110a and p110b) and p85 bind to RTKs, and both generate the same lipid products by using the same substrates. However, both isoforms of Class IA PI3Ks have very different roles in cell signaling, and the transformation of an oncogene. The p110a play an important role in the activation of the downstream signaling of the PI3K pathway after RTK activation [58]. Whereas p110b is responsible for the G-protein coupled receptor signaling in all cell types, including the immune system [59].

The presence of a complex mTOR feedback loop and pathway cross-talk is the second challenge. Previous findings showed less than 10% response in many tumor types, including glioma and advanced breast cancer after using mTOR inhibitors [49]. Activated mTOR can start a signaling cascade *via* p70S6k, which stimulates upstream feedback inhibition of signaling through insulin and IGF-1 receptors, which is responsible for downregulation of PI3K and downstream effectors. Akt activity may be increased by using mTOR inhibitors, which can finally contribute to the enhancement of growth of tumor [60].

Therefore, for the alleviation of the mTOR feedback loop, dual inhibitors of PI3K and mTOR have been developed. Maira *et al.* [61] reported that BEZ235 (an imidazoquinazoline derivative) inhibits the isoforms of Class I PI3K and kinase activity of mTOR by binding to the ATP-binding site of PI3K. These evidence indicate another complexity of feedback regulation for targeting this pathway, which is associated with cross-talk between PI3K pathway and many other important signaling pathways. Since both the PI3K and RAF-MAPK pathways may be activated by oncogene (*e.g.* RAS) or RTKs, therefore, upregulation in the signaling of the Ras/MAPK pathway could be achieved by blocking the PI3K pathway [62].

Recently, a tumor suppressor (LHHP) for HCC has been identified, but unfortunately, reactivation or restoration of tumor suppressors in patients is still challenging. Therefore, the development of a new agent that can restore tumor suppressor activity may be a future direction in HCC.

CONCLUSION AND FUTURE PERSPECTIVE

Hepatocellular carcinoma is the most common primary malignant tumor with poor prognosis and high mortality. Based on the studies discussed in this chapter, PI3K/Akt/mTOR signaling pathway has a very important role in HCC development. Many inhibitors have been investigated for targeting PI3K, Akt and mTOR in HCC models, but there are some limitations using compounds that target at one specific level of this signaling pathway. Both preclinical and clinical studies are promising for the target of the PI3K/Akt pathway in HCC. The concise information, based on the literature provided in this chapter, will help to improve the understanding of this signaling pathway for survival and growth of tumor in HCC. Furthermore, the improved medical profile of inhibitors against this pathway may create a new therapeutic opportunity for HCC. Therefore, the development of effective and appropriate diagnostic tools will be one of the future directions for the treatment of HCC.

CONSENT FOR PUBLICATION

Not applicable.

CONFLICT OF INTEREST

The author declares that there is no conflict of interest in this chapter.

ACKNOWLEDGEMENTS

Declared none.

REFERENCES

[1]   Mo Y, He L, Lai Z, *et al.* LINC01287 regulates tumorigenesis and invasion *via* miR-298/MYB in hepatocellular carcinoma. J Cell Mol Med 2018; 22(11): 5477-85.
        [http://dx.doi.org/10.1111/jcmm.13818] [PMID: 30133116]

[2]   Xue Y, Jia X, Li L, *et al.* DDX5 promotes hepatocellular carcinoma tumorigenesis *via* Akt signaling pathway. Biochem Biophys Res Commun 2018; 503(4): 2885-91.
        [http://dx.doi.org/10.1016/j.bbrc.2018.08.063] [PMID: 30119889]

[3]   Mancebo A, Varela M, González-Diéguez ML, *et al.* Incidence and risk factors associated with hepatocellular carcinoma surveillance failure. J Gastroenterol Hepatol 2018; 33(8): 1524-9.
        [http://dx.doi.org/10.1111/jgh.14108] [PMID: 29384236]

[4]   Quencer KB, Friedman T, Sheth R, Oklu R. Tumor thrombus: incidence, imaging, prognosis and treatment. Cardiovasc Diagn Ther 2017; 7 (Suppl. 3): S165-77.
        [http://dx.doi.org/10.21037/cdt.2017.09.16] [PMID: 29399520]

[5]   Roche B, Coilly A, Duclos-Vallee J C, Samuel D. The impact of treatment of hepatitis C with DAAs on the occurrence of HCC 2018; 38(Suppl 1): 139-45.
        [http://dx.doi.org/10.1111/liv.13659]

[6]   Chen ZH, Hong YF, Chen X, *et al.* Comparison of five staging systems in predicting the survival rate

of patients with hepatocellular carcinoma undergoing trans-arterial chemoembolization therapy. Oncol Lett 2018; 15(1): 855-62.
[PMID: 29403561]

[7]   He X, Guo X, Zhang H, Kong X, Yang F, Zheng C. Mechanism of action and efficacy of LY2109761, a TGF-β receptor inhibitor, targeting tumor microenvironment in liver cancer after TACE. Oncotarget 2017; 9(1): 1130-42.
[http://dx.doi.org/10.18632/oncotarget.23193] [PMID: 29416682]

[8]   Zou ZC, Dai M, Huang ZY, *et al.* MicroRNA-139-3p suppresses tumor growth and metastasis in hepatocellular carcinoma by repressing ANXA2R. Oncol Res 2018; 26(9): 1391-9.
[http://dx.doi.org/10.3727/096504018X15178798885361] [PMID: 29422116]

[9]   Ji K, Lin K, Wang Y, *et al.* TAZ inhibition promotes IL-2-induced apoptosis of hepatocellular carcinoma cells by activating the JNK/F-actin/mitochondrial fission pathway. Cancer Cell Int 2018; 18: 117.
[http://dx.doi.org/10.1186/s12935-018-0615-y] [PMID: 30127666]

[10]   Xiao L, Wang Y, Liang W, *et al.* LRH-1 drives hepatocellular carcinoma partially through induction of c-myc and cyclin E1, and suppression of p21. Cancer Manag Res 2018; 10: 2389-400.
[http://dx.doi.org/10.2147/CMAR.S162887] [PMID: 30122988]

[11]   Lapointe-Shaw L, Georgie F, Carlone D, *et al.* Identifying cirrhosis, decompensated cirrhosis and hepatocellular carcinoma in health administrative data: A validation study. PLoS One 2018; 13(8): e0201120.
[http://dx.doi.org/10.1371/journal.pone.0201120] [PMID: 30133446]

[12]   Thomas MB, Abbruzzese JL. Opportunities for targeted therapies in hepatocellular carcinoma. J Clin Oncol 2005; 23(31): 8093-108.
[http://dx.doi.org/10.1200/JCO.2004.00.1537] [PMID: 16258107]

[13]   Yang B, Zan RY, Wang SY, *et al.* Radiofrequency ablation *versus* percutaneous ethanol injection for hepatocellular carcinoma: a meta-analysis of randomized controlled trials. World J Surg Oncol 2015; 13(96): 96.
[http://dx.doi.org/10.1186/s12957-015-0516-7] [PMID: 25889181]

[14]   Baek YH, Kim KT, Lee SW, *et al.* Efficacy of hepatic arterial infusion chemotherapy in advanced hepatocellular carcinoma. World J Gastroenterol 2012; 18(26): 3426-34.
[http://dx.doi.org/10.3748/wjg.v18.i26.3426] [PMID: 22807613]

[15]   Kim JY, Chung SM, Choi BO, Kay CS. Hepatocellular carcinoma with portal vein tumor thrombosis: Improved treatment outcomes with external beam radiation therapy. Hepatol Res 2011; 41(9): 813-24.
[http://dx.doi.org/10.1111/j.1872-034X.2011.00826.x] [PMID: 21696524]

[16]   Johnson PJ. How do mechanisms of hepatocarcinogenesis (HBV, HCV and NASH) affect our understanding and approach to HCC?. ASCO Educational Book 2013; pp. 132-6.

[17]   Greten TF, Korangy F, Manns MP, Malek NP. Molecular therapy for the treatment of hepatocellular carcinoma. Br J Cancer 2009; 100(1): 19-23.
[http://dx.doi.org/10.1038/sj.bjc.6604784] [PMID: 19018262]

[18]   Marquardt JU, Andersen JB, Thorgeirsson SS. Functional and genetic deconstruction of the cellular origin in liver cancer. Nat Rev Cancer 2015; 15(11): 653-67.
[http://dx.doi.org/10.1038/nrc4017] [PMID: 26493646]

[19]   Schulze K, Imbeaud S, Letouzé E, *et al.* Exome sequencing of hepatocellular carcinomas identifies new mutational signatures and potential therapeutic targets. Nat Genet 2015; 47(5): 505-11.
[http://dx.doi.org/10.1038/ng.3252] [PMID: 25822088]

[20]   Llovet JM, Villanueva A, Lachenmayer A, Finn RS. Advances in targeted therapies for hepatocellular carcinoma in the genomic era. Nat Rev Clin Oncol 2015; 12(7): 408-24.
[http://dx.doi.org/10.1038/nrclinonc.2015.103] [PMID: 26054909]

[21] Moeini A, Cornellà H, Villanueva A. Emerging signaling pathways in hepatocellular carcinoma. Liver Cancer 2012; 1(2): 83-93.
[http://dx.doi.org/10.1159/000342405] [PMID: 24159576]

[22] Bader AG, Kang S, Zhao L, Vogt PK. Oncogenic PI3K deregulates transcription and translation. Nat Rev Cancer 2005; 5(12): 921-9.
[http://dx.doi.org/10.1038/nrc1753] [PMID: 16341083]

[23] Engelman JA, Luo J, Cantley LC. The evolution of phosphatidylinositol 3-kinases as regulators of growth and metabolism. Nat Rev Genet 2006; 7(8): 606-19.
[http://dx.doi.org/10.1038/nrg1879] [PMID: 16847462]

[24] Yap TA, Garrett MD, Walton MI, Raynaud F, de Bono JS, Workman P. Targeting the PI3K-AK-mTOR pathway: progress, pitfalls, and promises. Curr Opin Pharmacol 2008; 8(4): 393-412.
[http://dx.doi.org/10.1016/j.coph.2008.08.004] [PMID: 18721898]

[25] Dunlop EA, Tee AR. Mammalian target of rapamycin complex 1: signalling inputs, substrates and feedback mechanisms. Cell Signal 2009; 21(6): 827-35.
[http://dx.doi.org/10.1016/j.cellsig.2009.01.012] [PMID: 19166929]

[26] Mamane Y, Petroulakis E, LeBacquer O, Sonenberg N. mTOR, translation initiation and cancer. Oncogene 2006; 25(48): 6416-22.
[http://dx.doi.org/10.1038/sj.onc.1209888] [PMID: 17041626]

[27] Freeburn RW, Wright KL, Burgess SJ, Astoul E, Cantrell DA, Ward SG. Evidence that SHIP-1 contributes to phosphatidylinositol 3,4,5-trisphosphate metabolism in T lymphocytes and can regulate novel phosphoinositide 3-kinase effectors. J Immunol 2002; 169(10): 5441-50.
[http://dx.doi.org/10.4049/jimmunol.169.10.5441] [PMID: 12421919]

[28] Miao B, Skidan I, Yang J, *et al.* Small molecule inhibition of phosphatidylinositol-3,4,5-triphosphate (PIP3) binding to pleckstrin homology domains. Proc Natl Acad Sci USA 2010; 107(46): 20126-31.
[http://dx.doi.org/10.1073/pnas.1004522107] [PMID: 21041639]

[29] Zhou Q, Lui VW, Yeo W. Targeting the PI3K/Akt/mTOR pathway in hepatocellular carcinoma. Future Oncol 2011; 7(10): 1149-67.
[http://dx.doi.org/10.2217/fon.11.95] [PMID: 21992728]

[30] Sahin F, Kannangai R, Adegbola O, Wang J, Su G, Torbenson M. mTOR and P70 S6 kinase expression in primary liver neoplasms. Clin Cancer Res 2004; 10(24): 8421-5.
[http://dx.doi.org/10.1158/1078-0432.CCR-04-0941] [PMID: 15623621]

[31] Villanueva A, Chiang DY, Newell P, *et al.* Pivotal role of mTOR signaling in hepatocellular carcinoma. Gastroenterology 2008; 135(6): 1972-1983, 1983.e1-1983.e11.
[http://dx.doi.org/10.1053/j.gastro.2008.08.008] [PMID: 18929564]

[32] Sieghart W, Fuereder T, Schmid K, *et al.* Mammalian target of rapamycin pathway activity in hepatocellular carcinomas of patients undergoing liver transplantation. Transplantation 2007; 83(4): 425-32.
[http://dx.doi.org/10.1097/01.tp.0000252780.42104.95] [PMID: 17318075]

[33] Zhou L, Huang Y, Li J, Wang Z. The mTOR pathway is associated with the poor prognosis of human hepatocellular carcinoma. Med Oncol 2010; 27(2): 255-61.
[http://dx.doi.org/10.1007/s12032-009-9201-4] [PMID: 19301157]

[34] Daveau M, Scotte M, François A, *et al.* Hepatocyte growth factor, transforming growth factor alpha, and their receptors as combined markers of prognosis in hepatocellular carcinoma. Mol Carcinog 2003; 36(3): 130-41.
[http://dx.doi.org/10.1002/mc.10103] [PMID: 12619035]

[35] Tavian D, De Petro G, Benetti A, Portolani N, Giulini SM, Barlati S. *u-PA* and *c-MET* mRNA expression is co-ordinately enhanced while hepatocyte growth factor mRNA is down-regulated in human hepatocellular carcinoma. Int J Cancer 2000; 87(5): 644-9.

[http://dx.doi.org/10.1002 /1097 -0215 (20000901) 87:5<644:: AID-IJC4> 3.0.CO;2-W] [PMID: 10925356]

[36]   Sakata H, Takayama H, Sharp R, Rubin JS, Merlino G, LaRochelle WJ. Hepatocyte growth factor/scatter factor overexpression induces growth, abnormal development, and tumor formation in transgenic mouse livers. Cell Growth Differ 1996; 7(11): 1513-23.
       [PMID: 8930401]

[37]   Bader AG, Kang S, Vogt PK. Cancer-specific mutations in *PIK3CA* are oncogenic *in vivo.* Proc Natl Acad Sci USA 2006; 103(5): 1475-9.
       [http://dx.doi.org/10.1073/pnas.0510857103] [PMID: 16432179]

[38]   Samuels Y, Diaz LA Jr, Schmidt-Kittler O, *et al.* Mutant *PIK3CA* promotes cell growth and invasion of human cancer cells. Cancer Cell 2005; 7(6): 561-73.
       [http://dx.doi.org/10.1016/j.ccr.2005.05.014] [PMID: 15950905]

[39]   Zhao JJ, Liu Z, Wang L, Shin E, Loda MF, Roberts TM. The oncogenic properties of mutant p110alpha and p110beta phosphatidylinositol 3-kinases in human mammary epithelial cells. Proc Natl Acad Sci USA 2005; 102(51): 18443-8.
       [http://dx.doi.org/10.1073/pnas.0508988102] [PMID: 16339315]

[40]   Hu L, Zaloudek C, Mills GB, Gray J, Jaffe RB. *In vivo* and *in vitro* ovarian carcinoma growth inhibition by a phosphatidylinositol 3-kinase inhibitor (LY294002). Clin Cancer Res 2000; 6(3): 880-6.
       [PMID: 10741711]

[41]   Amaravadi R, Thompson CB. The survival kinases Akt and Pim as potential pharmacological targets. J Clin Invest 2005; 115(10): 2618-24.
       [http://dx.doi.org/10.1172/JCI26273] [PMID: 16200194]

[42]   Knight ZA, Gonzalez B, Feldman ME, *et al.* A pharmacological map of the PI3-K family defines a role for p110alpha in insulin signaling. Cell 2006; 125(4): 733-47.
       [http://dx.doi.org/10.1016/j.cell.2006.03.035] [PMID: 16647110]

[43]   Hilgard P, Klenner T, Stekar J, Nössner G, Kutscher B, Engel J. D-21266, a new heterocyclic alkylphospholipid with antitumour activity. Eur J Cancer 1997; 33(3): 442-6.
       [http://dx.doi.org/10.1016/S0959-8049(97)89020-X] [PMID: 9155530]

[44]   Campos Lt, Nemunaitis J. Phase II study of single agent perifosine in patients with hepatocellular carcinoma (HCC). J Clin Oncol 2009; 27(15): e15505.

[45]   Chen KF, Chen HL, Tai WT, *et al.* Activation of PI3K/AKT signaling pathway mediates acquired resistance to sorafenib in hepatocellular carcinoma cells. J Pharmacol Exp Ther 2011; 337(1): 155-61.
       [http://dx.doi.org/10.1124/jpet.110.175786] [PMID: 21205925]

[46]   Vézina C, Kudelski A, Sehgal SN. Rapamycin (AY-22,989), a new antifungal antibiotic. I. Taxonomy of the producing streptomycete and isolation of the active principle. J Antibiot (Tokyo) 1975; 28(10): 721-6.
       [http://dx.doi.org/10.7164/antibiotics.28.721] [PMID: 1102508]

[47]   Yatscoff RW, LeGatt DF, Kneteman NM. Therapeutic monitoring of rapamycin: a new immunosuppressive drug. Ther Drug Monit 1993; 15(6): 478-82.
       [http://dx.doi.org/10.1097/00007691-199312000-00004] [PMID: 8122280]

[48]   Hay N. The Akt-mTOR tango and its relevance to cancer. Cancer Cell 2005; 8(3): 179-83.
       [http://dx.doi.org/10.1016/j.ccr.2005.08.008] [PMID: 16169463]

[49]   Faivre S, Kroemer G, Raymond E. Current development of mTOR inhibitors as anticancer agents. Nat Rev Drug Discov 2006; 5(8): 671-88.
       [http://dx.doi.org/10.1038/nrd2062] [PMID: 16883305]

[50]   Guertin DA, Sabatini DM. Defining the role of mTOR in cancer. Cancer Cell 2007; 12(1): 9-22.
       [http://dx.doi.org/10.1016/j.ccr.2007.05.008] [PMID: 17613433]

[51] Sabatini DM. mTOR and cancer: insights into a complex relationship. Nat Rev Cancer 2006; 6(9): 729-34.
[http://dx.doi.org/10.1038/nrc1974] [PMID: 16915295]

[52] Lian Y, Xiao C, Yan C, *et al.* Knockdown of pseudogene derived from lncRNA DUXAP10 inhibits cell proliferation, migration, invasion, and promotes apoptosis in pancreatic cancer. J Cell Biochem 2018; 119(4): 3671-82.
[http://dx.doi.org/10.1002/jcb.26578] [PMID: 29286182]

[53] Llovet JM, Montal R, Sia D, Finn RS. Molecular therapies and precision medicine for hepatocellular carcinoma. Nat Rev Clin Oncol 2018; 15(10): 599-616.
[http://dx.doi.org/10.1038/s41571-018-0073-4] [PMID: 30061739]

[54] Masuda M. Hunting hidden pieces of signaling pathways in hepatocellular carcinoma. Hepatobiliary Surg Nutr 2019; 8(1): 74-6.
[http://dx.doi.org/10.21037/hbsn.2018.10.10] [PMID: 30881973]

[55] Hindupur SK, Colombi M, Fuhs SR, *et al.* The protein histidine phosphatase LHPP is a tumour suppressor. Nature 2018; 555(7698): 678-82.
[http://dx.doi.org/10.1038/nature26140] [PMID: 29562234]

[56] Llovet JM, Zucman-Rossi J, Pikarsky E, *et al.* Hepatocellular carcinoma. Nat Rev Dis Primers 2016; 2: 16018.
[http://dx.doi.org/10.1038/nrdp.2016.18] [PMID: 27158749]

[57] Masuda M, Chen WY, Miyanaga A, *et al.* Alternative mammalian target of rapamycin (mTOR) signal activation in sorafenib-resistant hepatocellular carcinoma cells revealed by array-based pathway profiling. Mol Cell Proteomics 2014; 13(6): 1429-38.
[http://dx.doi.org/10.1074/mcp.M113.033845] [PMID: 24643969]

[58] Zhao JJ, Cheng H, Jia S, *et al.* The p110alpha isoform of PI3K is essential for proper growth factor signaling and oncogenic transformation. Proc Natl Acad Sci USA 2006; 103(44): 16296-300.
[http://dx.doi.org/10.1073/pnas.0607899103] [PMID: 17060635]

[59] Guillermet-Guibert J, Bjorklof K, Salpekar A, *et al.* The p110beta isoform of phosphoinositide 3-kinase signals downstream of G protein-coupled receptors and is functionally redundant with p110gamma. Proc Natl Acad Sci USA 2008; 105(24): 8292-7.
[http://dx.doi.org/10.1073/pnas.0707761105] [PMID: 18544649]

[60] O'Reilly KE, Rojo F, She QB, *et al.* mTOR inhibition induces upstream receptor tyrosine kinase signaling and activates Akt. Cancer Res 2006; 66(3): 1500-8.
[http://dx.doi.org/10.1158/0008-5472.CAN-05-2925] [PMID: 16452206]

[61] Maira SM, Stauffer F, Brueggen J, *et al.* Identification and characterization of NVP-BEZ235, a new orally available dual phosphatidylinositol 3-kinase/mammalian target of rapamycin inhibitor with potent *in vivo* antitumor activity. Mol Cancer Ther 2008; 7(7): 1851-63.
[http://dx.doi.org/10.1158/1535-7163.MCT-08-0017] [PMID: 18606717]

[62] Moelling K, Schad K, Bosse M, Zimmermann S, Schweneker M. Regulation of Raf–AKT cross-talk. J Biol Chem 2002; 277(34): 31099-106.
[http://dx.doi.org/10.1074/jbc.M111974200] [PMID: 12048182]

[63] Martelli AM, Chiarini F, Evangelisti C, *et al.* The phosphatidylinositol 3-kinase/AKT/mammalian target of rapamycin signaling network and the control of normal myelopoiesis. Histol Histopathol 2010; 25(5): 669-80.
[http://dx.doi.org/10.1002/jcb.2657810.1002/jcb.26578] [PMID: 20238304]

CHAPTER 5

MAPK Signaling Pathway: A Central Target in Pancreatic Cancer Therapeutics

Sahdeo Prasad and **Sanjay K. Srivastava**[*]

Department of Immunotherapeutics and Biotechnology, and Center for Tumor Immunology and Targeted Cancer Therapy, Texas Tech University Health Sciences Center, Abilene, TX 79601, USA

Abstract: Pancreatic cancer remains one of the most clinically challenging cancer despite the advancement in molecular characterization of this disease. Malignancy of this disease is characterized by the constitutively activated mitogen-activated protein kinase (MAPK) pathway. The MAPK pathway is activated by growth factors, mitogens, hormones, cytokines and environmental factors. Activated MAPK induces expression of downstream genes and regulates cell proliferation, survival, differentiation, motility, receptor signaling, senescence and transport. Activation of MAPK in pancreatic cancer is associated with a poor prognosis and results in limited treatment options. This poor prognosis elicits a need for the development of effective therapeutic measures to treat and improve pancreatic cancer patient survival. MAPK targeted pancreatic cancer therapy has been developed in the last few decades with the use of a number of inhibitors. Inhibitors of RAS, MEK1/2 and ERK1/2 are the main drugs used pre-clinically and in clinical settings of pancreatic cancer treatment. Although these inhibitors have shown some clinical benefits, extensive research on the development of new MAPK signaling pathway inhibitors for the treatment of pancreatic cancer is warranted.

Keywords: Inhibitors, MAPK, Pancreatic cancer, Targeted therapy.

INTRODUCTION

Pancreatic cancer is the fourth leading cause of cancer-related deaths and one of the most lethal malignant neoplasms across the world. According to the American Cancer Society, about 55,770 people will be diagnosed with pancreatic cancer and about 45,750 people will die in 2019. Pancreatic cancer accounts for about 7% of all cancer deaths in the USA and about 3% of all cancers. The 5-year survival rate of people with pancreatic cancer is also very low (8%). Incidence rates are also observed 25% higher in black people than in white people. Although tremendous

[*] **Corresponding author Sanjay K. Srivastava:** Department of Immunotherapeutics and Biotechnology, Texas Tech University Health Sciences Center, Suite 1305, 1718 Pine Street, Abilene, Texas 79601 USA; Tel: 325-696-0464; E-mail: sanjay.srivastava@ttuhsc.edu

Manoj K. Pandey & Vijay P. Kale (Eds.)

efforts have been made to improve therapeutic intervention, the prognosis remains poor because the diagnosis of pancreatic cancer at an early stage is very difficult due to the lack of specificity and cost-effective screening tests. This cancer is usually diagnosed at an advanced stage and is also resistant to chemotherapy [1]. Despite the recent advancement in therapeutic techniques and medical management, the median survival time of pancreatic cancer patients is only 5-8 months because of tumor cell invasion, early metastasis, and resistance to standard chemotherapy.

This poor prognosis, metastasis and resistance to therapy lead to target specific molecules for effective therapy and improvement of pancreatic patient survival. Advanced studies are needed to understand the pathogenesis, signaling network and molecular targets that may provide clues for the treatment of pancreatic cancer. Although pancreatic cancer is a multifactorial disease, the mitogen-activated protein kinase (MAPK) pathway is found to be constitutively activated in this cancer. In this chapter, the relevance and mechanism of MAPK activation in the pathobiology of pancreatic cancer will be explored. The therapeutic approach of pancreatic cancer by targeting MAPK will also be discussed.

Activation of the MAPK Pathway

MAPK proteins are Ser/Thr kinases, which coordinately regulate signal transduction, cell division, proliferation, gene expression, metabolism, motility, transport, survival, apoptosis, and differentiation. Typically MAPKs include the extracellular signal-regulated kinases 1/2 (ERK1/2), c-Jun amino (N)-terminal kinases 1/2/3 (JNK1/2/3), p38 [2 - 4], but recent studies suggest that atypically ERK3/4, ERK5, ERK7, and nemo-like kinase (NLK) are also included [5]. ERK, JNK, and p38 isoforms are known to form a group based on their activation motif, structure and function [6]. p38 MAPK is classified into four types such as p38α, p38β, p38γ, and p38δ [7].

MAPKs consist of three sets of kinases including MAPK, MAPK kinase (MAPKK), and MAPKK kinase (MAPKKK). It has been found that the canonical MAPK/ERK pathway is composed of three types of MAPKKK that include A-RAF, B-RAF and RAF-1 or C-RAF kinases while MAPKK is composed of MAPK/ERK kinase (MEK)1 and MEK2. ERK1 and ERK2 are the downstream kinases and are the final effectors of the MAPK pathway [8]. MAPK is activated by a broad range of stimuli such as mitogens, growth factors, cytokines, environmental and other factors. Besides these, other factors such as chemokines, microRNA, kinases, and other proteins are associated with the activation of the MAPK signaling pathway (Fig. **1**). These stimuli first activate MAPKKK, which are protein Ser/Thr kinases, by phosphorylation. The activation of MAPKKK occurs *via* receptor-dependent and -independent mechanisms. In receptor-dependent mechanism, activation is initiated by the binding of an inducing ligand to the receptor tyrosine kinase (RTK) residing on the plasma membrane of the cells, which leads to the activation of RAS G-protein. In turn, RAS recruits and activates the serine/threonine protein kinase, RAF, a MAPKKK [9]. The activated MAPKKK phosphorylates and activates its downstream kinase MAPKK, which in turn phosphorylates Thr and Tyr residues and activates MAPKs. Activation of MAPKs further leads to the activation of specific MAPK-activated protein kinases (MAPKAPKs). The activation of MAPKAPKs results in a broad range of fundamental cellular activities including stress response, growth, proliferation, differentiation, survival, motility and apoptosis. However, events of MAPK phosphorylation are found to be inactivated by MAPK protein phosphatases (MKPs) that dephosphorylate both threonine and tyrosine residues on MAPKs [10].

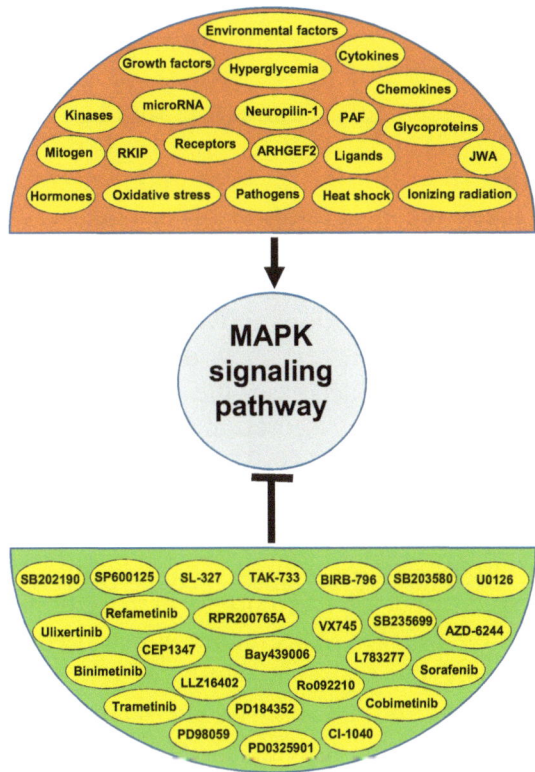

Fig. (1). Activators and inhibitors of the MAPK signaling pathway.

MAPK PATHWAY IN PANCREATIC CANCER PROGRESSION

Activated MAPK is a good prognostic marker in pancreatic cancer. MAPK cascade is critical for human pancreatic cancer cell growth, survival, and proliferation. The MAPK pathway receives signals internally or from external stimuli to get activated and further stimulates the proliferation of pancreatic cancer cells. Activated MAPK induces expression of downstream genes involved in cell division, signal transduction, motility, and transport [11, 12].

The importance of 38 MAPK in the proliferation of pancreatic cancer was demonstrated in various *in vitro* and animal models. In diabetic animals with pancreatic tumors, treatment with high glucose increased the phosphorylation of MAPK. However, p38 MAPK inhibitor decreased the growth and invasive nature of pancreatic cancer cells under high-glucose conditions [13]. Another study also supports that hyperglycemia activates the ERK and p38 MAPK pathways through increasing hydrogen peroxide (H_2O_2) mediated up-regulation of manganese superoxide dismutase (SOD2) expression. This H2O2 mediated activation of MAPK results in the invasion of pancreatic cancer cells. The involvement of H_2O_2/MAPK in the invasion of pancreatic cancer cells was confirmed by inhibiting MEK (PD98059), p38 MAPK inhibitor (SB203580), or the siRNA specific to SOD_2, which abolished the invasion and metastasis [14]. Activation of MAPK not only induces the proliferation of pancreatic cancer cells but also prevents apoptotic and autophagic cell death, which is evident by a study where suppression of MAPK by its inhibitor U0126 suppressed the growth of pancreatic cancer cells [15]. Besides proliferation, activation of MAPK signaling pathway regulates invasive and metastatic efficacy of pancreatic cancer cells. ERK inhibition by its specific inhibitor decreases the metastatic proteins urokinase-type plasminogen activator (uPA) secretion and expression of matrix metalloproteinases (MMP-2 and MMP-9). ERK pathway also regulates uPA secretion and metastasis mediated through the p38 MAPK pathway [16]. Apoptosis signal-regulating kinase 1 (ASK1, also known as MAP3K5), a member of mitogen-activated protein kinase kinase kinase family, remains in the active form by the suppressive effect of thioredoxin (Trx). Higher expression of Trx facilitates the association of TRX-ASK1 complex formation and increases the proliferation of pancreatic cancer cells while reduces the expression of Trx, dissociates Trx-ASK1 complex and induces apoptosis [17].

Mutations in the KRAS gene have been found in the vast majority (95%) of pancreatic cancers [18]; however, some pancreatic cancers harbor mutations of BRAF rather than KRAS [19]. In pancreatic cancers, mutations of KRAS and BRAF are mutually exclusive. These activated mutations of KRAS and BRAF lead to the activation of the MAPK signaling pathway. RAS molecules also induce reactive oxygen species (ROS) production primarily mediated by NADPH oxidase (NOX) enzymes and mitochondrial respiratory chain enzymatic complexes [18, 20]. The production of ROS causes initiation, progression, metastasis and maintenance of pancreatic tumor environment [18].

Neuropilin-1, a co-receptor, is highly expressed in malignant pancreatic cancer. Neuropilin-1 overexpression increases constitutive MAPK signaling, possibly *via* an autocrine loop. This overexpression further enhances resistance to anoikis and chemotherapeutic drugs. Neuropilin-1 mediated activation of MAPK increases the survival of pancreatic cancer cells by increased expression of the antiapoptotic regulator, Mcl-1 [21]. Another molecule RHO guanine exchange factor ARHGEF2 regulates the MAPK signaling pathway. In a study, forced expression of ARHGEF2 desensitizes cells to pharmacological MEK inhibition and initiates a positive feedback loop, which activates ERK phosphorylation and the downstream ARHGEF2 promoter. Thus, ARHGEF2 mediated MAPK signaling promotes the growth and survival of RAS-transformed pancreatic tumors [22]. MAPK signaling is reported to regulate a putative oncogene Zinc finger protein X-linked (ZFX). Although the role of ZFX in pancreatic tumorigenesis is not clear, it promotes tumor growth and survival of pancreatic tumors in animals. It is reported that as compared to ZFX-negative, patients with ZFX-positive tumors exhibit very low overall survival. However, the knocking down of ZFX inhibits cell proliferation through stimulation of cell cycle arrest and increases apoptosis and suppresses invasion [23]. MAPK is known to be regulated by upstream kinase TAK1 that induces proliferation and migration of pancreatic cancer cells. Inhibition of TAK1 suppresses cell growth and migration, and induces cell apoptosis *in vitro* and *in vivo* [24].

P38-MAPK signaling is also activated by the interaction of apoptosis signal-regulating kinase 1 and thioredoxin, which leads to the proliferation of pancreatic cancer cells [17, 25]. Thus, inhibition of the interaction between signal-regulating kinase 1 and thioredoxin or suppression of either signal-regulating kinase 1 or MAPK attenuates pancreatic cancer cell proliferation [26]. A JWA gene regulates the activation of the MAPK signaling pathway as silencing of JWA inhibited the activation of ERK1/2 of the MAPK pathway without affecting the expression levels of ERK1/2, JNK, p38, and activation of JNK and p38. Forced expression of JWA is also reported to increase the invasion and metastasis of the pancreatic cancer cells. Thus, JWA regulates apoptosis, growth, proliferation, invasion and metastasis of pancreatic cancer cells, which is attributed to the activation of ERK1/2 in the MAPK pathway [27]. The proliferation of pancreatic cancer cells is also accompanied by PCNA-associated factor (PAF)-induced ERK phosphorylation. PAF transcriptionally activates the expression of MAPK, which hyperphosphorylates MEK and ERK and is necessary for pancreatic cancer cell proliferation [28]. The proliferation of pancreatic cancer cells is also reported to be mediated by MAPK-associated gene SON. SON expression is prominent in pancreatic adenocarcinomas. It has been reported that knockdown of SON induces G2/M arrest and apoptosis in pancreatic cancer cells [29]. Although various studies have shown that p38 MAPK is significantly activated in pancreatic adenocarcinoma [13, 30], some reports revealed that functional p38 MAPK is correlated with improved survival of pancreatic cancer patients [31] and increases anticancer effects of the therapeutic drugs [32]. Zhong *et al.* further showed that inhibition of functional p38 MAPK by SB202190 increases the proliferation of pancreatic cancer cells. These findings indicate that p38MAPK acts as a double-edged sword [33].

The proliferation of pancreatic cancer is directly or indirectly mediated by MAPK signaling pathways. Certain kinases or proteins activate the MAPK pathway and further induce growth and proliferation of pancreatic cancer. Interaction of stromal cell-derived factor (SDF)-1α with C-X-C chemokine receptor (CXCR)-4 is known to play an important role in tumor growth, invasion, metastasis, and angiogenesis of pancreatic cancer. How SDF-1 induces pancreatic cancer tumorigenesis is mechanistically not clear. However, a study showed that SDF-1α induces p38 MAPK phosphorylation and MMP-2 and MMP-9 upregulation, which was associated with increased pancreatic cancer cell proliferation and invasion [34]. The chemokine leukotriene B4 activates MEK and ERK1/2 through the induction of ROS generation. This leukotriene B4 participates in cell survival signaling by increasing expression of Bcl-2, cyclooxygenase (COX)-2, and β-catenin, and also it reduces apoptosis. However, inhibition of MEK and ERK1/2 activation by PD98059 and U0126 reduces the anti-apoptotic effects of leukotriene B4, indicating that leukotriene B4 mediates survival and proliferation of pancreatic cancer cells through activation of MEK and ERK1/2 [35].

Stress hormone norepinephrine induces proliferation, invasion and metastasis of human pancreatic cancer cells. Norepinephrine hormone elevates the P38/MAPK phosphorylation level, which stimulates growth and tumorigenesis of pancreatic cancer. This is evident by a fact that β-adrenergic-receptor antagonist propranolol or P38/MAPK inhibitor SB203580 inhibits stimulatory effects of norepinephrine hormone [36]. Trop2, a cell-surface glycoprotein overexpressed in pancreatic tumor cells, phosphorylates ERK1/2 and activates MAPK signaling pathway. This activation leads to pancreatic cancer cell cycle progression by increasing the expression of mitotic proteins cyclin D1 and cyclin E as well as downregulating p27 [37]. This study indicates that Trop2 mediated activation of the MAPK signaling pathway has important implications for pancreatic cancer cell growth and survival. MAPK also increases the proliferation of pancreatic cancer cells by increasing sensitivity to Ca^{2+}. Transfecting pancreatic cancer cells with a p38

MAPK expression construct prominently enhances their sensitivity to Ca^{2+}. However, suppression of p38 MAPK reduces Ca^{2+} sensitivity and further inhibition in proliferation [38].

Over 90% of pancreatic cancer cells have mutations in the *KRAS* gene, which result in constitutively active RAS. This activated RAS further activates ERK1/2 and MAPK signaling pathways [39 - 41]. KRAS expression also inversely regulates the expression of RAF kinase inhibitory protein (RKIP) tumor repressor protein in pancreatic cancer cells regardless of the KRAS mutant status. RKIP inhibits the RAF-MEK-ERK pathway and results in suppression of pancreatic cancer malignancy. The knockdown of KRAS protein results in increased RKIP expression that leads to inhibition of metastasis and chemoresistance [42]. Mutation of KRAS (G12D) causes resistance to tumor necrosis factor-relate--apoptosis-inducing-ligand (TRAIL). We have shown TRAIL-induced apoptosis in pancreatic cancer BxPC-3 (wild type G12) cell lines, while Panc-1 pancreatic cancer cell lines having a mutated (G12D) KRAS genotype were found to be resistant to the actions of TRAIL [43]. The role of the MAPK signaling pathway in angiogenesis, metastasis and chemoresistance of pancreatic cancer is demonstrated through specificity protein (SP1) expression. Activated p38 MAPK induces expression of SP1 that further results in increased expression of COX-2 and vascular endothelial growth factor (VEGF). In contrast, inhibition of p38-MAPK signaling by specific inhibitor results in reduced SP1 activation as well as decreased expression of COX-2 and VEGF [44]. Thus, the MAPK signaling pathway plays a central role in pancreatic cancer survival, proliferation, metastasis and chemoresistance.

MAPK-associated microRNAs such as miR-7, miR-34a, miR-181d, and miR-193b are also found to be associated with pancreatic cancer malignancy. The expression of these miRNAs was reported to be altered significantly with the upregulation of the MAPK signaling pathway. In a study, significantly higher levels of miR-7, miR-34a, miR-181d, and miR-193b serum MAPK-associated miRNAs were observed in pancreatic cancer patients than autoimmune pancreatitis patients. These serum miRNA especially miR-181d was found to be associated with metastasis of pancreatic cancer in patients [45].

ROLE OF MAPK INHIBITORS IN PANCREATIC CANCER THERAPEUTICS

As reported, 90% pancreatic cancer cells have mutated KRAS that leads to sustainable tumor growth and also confer resistance to therapeutic agents through constitutive activation of the RAF-MEK-MAPK pathway. Intense efforts have been undertaken to develop MAPK pathways inhibitory compounds for the treatment of pancreatic cancer (Fig. **1**). Inhibitor of MEK, an upstream kinase of MAPK, have been developed against pancreatic cancer. In several preclinical and clinical studies, MEK inhibitors have shown promising anti-tumor responses against multiple cancer types including pancreatic cancer. CI-1040 (PD184352) is discovered as a highly specific, small-molecule inhibitor of MEK1/MEK2. It inhibits MEK1/MEK2, thereby prominently suppressing the activation of ERK and MAPK signaling pathways. In phase I clinical study with pancreatic cancer patients, MEK inhibitor CI-1040 showed partial response [46]. However, in the phase II clinical study, CI-1040 did not result in favorable response to the pancreatic cancer patients but stabilized the disease lasting a median of 4.4 months. However, the treatment appeared to be well-tolerated, with mild toxicity [47].

MEK inhibitor PD98059 has shown to modulate the survival of the pancreatic cancer MIAPaCa-2 cells. PD98059 treatment results in the inhibition of ERK1/2 activities and induction of apoptosis by cell cycle arrest, cleavage of caspases and PARP, and down-regulation of Bcl-2, Mcl-1, and Bcl-xL without affecting the expression of pro-apoptotic proteins Bak and Bax [48]. Another MEK inhibitor PD0325901 exhibits anticancer activity in the KRAS mutant tumors *in vitro* and *in vivo* by decreasing MEK/ERK signaling and destabilizes cyclin D1 [49]. PD0325901 not only suppresses pancreatic tumors but also exhibits radiosensitization alone and in combination. PD0325901 has shown to decrease phosphorylated ERK1/2 and Akt in radio-resistant MIAPaCa-2 pancreatic cancer cells *in vitro* and in a xenograft mouse model. MEK inhibitor induces radiosensitization in both *in vitro* and *in vivo* models [50]. MEK inhibitor PD0325901 also inhibits oncogenic microRNA such as miR-17-92 cluster and suppresses cell growth with G1-phase arrest in MIAPaCa-2 cells [51]. Thus, MEK inhibitors suppress growth, induce apoptosis, inhibit oncogenic miRNA and exhibit radiosensitization in pancreatic tumor models.

Trametinib (GSK1120212) is an FDA-approved MEK inhibitor, which is being used for the treatment of multiple cancers including pancreatic cancer. In preclinical models, treatment of established and patient-derived pancreatic cancer cell lines with trametinib inhibits the growth and proliferation. It also enhances the antitumor efficacy of EGFR/HER2 inhibitor lapatinib in both *in vitro* and in the orthotopic xenograft model [52]. Trametinib also enhances the therapeutic efficacy of other drugs such as gemcitabine. In a study, treatment of trametinib with gemcitabine in combination effectively suppressed the growth of patient-derived tumors implanted in mice as compared to the individual drug [53]. In animal models, MEK inhibitors, cobimetinib and trametinib, regressed patient-derived human tumor growth. Thus, it shows potential for individualizing pancreatic-cancer therapy [54]. Binimetinib (MEK162), another MEK inhibitor, has shown potential in treating pancreatic cancer patients. MEK162 not only blocks ERK1/2 but also inhibits phosphoinositide 3-kinase (PI3K) and S6 and increases p27KIP1 levels in pancreatic cancer lines [55].

MAP kinase kinase kinase (or MAP3K or MEKK) is a serine/threonine-specific protein kinase which acts upon MAP kinase kinase also known as RAF. Sorafenib, a RAF (RAF-1, A-RAF, and B-RAF) inhibitor, has shown to be effective against pancreatic cancer. *In vitro* study revealed that sorafenib has strong anti-proliferative effects in pancreatic cancer cells. It induces apoptosis and inhibits the growth of pancreatic cancer cells by suppressing constitutive STAT3 phosphorylation (Tyr705) and inhibiting Mcl-1 and Bcl-xL proteins. Sorafenib also enhances TRAIL-induced apoptosis by releasing mitochondrial cytochrome c, activating caspase-3, caspase-9 cleavage, and Bax/Bak activation [56]. Another study showed that sorafenib has strong synergistic interaction with docetaxel, which results in effective pancreatic tumor regression. Sorafenib treated with docetaxel decreases and delays the growth of human pancreatic tumors implanted in nude mice. The suppression of tumor growth was accompanied by stimulation of apoptosis, inhibition angiogenesis and downregulation of ERK signaling pathway. Consequently, the treatment of sorafenib with docetaxel results in increased overall survival of mice [57].

Sorafenib alone or in combination with gemcitabine exhibits antitumor activity in pancreatic cancer patients. About 10.5% of patients had decreased tumors while 56.5% of patients achieved disease stabilization in the pancreatic cancer patient cohort [58]. However, in phase II clinical trial, sorafenib plus gemcitabine was found to be ineffective in advanced pancreatic cancer. The median overall survival of pancreatic cancer patients was 4.0 months and median progression-free survival was 3.2 months [59]. In another study, patients with metastatic pancreatic cancer were either treated with sorafenib alone or sorafenib with gemcitabine. Median progression-free survival and overall survival were 2.3 and 4.3 months, respectively with sorafenib treatment, whereas median progression-free survival and overall survival were 2.9 and 6.5 months, respectively with the treatment of sorafenib and gemcitabine combination [60]. Thus, in these phase II clinical studies, neither sorafenib alone nor sorafenib in combination with gemcitabine showed promising activity in metastatic pancreatic cancer, however, it showed a promising effect in preclinical studies.

Ulixertinib (or BVD-523) is an ERK-specific inhibitor that has demonstrated promising antitumor activity in phase I clinical trial for advanced solid tumors. Ulixertinib also effectively inhibits the *in vitro* growth of various pancreatic cancer cell lines and potentiates the cytotoxic effects of gemcitabine. Mechanistically, it upregulates the PI3K-Akt pathway through activating

HER/ErbB family proteins, which results in suppression of pancreatic cancer cell growth *in vitro* and *in vivo* [61]. Another ERK inhibitor AZD-6244 increases the sensitivity of pancreatic cancer cells to glycosphingolipid biosynthesis inhibitor PDMP. Co-administration of AZD-6244 and PDMP induced massive pancreatic cancer cell death and apoptosis more potently than either drug alone. The antitumor effect of these drugs was mediated through the inactivation of ERK1/2 and Akt-mTOR signaling simultaneously in pancreatic cancer cells since either agent alone only affected one signaling [62]. U0126 another known inhibitor of ERK1/2 also inhibits the proliferation of pancreatic cancer cells. In a study, CXCR4-induced proliferation of pancreatic cancer cells was mediated by both Akt and ERK signaling but pretreatment with U0126 resulted in complete abrogation of CXCR4-enhanced proliferation in all the cell lines [63].

CONCLUSION

Pancreatic cancer is characterized by mutated KRAS, which results in constitutive activation of MAPK signaling pathway. Extensive preclinical and clinical studies suggest that the MAPK signaling pathway has a very important role in pancreatic cancer malignancy. Upon activation by growth factors and upstream kinases, MAPK signaling induces a variety of downstream genes involved in multiple critical cellular functions including proliferation, growth and senescence in pancreatic cancer. Because of its constitutive activation, MAPK pathway is a potential therapeutic target in pancreatic cancer. Thus, the development of drugs targeting RAS-RAF-MAPK-ERK and their downstream genes may provide a novel therapeutic option for pancreatic cancer. A variety of MAPK signaling inhibitors have been developed, which are effective in preclinical models. In general, these inhibitors appear to be well-tolerated with only mild common side effects. However, these inhibitors are not prominently effective in clinical settings. Therefore, the development of specific inhibitors of the MAPK signaling pathway is required which, can be useful in regressing pancreatic as well as tumors of other types.

CONSENT FOR PUBLICATION

Not applicable.

CONFLICT OF INTEREST

The author declares that there is no conflict of interest in this chapter.

ACKNOWLEDGEMENTS

This work was supported in part by R01 grant CA129038 (to Sanjay K.

Srivastava) awarded by the National Cancer Institute, NIH.

REFERENCES

[1]   Ryan DP, Hong TS, Bardeesy N. Pancreatic adenocarcinoma. N Engl J Med 2014; 371(11): 1039-49.
        [http://dx.doi.org/10.1056/NEJMra1404198] [PMID: 25207767]

[2]   Chen Z, Gibson TB, Robinson F, *et al.* MAP kinases. Chem Rev 2001; 101(8): 2449-76.
        [http://dx.doi.org/10.1021/cr000241p] [PMID: 11749383]

[3]   Kyriakis JM, Avruch J. Mammalian mitogen-activated protein kinase signal transduction pathways
        activated by stress and inflammation. Physiol Rev 2001; 81(2): 807-69.
        [http://dx.doi.org/10.1152/physrev.2001.81.2.807] [PMID: 11274345]

[4]   Pearson G, Robinson F, Beers Gibson T, *et al.* Mitogen-activated protein (MAP) kinase pathways:
        regulation and physiological functions. Endocr Rev 2001; 22(2): 153-83.
        [PMID: 11294822]

[5]   Coulombe P, Meloche S. Atypical mitogen-activated protein kinases: structure, regulation and
        functions. Biochim Biophys Acta 2007; 1773(8): 1376-87.
        [http://dx.doi.org/10.1016/j.bbamcr.2006.11.001] [PMID: 17161475]

[6]   Raman M, Chen W, Cobb MH. Differential regulation and properties of MAPKs. Oncogene 2007;
        26(22): 3100-12.
        [http://dx.doi.org/10.1038/sj.onc.1210392] [PMID: 17496909]

[7]   Wagner EF, Nebreda AR. Signal integration by JNK and p38 MAPK pathways in cancer development.
        Nat Rev Cancer 2009; 9(8): 537-49.
        [http://dx.doi.org/10.1038/nrc2694] [PMID: 19629069]

[8]   Robinson MJ, Cobb MH. Mitogen-activated protein kinase pathways. Curr Opin Cell Biol 1997; 9(2):
        180-6.
        [http://dx.doi.org/10.1016/S0955-0674(97)80061-0] [PMID: 9069255]

[9]   Avruch J, Khokhlatchev A, Kyriakis JM, *et al.* Ras activation of the Raf kinase: tyrosine kinase
        recruitment of the MAP kinase cascade. Recent Prog Horm Res 2001; 56: 127-55.
        [http://dx.doi.org/10.1210/rp.56.1.127] [PMID: 11237210]

[10]   Liu Y, Shepherd EG, Nelin LD. MAPK phosphatases--regulating the immune response. Nat Rev
        Immunol 2007; 7(3): 202-12.
        [http://dx.doi.org/10.1038/nri2035] [PMID: 17318231]

[11]   Furukawa T, Kanai N, Shiwaku HO, Soga N, Uehara A, Horii A. AURKA is one of the downstream
        targets of MAPK1/ERK2 in pancreatic cancer. Oncogene 2006; 25(35): 4831-9.
        [http://dx.doi.org/10.1038/sj.onc.1209494] [PMID: 16532023]

[12]   Kandala PK, Wright SE, Srivastava SK. Blocking epidermal growth factor receptor activation by 3,3′-
        diindolylmethane suppresses ovarian tumor growth *in vitro* and *in vivo*. J Pharmacol Exp Ther 2012;
        341(1): 24-32.
        [http://dx.doi.org/10.1124/jpet.111.188706] [PMID: 22205686]

[13]   Wang L, Bai YY, Yang Y, *et al.* Diabetes mellitus stimulates pancreatic cancer growth and epithelial-
        mesenchymal transition-mediated metastasis *via* a p38 MAPK pathway. Oncotarget 2016; 7(25):
        38539-50.
        [http://dx.doi.org/10.18632/oncotarget.9533] [PMID: 27413117]

[14]   Li W, Ma Z, Ma J, *et al.* Hydrogen peroxide mediates hyperglycemia-induced invasive activity *via*
        ERK and p38 MAPK in human pancreatic cancer. Oncotarget 2015; 6(31): 31119-33.
        [http://dx.doi.org/10.18632/oncotarget.5045] [PMID: 26439801]

[15]   Papademetrio DL, Lompardía SL, Simunovich T, *et al.* Inhibition of Survival Pathways MAPK and
        NF-kB Triggers Apoptosis in Pancreatic Ductal Adenocarcinoma Cells *via* Suppression of Autophagy.

Target Oncol 2016; 11(2): 183-95.
[http://dx.doi.org/10.1007/s11523-015-0388-3] [PMID: 26373299]

[16]   Lee KH, Hyun MS, Kim JR. Growth factor-dependent activation of the MAPK pathway in human pancreatic cancer: MEK/ERK and p38 MAP kinase interaction in uPA synthesis. Clin Exp Metastasis 2003; 20(6): 499-505.
[http://dx.doi.org/10.1023/A:1025824816021] [PMID: 14598883]

[17]   Pramanik KC, Srivastava SK. Apoptosis signal-regulating kinase 1-thioredoxin complex dissociation by capsaicin causes pancreatic tumor growth suppression by inducing apoptosis. Antioxid Redox Signal 2012; 17(10): 1417-32.
[http://dx.doi.org/10.1089/ars.2011.4369] [PMID: 22530568]

[18]   Durand N, Storz P. Targeting reactive oxygen species in development and progression of pancreatic cancer. Expert Rev Anticancer Ther 2017; 17(1): 19-31.
[http://dx.doi.org/10.1080/14737140.2017.1261017] [PMID: 27841037]

[19]   Calhoun ES, Jones JB, Ashfaq R, *et al.* BRAF and FBXW7 (CDC4, FBW7, AGO, SEL10) mutations in distinct subsets of pancreatic cancer: potential therapeutic targets. Am J Pathol 2003; 163(4): 1255-60.
[http://dx.doi.org/10.1016/S0002-9440(10)63485-2] [PMID: 14507635]

[20]   Doppler W, Jansen-Dürr P. Regulation of mitochondrial ROS production by HIC-5: a common feature of oncogene-induced senescence and tumor invasiveness? FEBS J 2019; 286(3): 456-8.
[http://dx.doi.org/10.1111/febs.14746] [PMID: 30680933]

[21]   Wey JS, Gray MJ, Fan F, *et al.* Overexpression of neuropilin-1 promotes constitutive MAPK signalling and chemoresistance in pancreatic cancer cells. Br J Cancer 2005; 93(2): 233-41.
[http://dx.doi.org/10.1038/sj.bjc.6602663] [PMID: 15956974]

[22]   Kent OA, Sandi MJ, Rottapel R. Co-dependency between KRAS addiction and ARHGEF2 promotes an adaptive escape from MAPK pathway inhibition. Small GTPases 2017; 1-8.
[PMID: 28656876]

[23]   Song X, Zhu M, Zhang F, *et al.* ZFX Promotes proliferation and metastasis of pancreatic cancer cells *via* the MAPK pathway. Cell Physiol Biochem 2018; 48(1): 274-84.
[http://dx.doi.org/10.1159/000491727] [PMID: 30007968]

[24]   Huang FT, Peng JF, Cheng WJ, *et al.* MiR-143 targeting TAK1 attenuates pancreatic ductal adenocarcinoma progression *via* MAPK and NF-κB pathway *In vitro*. Dig Dis Sci 2017; 62(4): 944-57.
[http://dx.doi.org/10.1007/s10620-017-4472-7] [PMID: 28194669]

[25]   Junn E, Han SH, Im JY, *et al.* Vitamin D3 up-regulated protein 1 mediates oxidative stress *via* suppressing the thioredoxin function. J Immunol 2000; 164(12): 6287-95.
[http://dx.doi.org/10.4049/jimmunol.164.12.6287] [PMID: 10843682]

[26]   Cheng X, Holenya P, Can S, *et al.* A TrxR inhibiting gold(I) NHC complex induces apoptosis through ASK1-p38-MAPK signaling in pancreatic cancer cells. Mol Cancer 2014; 13: 221.
[http://dx.doi.org/10.1186/1476-4598-13-221] [PMID: 25253202]

[27]   Wu YY, Ma TL, Ge ZJ, *et al. JWA* gene regulates PANC-1 pancreatic cancer cell behaviors through MEK-ERK1/2 of the MAPK signaling pathway. Oncol Lett 2014; 8(4): 1859-63.
[http://dx.doi.org/10.3892/ol.2014.2329] [PMID: 25202426]

[28]   Jun S, Lee S, Kim HC, *et al.* PAF-mediated MAPK signaling hyperactivation *via* LAMTOR3 induces pancreatic tumorigenesis. Cell Rep 2013; 5(2): 314-22.
[http://dx.doi.org/10.1016/j.celrep.2013.09.026] [PMID: 24209743]

[29]   Furukawa T, Tanji E, Kuboki Y, *et al.* Targeting of MAPK-associated molecules identifies SON as a prime target to attenuate the proliferation and tumorigenicity of pancreatic cancer cells. Mol Cancer 2012; 11: 88.

[http://dx.doi.org/10.1186/1476-4598-11-88] [PMID: 23227827]

[30]   Yang L, Sun X, Ye Y, *et al.* p38α Mitogen-activated protein kinase is a druggable target in pancreatic adenocarcinoma. Front Oncol 2019; 9: 1294.
[http://dx.doi.org/10.3389/fonc.2019.01294] [PMID: 31828036]

[31]   Zhong Y, Naito Y, Cope L, *et al.* Functional p38 MAPK identified by biomarker profiling of pancreatic cancer restrains growth through JNK inhibition and correlates with improved survival. Clin Cancer Res 2014; 20(23): 6200-11.
[http://dx.doi.org/10.1158/1078-0432.CCR-13-2823] [PMID: 24963048]

[32]   Habiro A, Tanno S, Koizumi K, *et al.* Involvement of p38 mitogen-activated protein kinase in gemcitabine-induced apoptosis in human pancreatic cancer cells. Biochem Biophys Res Commun 2004; 316(1): 71-7.
[http://dx.doi.org/10.1016/j.bbrc.2004.02.017] [PMID: 15003513]

[33]   García-Cano J, Roche O, Cimas FJ, *et al.* p38MAPK and Chemotherapy: We Always Need to Hear Both Sides of the Story. Front Cell Dev Biol 2016; 4: 69.
[http://dx.doi.org/10.3389/fcell.2016.00069] [PMID: 27446920]

[34]   Pan F, Ma S, Cao W, *et al.* SDF-1α upregulation of MMP-2 is mediated by p38 MAPK signaling in pancreatic cancer cell lines. Mol Biol Rep 2013; 40(7): 4139-46.
[http://dx.doi.org/10.1007/s11033-012-2225-4] [PMID: 23712777]

[35]   Tong WG, Ding XZ, Talamonti MS, Bell RH, Adrian TE. LTB4 stimulates growth of human pancreatic cancer cells *via* MAPK and PI-3 kinase pathways. Biochem Biophys Res Commun 2005; 335(3): 949-56.
[http://dx.doi.org/10.1016/j.bbrc.2005.07.166] [PMID: 16105664]

[36]   Huang XY, Wang HC, Yuan Z, Huang J, Zheng Q. Norepinephrine stimulates pancreatic cancer cell proliferation, migration and invasion *via* β-adrenergic receptor-dependent activation of P38/MAPK pathway. Hepatogastroenterology 2012; 59(115): 889-93.
[PMID: 22020907]

[37]   Cubas R, Zhang S, Li M, Chen C, Yao Q. Trop2 expression contributes to tumor pathogenesis by activating the ERK MAPK pathway. Mol Cancer 2010; 9: 253.
[http://dx.doi.org/10.1186/1476-4598-9-253] [PMID: 20858281]

[38]   Morgan R, Fairfax B, Pandha HS. Calcium insensitivity of FA-6, a cell line derived from a pancreatic cancer associated with humoral hypercalcemia, is mediated by the significantly reduced expression of the Calcium Sensitive Receptor transduction component p38 MAPK. Mol Cancer 2006; 5: 51.
[http://dx.doi.org/10.1186/1476-4598-5-51] [PMID: 17078869]

[39]   Bardeesy N, DePinho RA. Pancreatic cancer biology and genetics. Nat Rev Cancer 2002; 2(12): 897-909.
[http://dx.doi.org/10.1038/nrc949] [PMID: 12459728]

[40]   Shields JM, Pruitt K, McFall A, Shaub A, Der CJ. Understanding Ras: 'it ain't over 'til it's over'. Trends Cell Biol 2000; 10(4): 147-54.
[http://dx.doi.org/10.1016/S0962-8924(00)01740-2] [PMID: 10740269]

[41]   Rozenblum E, Schutte M, Goggins M, *et al.* Tumor-suppressive pathways in pancreatic carcinoma. Cancer Res 1997; 57(9): 1731-4.
[PMID: 9135016]

[42]   Yang K, Li Y, Lian G, *et al.* KRAS promotes tumor metastasis and chemoresistance by repressing RKIP *via* the MAPK-ERK pathway in pancreatic cancer. Int J Cancer 2018; 142(11): 2323-34.
[http://dx.doi.org/10.1002/ijc.31248] [PMID: 29315556]

[43]   Sahu RP, Batra S, Kandala PK, Brown TL, Srivastava SK. The role of K-ras gene mutation in TRAIL-induced apoptosis in pancreatic and lung cancer cell lines. Cancer Chemother Pharmacol 2011; 67(2): 481-7.

[http://dx.doi.org/10.1007/s00280-010-1463-1] [PMID: 20848283]

[44]   Hu H, Han T, Zhuo M, *et al.* Elevated COX-2 expression promotes angiogenesis through EGFR/p38-MAPK/Sp1-dependent signalling in pancreatic cancer. Sci Rep 2017; 7(1): 470.
[http://dx.doi.org/10.1038/s41598-017-00288-4] [PMID: 28352075]

[45]   Akamatsu M, Makino N, Ikeda Y, *et al.* Specific MAPK-associated micrornas in serum differentiate pancreatic cancer from autoimmune pancreatitis. PLoS One 2016; 11(7): e0158669.
[http://dx.doi.org/10.1371/journal.pone.0158669] [PMID: 27380024]

[46]   Allen LF, Sebolt-Leopold J, Meyer MB. CI-1040 (PD184352), a targeted signal transduction inhibitor of MEK (MAPKK). Semin Oncol 2003; 30(5) (Suppl. 16): 105-16.
[http://dx.doi.org/10.1053/j.seminoncol.2003.08.012] [PMID: 14613031]

[47]   Rinehart J, Adjei AA, Lorusso PM, *et al.* Multicenter phase II study of the oral MEK inhibitor, CI-1040, in patients with advanced non-small-cell lung, breast, colon, and pancreatic cancer. J Clin Oncol 2004; 22(22): 4456-62.
[http://dx.doi.org/10.1200/JCO.2004.01.185] [PMID: 15483017]

[48]   Boucher MJ, Morisset J, Vachon PH, Reed JC, Lainé J, Rivard N. MEK/ERK signaling pathway regulates the expression of Bcl-2, Bcl-X(L), and Mcl-1 and promotes survival of human pancreatic cancer cells. J Cell Biochem 2000; 79(3): 355-69.
[http://dx.doi.org/10.1002/1097-4644(20001201)79:3<355::AID-JCB20>3.0.CO;2-0]   [PMID: 10972974]

[49]   Halilovic E, She QB, Ye Q, *et al.* PIK3CA mutation uncouples tumor growth and cyclin D1 regulation from MEK/ERK and mutant KRAS signaling. Cancer Res 2010; 70(17): 6804-14.
[http://dx.doi.org/10.1158/0008-5472.CAN-10-0409] [PMID: 20699365]

[50]   Williams TM, Flecha AR, Keller P, *et al.* Cotargeting MAPK and PI3K signaling with concurrent radiotherapy as a strategy for the treatment of pancreatic cancer. Mol Cancer Ther 2012; 11(5): 1193-202.
[http://dx.doi.org/10.1158/1535-7163.MCT-12-0098] [PMID: 22411900]

[51]   Tanaka R, Tomosugi M, Sakai T, Sowa Y. MEK Inhibitor Suppresses Expression of the miR-17-92 Cluster with G1-Phase Arrest in HT-29 Human Colon Cancer Cells and MIA PaCa-2 Pancreatic Cancer Cells. Anticancer Res 2016; 36(9): 4537-43.
[http://dx.doi.org/10.21873/anticanres.11001] [PMID: 27630293]

[52]   Walters DM, Lindberg JM, Adair SJ, *et al.* Inhibition of the growth of patient-derived pancreatic cancer xenografts with the MEK inhibitor trametinib is augmented by combined treatment with the epidermal growth factor receptor/HER2 inhibitor lapatinib. Neoplasia 2013; 15(2): 143-55.
[http://dx.doi.org/10.1593/neo.121712] [PMID: 23441129]

[53]   Kawaguchi K, Igarashi K, Miyake K, *et al.* MEK inhibitor trametinib in combination with gemcitabine regresses a patient-derived orthotopic xenograft (PDOX) pancreatic cancer nude mouse model. Tissue Cell 2018; 52: 124-8.
[http://dx.doi.org/10.1016/j.tice.2018.05.003] [PMID: 29857821]

[54]   Kawaguchi K, Igarashi K, Murakami T, *et al.* MEK inhibitors cobimetinib and trametinib, regressed a gemcitabine-resistant pancreatic-cancer patient-derived orthotopic xenograft (PDOX). Oncotarget 2017; 8(29): 47490-6.
[http://dx.doi.org/10.18632/oncotarget.17667] [PMID: 28537897]

[55]   Hamidi H, Lu M, Chau K, *et al.* KRAS mutational subtype and copy number predict *In vitro* response of human pancreatic cancer cell lines to MEK inhibition. Br J Cancer 2014; 111(9): 1788-801.
[http://dx.doi.org/10.1038/bjc.2014.475] [PMID: 25167228]

[56]   Huang S, Sinicrope FA. Sorafenib inhibits STAT3 activation to enhance TRAIL-mediated apoptosis in human pancreatic cancer cells. Mol Cancer Ther 2010; 9(3): 742-50.
[http://dx.doi.org/10.1158/1535-7163.MCT-09-1004] [PMID: 20197401]

[57]   Ulivi P, Arienti C, Zoli W, *et al*. *In vitro* and *in vivo* antitumor efficacy of docetaxel and sorafenib combination in human pancreatic cancer cells. Curr Cancer Drug Targets 2010; 10(6): 600-10.
[http://dx.doi.org/10.2174/156800910791859489] [PMID: 20491617]

[58]   Siu LL, Awada A, Takimoto CH, *et al*. Phase I trial of sorafenib and gemcitabine in advanced solid tumors with an expanded cohort in advanced pancreatic cancer. Clin Cancer Res 2006; 12(1): 144-51.
[http://dx.doi.org/10.1158/1078-0432.CCR-05-1571] [PMID: 16397036]

[59]   Kindler HL, Wroblewski K, Wallace JA, *et al*. Gemcitabine plus sorafenib in patients with advanced pancreatic cancer: a phase II trial of the University of Chicago Phase II Consortium. Invest New Drugs 2012; 30(1): 382-6.
[http://dx.doi.org/10.1007/s10637-010-9526-z] [PMID: 20803052]

[60]   El-Khoueiry AB, Ramanathan RK, Yang DY, *et al*. A randomized phase II of gemcitabine and sorafenib *versus* sorafenib alone in patients with metastatic pancreatic cancer. Invest New Drugs 2012; 30(3): 1175-83.
[http://dx.doi.org/10.1007/s10637-011-9658-9] [PMID: 21424698]

[61]   Jiang H, Xu M, Li L, *et al*. Concurrent HER or PI3K inhibition potentiates the antitumor effect of the erk inhibitor ulixertinib in preclinical pancreatic cancer models. Mol Cancer Ther 2018; 17(10): 2144-55.
[http://dx.doi.org/10.1158/1535-7163.MCT-17-1142] [PMID: 30065098]

[62]   Wang T, Wei J, Wang N, Ma JL, Hui PP. The glucosylceramide synthase inhibitor PDMP sensitizes pancreatic cancer cells to MEK/ERK inhibitor AZD-6244. Biochem Biophys Res Commun 2015; 456(3): 821-6.
[http://dx.doi.org/10.1016/j.bbrc.2014.12.019] [PMID: 25498501]

[63]   Shen X, Artinyan A, Jackson D, Thomas RM, Lowy AM, Kim J. Chemokine receptor CXCR4 enhances proliferation in pancreatic cancer cells through AKT and ERK dependent pathways. Pancreas 2010; 39(1): 81-7.
[http://dx.doi.org/10.1097/MPA.0b013e3181bb2ab7] [PMID: 19820417]

CHAPTER 6

Role of NF-κB Activation in Multiple Myeloma and Other Hematological Malignancies

Loukik Arora[1], Frank Arfuso[2], Alan Prem Kumar[1] and Gautam Sethi[1,*]

[1] *Department of Pharmacology, Yong Loo Lin School of Medicine, National University of Singapore, Singapore*

[2] *Stem Cell and Cancer Biology Laboratory, School of Pharmacy and Biomedical Sciences, Curtin Health Innovation Research Institute, Curtin University, Perth, Australia*

Abstract: NF-κB (nuclear factor kappa-light-chain-enhancer of activated B cells) is a rapid-acting transcription factor. It is present in almost all cell types and is one of the primary responders to several stimuli such as stress, cytokines, radiation, chemotherapeutic drugs, bacterial, and viral antigens. Aberrant regulation and activation of NF-κB have been implicated in several cancers, inflammatory and autoimmune disorders, viral infections, and erroneous immune system development. This chapter summarizes the role of NF-κB activation specifically in hematological malignancies and various strategies developed for its potential pharmacological intervention to abrogate the process of carcinogenesis.

Keywords: Leukemia, Lymphoma, Myeloma, NF-κB, IKKs.

INTRODUCTION

NF-κB (Nuclear factor kappa-light-chain-enhancer of B cells) is a nucleo-cytoplasmic protein complex involved in controlling transcription, production of cytokines, and regulating cell survival [1 - 5]. NF-κB is ubiquitously present in almost all human tissue types and responds to various stress stimuli such as cytokines, growth factors, radiation, oxidative stress, free radicals, *etc*. It also plays an important role in regulating the immune response to infections [2, 6 - 8]. Five members have discovered and classified in the mammalian NF-κB family so far. They are NF-κB1 NF-κB2, Rel A, Rel B, and c-Rel [9 - 11] (Table **1**). Fig. (**1**) shows the downstream target genes modulated by NF-κB to regulate a myriad of cellular responses.

---

* **Corresponding author Gautam Sethi:** Department of Pharmacology, Yong Loo Lin School of Medicine, National University of Singapore, Singapore 117600; Tel: +65 65163267; Fax: +65 68737690; Email: phcgs@nus.edu.sg

Manoj K. Pandey & Vijay P. Kale (Eds.)

Table 1. Human NF-κB proteins.

Class	Protein	Gene
Class I	NF-κB1 (p50)	*NFKB1*
	NF-κB2 (p52)	*NFKB2*
Class II	RelA (p65)	*RELA*
	RelB	*RELB*
	c-Rel	*REL*

Theoretically, about 15 unique homo- and heterodimer combinations can be derived from the dimerization of five NF-κB subunits; of which 12 have been identified *in vivo*. The interactions between these subunits are based on the general principles of interaction between protein-protein complexes and this explains why RelA-p50 and RelB-p52 can form the most stable dimers among12 of them [12].

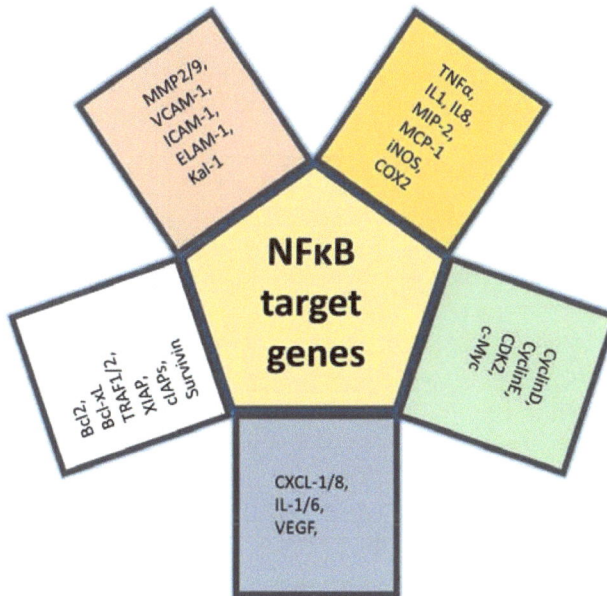

Fig. (1). A list of selected genes regulated by transcription factor NF-κB.

STRUCTURE AND SIGNALING CASCADE OF NF-κB PROTEINS

NF-κB Activation and Signaling

NF-κBs are classified as rapid-acting transcription factors; *i.e.* they are present in the cell in an inactive state and are not dependent on *de novo* protein synthesis for their activation [13 - 15]. The NF-κB pathway can be primarily activated by two different processes, namely the canonical/classical pathway and the non-canonical pathway [16, 17] as briefly summarized in Fig. (**2**).

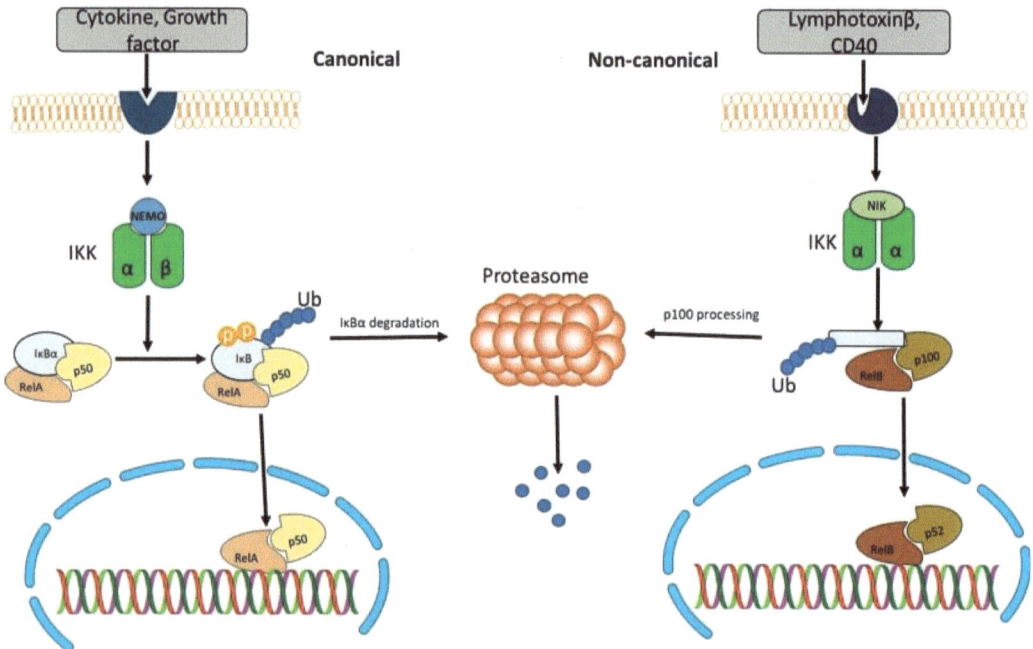

Fig. (2). A schematic representation of canonical and non-canonical NF-κB activation pathways.

Canonical or Classical Pathway

In the resting or unstimulated cell, the NF-κB heterodimer (RelA-p50) are sequestered in the cytoplasm as the nuclear localisation signal is masked by Inhibitors of κB (IκB). In canonical signaling, the ligand binding (cytokines, growth factors, lipopolysaccharides) to their respective receptors can induce the phosphorylation of the IKK (IκB Kinase) complex, which consists of IKKα, IKKβ, and NF-κB essential modulator (NEMO). The phosphorylation of IKKs leads them to phosphorylate IκBα. The phosphorylated IκBα after ubiquitination, undergoes proteasomal degradation, thereby freeing the p50-RelA heterodimer. This heterodimer translocates to the nucleus and initiates the transcription of NF-κB downstream effector genes [18]. It has been found that ubiquitination can activate NF-κB pathway independent of the proteasome. As the regulator of IKK complex, NEMO has been suggested to modulate this proteasome independent ubiquitination mediated by K63 polyubiquitin chains [19].

Non-canonical Pathway

The non-canonical pathway is activated by diverse stimuli such as CD40 and lymphotoxin-β. Unlike the canonical pathway, the non-canonical pathway is predominantly dependent only on IKKα activation but not on other IKKs. IKKα is phosphorylated and activated by NF-κB inducing kinase (NIK), and in turn phosphorylates p100, specifically p100 bound to RelB, leading to its cleavage and formation of the active p52 subunit [20, 21]. The RelB-p52 thus formed then translocates to the nucleus and induces the transcription of genes controlled by NF-κB promoters [21]. Although the regulation of canonical and non-canonical pathways is distinct, and they were at one point thought to be independent of each other, recent studies have indicated that they are mechanistically interlinked in the cellular environment [22].

Inhibition of the NF-κB Pathway

NF-κB forms an autoregulation feedback loop as it induces the synthesis of its own repressor IκBα. This *de novo* synthesised IκBα re-inhibits NF-κB, thereby regulating its activity [23]. Apart from this, there are currently two known protein inhibitors of NF-κB, *viz.* IFRD1 (Interferon-related developmental regulator 1) and SIRT 1 (Sirtuin1). Both proteins may inhibit NF-κB activity by promoting the deacetylation of the RelA/p65 subunit at lysine 310 [24, 25].

Ubiquitination, apart from playing a critical role in the activation of NF-κB also can mediate the degradation of the p65 subunit thus tightly regulating NF-κB activity. Also, a major part of the negative regulation of NF-κB is brought about by different deubiquitinating enzymes (DUBs), A20 and CYLD, in particular. E3 ligase has also been proposed to play a part in the ubiquitin- proteasome-induced inhibition of NF-κB [26, 27].

ROLE OF NF-κB IN SOLID TUMORS AND HEMATOLOGICAL MALIGNANCIES

NF-κB can mediate critical several steps of carcinogenesis. The transcription factor has been shown to regulate genes involved in cell proliferation (*Cyclin D1*, *Cyclin E*, *c-MYC*), cell survival (*Bcl-2*, *XIAP*, *c-IAP1/2*), promoting angiogenesis (*VEGF*, *TNF*), and tumor cell invasion and metastasis (*MMP2/9*, *ICAM1*) [28]. Furthermore, constitutive activation of NF-κB has been reported in many cancer cell lines and patient-derived tumor samples [29, 30]. As also shown in Fig. (**3**), Bassères *et al.* also highlighted constitutive activation of NF-κB in a number of human cancers including solid tumors and hematological malignancies [16, 31]. Both canonical and non-canonical pathways contribute to total NF-κB activity; however, either of the pathways may be dominant over the other or they may [32] contribute equally to carcinogenesis under different conditions in diverse models [33 - 35].

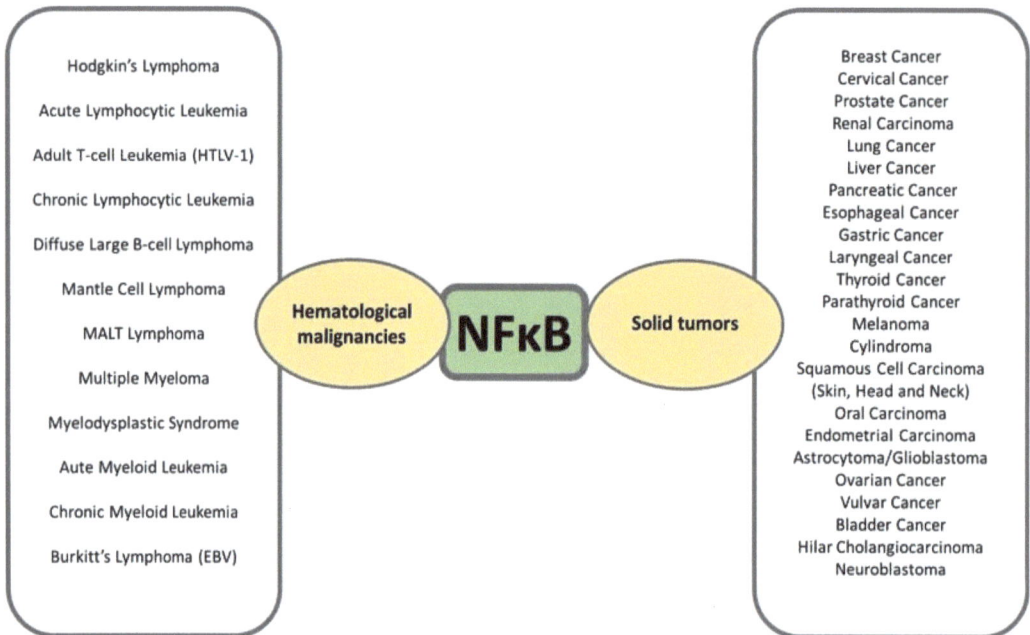

Fig. (3). A figure demonstrating constitutive activation of NF-κB in various human solid tumors and hematological malignancies.

Role of NF-κB in Multiple Myeloma

Multiple Myeloma (MM), which is marked by abnormal clonal B cells, accounts for 1% of all cancers and 10% of all hematological malignancies. Despite the recent advances in treatment options, it remains largely incurable [36]. MM exhibits uncontrolled growth and accumulation of plasma B cells, predominantly driven by resistance to apoptosis and alterations in cell-cycle regulation [37]. The bone marrow microenvironment can act as an important factor in the pathogenesis of MM [38]. Several pathways have been implicated in MM including NF-κB, JAK-STAT, and PI3K/AKT, and NF-κB has also emerged as one of the important contributors to MM tumorigenesis [36, 39].

NF-κB has been reported to be constitutively active (nuclear activity) in several human MM cell lines and primary myeloma cells [40], and its abrogation by pharmacological interventions (including proteasome inhibitors and IKK inhibitors) has been shown to inhibit growth and induce apoptosis in diverse MM cell lines [41 - 43]. The inhibition of NF-κB has been strongly correlated to decreased expression of various NF-κB target genes responsible for anti-apoptosis

(*Bcl-xL*, *XIAP*) and proliferative (*Cyclin D1*) activity. Indirectly, NF-κB activation in bone marrow cells also contributes to MM survival and progression [36]. NF-κB activation can also control the clinical manifestations of MM such as osteolytic lesions (reported in ~ 70% patients), which further promote bone metastases and MM cell survival and proliferation [44]. Additionally, gene expression profiling data from Bortezomib clinical trials have shown that the MM subgroup with characteristic NF-κB activity of myeloma cells may be more sensitive to bortezomib [45].

Furthermore, two multi-pronged studies have identified several genetic mutations in NF-κB pathway regulators, highlighting the role of this pathway in MM pathogenesis. The studies have reported a gain of function mutations in genes that enhance the activity of NF-κB (NIK, NF-κB 1/2) and three receptors involved in NF-κB signaling (CD40, LTβR, and TACI). On the other hand, loss-of-function mutations were reported in negative regulators of NF-κB (TRAF2/3, cIAP1/2). These genetic alterations lead to the activation of both canonical and non-canonical pathways and subsequent increased expression of NF-κB target genes [46, 47]. Another major consequence of these mutations and the suggested cause of NF-κB hyperactivation is the stabilisation of NIK, leading to its overexpression as its degradation is inhibited. The stabilisation induces strong NF-κB activation and consequent tumorigenesis [36].

NF-κB Activation in Leukemia and Lymphoma

Initially discovered to be constitutively activated in Hodgkin's Lymphoma (HL), aberrant NF-κB signaling has since been reported in many lymphoid malignancies and leukemias [5, 48]. c-Rel amplifications (in HL and DLBCL) are reported to be more frequent than c-Rel rearrangements (B cell lymphomas) in association with driving constitutive NF-κB activation. Conversely, RelA and RelB appear to be less consistently reported as drivers of constitutive NF-κB signaling. Furthermore, several B- and T-cell lymphomas, chronic lymphocytic lymphoma (CLL), and HL have been found to have constitutive NF-κB activity due to mutations in the *NF-κB2* gene, rather than *NF-κB1* and inactivating mutations of the IκB gene [5, 48]. Another major cause of active NF-κB signaling in leukemia and lymphomas is reported to be anomalistic activation of receptors and upstream mediators of the pathway [49].

Leukemias and lymphomas associated with viral infections such as adult T-cell leukemia (ATL caused by the human T-cell leukemia virus type 1 (HTLV-1) or Hodgkin's lymphoma, Burkitt's lymphoma, and B-cell lymphomas associated with Epstein–Barr virus (EBV)) can cause constitutive NF-κB activation. HTLV-1 promotes Tax oncoprotein/IKK complex formation, which activates both canonical and non-canonical pathways [50]. EBV induces non-ligand dependent activation of the NF-κB pathway by producing LMP1 protein, which acts as a member of the TNF receptor superfamily [51].

Bcr-Abl, an oncoprotein exhibiting strong association with chronic myelogenous leukemia (CML) and acute lymphoblastic leukemia (ALL), has been shown to be an activator of NF-κB signaling as well as being capable of transforming primary bone marrow cells. It has been shown that Bcr-Abl induced transformation and tumor growth can be impaired by inhibiting NF-κB signaling [52].

Potential Pharmacological Targeting of NF-κB Pathway

Taking the above into account, NF-κB appears to be an important therapeutic target [16], and after the approval of the proteasome inhibitor Bortezomib, several attempts have been made to develop potent NF-κB inhibitors. NF-κB blockage, however, is complex and tricky and may even promote tumorigenesis under certain circumstances [53]. Multiple pre-clinical studies have demonstrated the potential of NF-κB inhibitors as adjuvant therapies, promoting the development and promotion of more specific and rationally designed inhibitors [54 - 56]. Most of these inhibitors target one or more of the following major events in the NF-κB signaling pathway. Few important classes of blockers can target: 1) The upstream signaling (upstream of IKK); 2) IKKs; 3) Proteasomal activity; 4) Ubiquitination; or 5) NF-κB dimerization, and hence, nuclear function [42, 57]. These inhibitors encompass many categories of bioactive molecules including natural products, antioxidants, non-steroidal anti-inflammatory drugs (NSAIDs), peptides, anti-sense RNAs, glucocorticoids, and biologics.

Receptor Blockers and Upstream Signaling Inhibitors

NF-κB signaling may be activated by several cellular receptors, and hence, inhibiting or blocking these receptors presents a viable strategy for abrogating NF-κB signaling. One approach is the use of TNF receptors blockers such as Infliximab (chimeric anti-TNF-antibody) or Etanercept (receptor-antibody fusion protein), which has shown mitigation of TNF induced NF-κB activation [58]. Similarly, an interleukin-1 receptor antagonist (anakinra) has been FDA approved for the treatment of rheumatoid arthritis [42]. Toll-like receptor (TLR) signaling is often aberrantly activated in hematological malignancies due to genetic mutation of genes coding for the adapter protein MYD88. Recently, IMO 8400, an anti-sense oligonucleotide, has shown to act as a TLR 7,8,9 antagonist and proven efficacious in clinical trials, without any serious or severe adverse effects [59]. Another example of blocking upstream kinases is using Ibrutinib to block phosphorylation (at Tyr223) of Bruton's tyrosine kinase (BTK), which is stimulated in response to B cell antigen receptor (BCR). Inhibition of this phosphorylation can severely limit BTK induced NF-κB activity [60].

IKK Inhibitors

As explained earlier, the formation of the IKK complex is an important step in NF-κB signaling in both the canonical and non-canonical pathways, and hence, makes an attractive target for therapeutics development. IKK inhibitors have been shown to act through mainly three mechanisms, *viz.* competitive ATP inhibition (β-carboline and its synthetic derivatives), allosteric modification of the IKK complex (BMS-345541), and interference with kinase activity of the IKK complex, such as preventing IKK interaction with NEMO (Phenothiazine 22) [58]. However, despite promising pre-clinical results, only a few IKK inhibitors have been validated in clinical trials and none have been approved for clinical use till now [61, 62].

Ubiquitination and Proteasome Inhibitors

As we have seen earlier, ubiquitination and subsequent proteasomal degradation of inhibitory proteins form the key steps post IKK phosphorylation. These steps have, therefore, been of therapeutic interest. Amongst ubiquitination inhibitors, Ro 106-9920 has shown promising activity in pre-clinical models [63]. However, there are currently no ubiquitination inhibitors approved for clinical use. On the other hand, there has been extensive research on proteasome inhibitors, and lately, agents such as Bortezomib (26S proteasome inhibitor) and Carfilzomib (synthetic peptide) have been approved for clinical use in various hematological malignancies. Another structurally related analogue of Bortezomib, namely delazomib, is under clinical trials [57, 64, 65]. Another class of chemical compounds being explored as proteasome inhibitors are β lactones and marizomib, a marine β lactone, which is currently under clinical trials for several hematological malignancies [66].

Direct NF-κB and Nuclear Activity Inhibitors

One targeted approach of inhibiting NF-κB signaling is to directly inhibit NF-κB translocation or its DNA binding activity [55, 67]. Isolated from a fungal extract, dehydroxymethylepoxyquinomicin (DHMEQ) has been reported to exhibit potent inhibition of NF-κB translocation. Also, chromane derivatives including KL-1156, and several structural analogues, such as dihydronapthopyrans and benzofurans [57], have also been demonstrated to be active against a panel of human cancer cell lines and primary tumor cells. The examples of NF-κB DNA binding inhibitors include compounds such as parthenolide, which is a sesquiterpene lactone that has shown considerable abrogation of NF-κB binding to DNA [68]. Other compounds exhibiting considerable NF-κB DNA binding inhibition are: a triazine derivative called NI241, which interacts with p50 and prevents DNA binding [69]; retinoid named fenretinide [70]; and psoralen derivatives [71].

Non-steroidal Anti-inflammatory Drugs

Non-steroidal anti-inflammatory drugs "NSAIDs" can be used to treat a plethora of inflammatory disorders. Their action is attributable to the inhibition of the cyclooxygenase enzyme. However, it has recently been shown that NSAIDs, especially salicylates, can modulate NF-κB activity by acting as ATP competitors [54, 72]. Sulindac has also been reported to exhibit NF-κB abrogation [73]. Moreover, the co-administration of NSAIDs with tumor-inducing 1,2-dimethylhydrazine dihydrochloride significantly reduced the expression of NF-κB in pre-clinical colorectal cancer models [74].

Glucocorticoids and Immunomodulators

Another one of the most commonly prescribed class of therapeutics, glucocorticoids, is used in the treatment of diverse disorders ranging from allergy to cancer. Specifically, Dexamethasone, prednisone, and methyl prednisone have exhibited substantial mitigation of NF-κB signaling, and this has been postulated as partially being the mechanism behind their anti-inflammatory activity [75].

Natural Products

Several compounds and products of natural origin have been reported to demonstrate anti-inflammatory and anti-tumor effects [76] *via* modulating the activation of various oncogenic transcription factors, including NF-κB [67, 77, 78]. Some of these natural agents showing notable activity are thymoquinone [79], curcumin [80], celastrol [81], diosgenin [82], oleuropein [83], emodin [84], garcinol [85], pinitol [86], plumbagin, resveratrol, guggulsterone, thymoquinone, capsaicin, and ursolic acid [87 - 89]. The list of bioactive NF-κB inhibitors also includes thiacremonone [90], isoflavones [57], and hydroxytyrosol [91]. These natural agents may inhibit distinct or multiple steps in the signaling cascade of NF-κB [55, 92]. Amongst these agents, curcumin has been found to especially potent, and hence, several analogues of the parent molecule have been synthesised to improve pharmacokinetics and bioavailability. Also, curcumin has been shown to inhibit 26S proteasomal activity and is under clinical trials for several malignancies [42, 93, 94].

CONCLUSION

As highlighted briefly above, NF-κB has been shown to play a significant role in tumorigenesis. The aberrant activation of otherwise this tightly regulated transcription factor has been found to have a major implication in a large number of cancer types; solid tumors and hematological malignancies. However, further research into the detailed mechanism(s) of NF-κB regulation in appropriate models is warranted as the pathway may function as a double-edged sword and its inhibition in some cases may promote tumorigenesis [36]. The presence of several druggable components within this pathway can be exploited to design officious and safe pharmacological modulators. The design and development of specific drug candidates with improved pharmacotherapeutic and pharmacokinetic profiles will be a major step in providing new clinical intervention for several malignancies. Finally, many ongoing and oncoming research in both pathway elucidation and drug development will pave way for unprecedented and effective remedies targeting deregulated NF-κB activation in different cancers.

LIST OF ABBREVIATIONS

ALL	Acute lymphoblastic leukemia
AP-1	Activator protein-1
ATL	Adult T-cell leukemiaM
cIAP	cellular Inhibitors of apoptosis
CLL	Chronic lymphocytic leukemia
CML	Chronic myelogenous leukemia
COX	Cyclooxygenase
CXCR4	CXC-chemokine receptor 4
DLBCL	Diffuse large B-cell lymphoma
EBV	Epstein Barr virus
HBV	Hepatitis B virus
HL	Hodgkin's lymphoma
HTLV-1	Human T-cell leukemia virus type 1
ICAM-1	Intercellular adhesion molecule-1
IKK	IκB kinase
IL-1	Interleukin-1
IκBα	Inhibitor of kappa B-α
MMP	Matrix metalloproteinase
NF-κB	Nuclear factor kappa B
NIK	NF-κB-inducing kinase
NSAID	Nonsteroidal anti-inflammatory drug
PI3K	PI3-kinase
STAT3	Signal transducer and activator of transcription 3

TLR	Toll-like receptor
TNF	Tumor necrosis factor
TNFR	TNF receptorM
TRAF	TNFR-associated factor
VCAM-1	Vascular cell adhesion molecule-1
VEGF	Vascular endothelial growth factor

CONSENT FOR PUBLICATION

All authors give consent for the publication of the manuscript.

CONFLICT OF INTEREST

The authors confirm that they have no conflict of interest to declare for this publication.

ACKNOWLEDGEMENTS

Dr. Alan Prem Kumar is supported by a grant from the National Medical Research Council of Singapore. He is also supported by the National Medical Research Council of Singapore and the Singapore Ministry of Education under its Research Centres of Excellence initiative to Cancer Science Institute of Singapore, National University of Singapore.

REFERENCES

[1]   Gilmore TD. Introduction to NF-kappaβ: players, pathways, perspectives. Oncogene 2006; 25(51): 6680-4.
[http://dx.doi.org/10.1038/sj.onc.1209954] [PMID: 17072321]

[2]   Sethi G, Shanmugam MK, Ramachandran L, Kumar AP, Tergaonkar V. Multifaceted link between cancer and inflammation. Biosci Rep 2012; 32(1): 1-15.
[http://dx.doi.org/10.1042/BSR20100136] [PMID: 21981137]

[3]   Shin EM, Hay HS, Lee MH, *et al*. DEAD-box helicase DP103 defines metastatic potential of human breast cancers. J Clin Invest 2014; 124(9): 3807-24.
[http://dx.doi.org/10.1172/JCI73451] [PMID: 25083991]

[4]   Puar YR, Shanmugam MK, Fan L, Arfuso F, Sethi G, Tergaonkar V. Evidence for the involvement of the master transcription factor nf-κb in cancer initiation and progression. Biomedicines 2018; 6(3): 82.
[http://dx.doi.org/10.3390/biomedicines6030082] [PMID: 30060453]

[5]   Li F, Zhang J, Arfuso F, *et al*. NF-κB in cancer therapy. Arch Toxicol 2015; 89(5): 711-31.
[http://dx.doi.org/10.1007/s00204-015-1470-4] [PMID: 25690730]

[6]   Brasier AR. The NF-kappaβ regulatory network. Cardiovasc Toxicol 2006; 6(2): 111-30.
[http://dx.doi.org/10.1385/CT:6:2:111] [PMID: 17303919]

[7]   Shanmugam MK, Manu KA, Ong TH, *et al*. Inhibition of CXCR4/CXCL12 signaling axis by ursolic acid leads to suppression of metastasis in transgenic adenocarcinoma of mouse prostate model. Int J Cancer 2011; 129(7): 1552-63.

[http://dx.doi.org/10.1002/ijc.26120] [PMID: 21480220]

[8]   Manu KA, Shanmugam MK, Ramachandran L, *et al.* First evidence that gamma-tocotrienol inhibits the growth of human gastric cancer and chemosensitizes it to capecitabine in a xenograft mouse model through the modulation of nf-kappaβ pathway. Clinical cancer research : an official journal of the American Association for Cancer Research 2012; 18: 2220-9.

[9]   Nabel GJ, Verma IM. Proposed NF-kappa B/I kappa B family nomenclature. Genes Dev 1993; 7(11): 2063.
        [http://dx.doi.org/10.1101/gad.7.11.2063] [PMID: 8224837]

[10]   Ahn KS, Sethi G, Aggarwal BB. Reversal of chemoresistance and enhancement of apoptosis by statins through down-regulation of the NF-kappaβ pathway. Biochem Pharmacol 2008; 75(4): 907-13.
        [http://dx.doi.org/10.1016/j.bcp.2007.10.010] [PMID: 18036510]

[11]   Ahn KS, Sethi G, Chaturvedi MM, Aggarwal BB. Simvastatin, 3-hydroxy-3-methylglutaryl coenzyme A reductase inhibitor, suppresses osteoclastogenesis induced by receptor activator of nuclear factor-kappaβ ligand through modulation of NF-kappaβ pathway. Int J Cancer 2008; 123(8): 1733-40.
        [http://dx.doi.org/10.1002/ijc.23745] [PMID: 18688862]

[12]   Huxford T, Ghosh G. A structural guide to proteins of the NF-kappaβ signaling module. Cold Spring Harb Perspect Biol 2009; 1(3): a000075-5.
        [http://dx.doi.org/10.1101/cshperspect.a000075] [PMID: 20066103]

[13]   Gilmore TD. Introduction to NF-kappaβ: players, pathways, perspectives. Oncogene 2006; 25(51): 6680-4.
        [http://dx.doi.org/10.1038/sj.onc.1209954] [PMID: 17072321]

[14]   Sawhney M, Rohatgi N, Kaur J, *et al.* Expression of NF-kappaβ parallels COX-2 expression in oral precancer and cancer: association with smokeless tobacco. Int J Cancer 2007; 120(12): 2545-56.
        [http://dx.doi.org/10.1002/ijc.22657] [PMID: 17354234]

[15]   Manna SK, Aggarwal RS, Sethi G, Aggarwal BB, Ramesh GT. Morin (3,5,7,2,4-pentahydroxyflavone) abolishes nuclear factor-kappaβ activation induced by various carcinogens and inflammatory stimuli, leading to suppression of nuclear factor-kappaβ-regulated gene expression and up-regulation of apoptosis Clinical cancer research : an official journal of the American Association for Cancer Research 2007; 13: 2290-7.

[16]   Li F, Sethi G. Targeting transcription factor NF-kappaβ to overcome chemoresistance and radioresistance in cancer therapy. Biochim Biophys Acta 2010; 1805(2): 167-80.
        [PMID: 20079806]

[17]   Nair AS, Shishodia S, Ahn KS, Kunnumakkara AB, Sethi G, Aggarwal BB. Deguelin, an akt inhibitor, suppresses ikappaβalpha kinase activation leading to suppression of nf-kappaβ-regulated gene expression, potentiation of apoptosis, and inhibition of cellular invasion. J immunology (Baltimore, Md : 1950) 2006; 177: 5612-22.

[18]   Kaltschmidt B, Greiner JFW, Kadhim HM, Kaltschmidt C. Subunit-specific role of nf-κb in cancer. Biomedicines 2018; 6(2): 44.
        [http://dx.doi.org/10.3390/biomedicines6020044] [PMID: 29673141]

[19]   Chen J, Chen ZJ. Regulation of NF-κB by ubiquitination. Curr Opin Immunol 2013; 25(1): 4-12.
        [http://dx.doi.org/10.1016/j.coi.2012.12.005] [PMID: 23312890]

[20]   Oeckinghaus A, Ghosh S. The NF-kappaβ family of transcription factors and its regulation. Cold Spring Harb Perspect Biol 2009; 1(4): a000034-4.
        [http://dx.doi.org/10.1101/cshperspect.a000034] [PMID: 20066092]

[21]   Sun S-C. Non-canonical NF-κB signaling pathway. Cell Res 2011; 21(1): 71-85.
        [http://dx.doi.org/10.1038/cr.2010.177] [PMID: 21173796]

[22]   Basak S, Shih VF, Hoffmann A. Generation and activation of multiple dimeric transcription factors within the NF-kappaβ signaling system. Mol Cell Biol 2008; 28(10): 3139-50.

[http://dx.doi.org/10.1128/MCB.01469-07] [PMID: 18299388]

[23]   Nelson DE, Ihekwaba AE, Elliott M, *et al.* Oscillations in NF-kappaβ signaling control the dynamics of gene expression. Science 2004; 306(5696): 704-8.
[http://dx.doi.org/10.1126/science.1099962] [PMID: 15499023]

[24]   Micheli L, Leonardi L, Conti F, *et al.* PC4/Tis7/IFRD1 stimulates skeletal muscle regeneration and is involved in myoblast differentiation as a regulator of MyoD and NF-kappaβ. J Biol Chem 2011; 286(7): 5691-707.
[http://dx.doi.org/10.1074/jbc.M110.162842] [PMID: 21127072]

[25]   Yeung F, Hoberg JE, Ramsey CS, *et al.* Modulation of NF-kappaβ-dependent transcription and cell survival by the SIRT1 deacetylase. EMBO J 2004; 23(12): 2369-80.
[http://dx.doi.org/10.1038/sj.emboj.7600244] [PMID: 15152190]

[26]   Wertz IE, Dixit VM. Signaling to NF-kappaβ: regulation by ubiquitination. Cold Spring Harb Perspect Biol 2010; 2(3): a003350-0.
[http://dx.doi.org/10.1101/cshperspect.a003350] [PMID: 20300215]

[27]   Xu H, You M, Shi H, Hou Y. Ubiquitin-mediated NFκB degradation pathway. Cell Mol Immunol 2015; 12(6): 653-5.
[http://dx.doi.org/10.1038/cmi.2014.99] [PMID: 25345807]

[28]   Edna Zhi Pei Chai, Kodappully Sivaraman Siveen, Muthu K. Shanmugam, Frank Arfuso, Gautam Sethi; Analysis of the intricate relationship between chronic inflammation and cancer. Biochem J 15 May 2015; 468 (1): 1–15.
[http://dx.doi.org/10.1042/BJ20141337]

[29]   Sethi G, Sung B, Aggarwal BB. Nuclear factor-kappaβ activation: from bench to bedside. Exp Biol Med (Maywood) 2008; 233(1): 21-31.
[http://dx.doi.org/10.3181/0707-MR-196] [PMID: 18156302]

[30]   Ahn KS, Sethi G, Aggarwal BB. Nuclear factor-kappa B: from clone to clinic. Curr Mol Med 2007; 7(7): 619-37.
[http://dx.doi.org/10.2174/156652407782564363] [PMID: 18045141]

[31]   Bassères DS, Baldwin AS. Nuclear factor-kappaβ and inhibitor of kappaβ kinase pathways in oncogenic initiation and progression. Oncogene 2006; 25(51): 6817-30.
[http://dx.doi.org/10.1038/sj.onc.1209942] [PMID: 17072330]

[32]   Kendellen M, Bradford J, Lawrence C, Clark K, Baldwin A. Canonical and non-canonical NF-κB signaling promotes breast cancer tumor-initiating cells. Oncogene 2013; 33(10): 1297-305.
[PMID: 23474754]

[33]   Fabre C, Mimura N, Bobb K, *et al.*   Dual inhibition of canonical and noncanonical nf-kappaβ pathways demonstrates significant antitumor activities in multiple myeloma Clinical cancer research : an official journal of the American Association for Cancer Research 2012; 18: 4669-81.

[34]   Fuchs O. Targeting of NF-kappaβ signaling pathway, other signaling pathways and epigenetics in therapy of multiple myeloma. Cardiovasc Hematol Disord Drug Targets 2013; 13(1): 16-34.
[http://dx.doi.org/10.2174/1871529X11313010003] [PMID: 23534949]

[35]   Espinoza-Sánchez NA, Győrffy B, Fuentes-Pananá EM, Götte M. Differential impact of classical and non-canonical NF-κB pathway-related gene expression on the survival of breast cancer patients. J Cancer 2019; 10(21): 5191-211.
[http://dx.doi.org/10.7150/jca.34302] [PMID: 31602271]

[36]   Baud V, Karin M. Is NF-kappaβ a good target for cancer therapy? Hopes and pitfalls. Nat Rev Drug Discov 2009; 8(1): 33-40.
[http://dx.doi.org/10.1038/nrd2781] [PMID: 19116625]

[37]   Kyle RA, Rajkumar SV. Multiple myeloma. N Engl J Med 2004; 351(18): 1860-73.
[http://dx.doi.org/10.1056/NEJMra041875] [PMID: 15509819]

[38] Podar K, Richardson PG, Hideshima T, Chauhan D, Anderson KC. The malignant clone and the bone-marrow environment. Best Pract Res Clin Haematol 2007; 20(4): 597-612.
[http://dx.doi.org/10.1016/j.beha.2007.08.002] [PMID: 18070708]

[39] Arora L, Kumar AP, Arfuso F, Chng WJ, Sethi G. The role of signal transducer and activator of transcription 3 (stat3) and its targeted inhibition in hematological malignancies. Cancers (Basel) 2018; 10(9): 327.
[http://dx.doi.org/10.3390/cancers10090327] [PMID: 30217007]

[40] Bharti AC, Donato N, Singh S, Aggarwal BB. Curcumin (diferuloylmethane) down-regulates the constitutive activation of nuclear factor–κB and IκBα kinase in human multiple myeloma cells, leading to suppression of proliferation and induction of apoptosis. Blood 2003; 101(3): 1053-62.
[http://dx.doi.org/10.1182/blood-2002-05-1320] [PMID: 12393461]

[41] Hideshima T, Neri P, Tassone P, *et al.* MLN120B, a novel IkappaB kinase kinase beta inhibitor, blocks multiple myeloma cell growth *in vitro* and *in vivo* Clin Cancer Res 2006; 12: 5887-94.

[42] Sethi G, Tergaonkar V. Potential pharmacological control of the NF-κB pathway. Trends Pharmacol Sci 2009; 30(6): 313-21.
[http://dx.doi.org/10.1016/j.tips.2009.03.004] [PMID: 19446347]

[43] Jourdan M, Moreaux J, Vos JD, *et al.* Targeting NF-kappaβ pathway with an IKK2 inhibitor induces inhibition of multiple myeloma cell growth. Br J Haematol 2007; 138(2): 160-8.
[http://dx.doi.org/10.1111/j.1365-2141.2007.06629.x] [PMID: 17542984]

[44] Feng R, Anderson G, Xiao G, *et al.* SDX-308, a nonsteroidal anti-inflammatory agent, inhibits NF-kappaβ activity, resulting in strong inhibition of osteoclast formation/activity and multiple myeloma cell growth. Blood 2007; 109(5): 2130-8.
[http://dx.doi.org/10.1182/blood-2006-07-027458] [PMID: 17095620]

[45] Mulligan G, Mitsiades C, Bryant B, *et al.* Gene expression profiling and correlation with outcome in clinical trials of the proteasome inhibitor bortezomib. Blood 2007; 109(8): 3177-88.
[http://dx.doi.org/10.1182/blood-2006-09-044974] [PMID: 17185464]

[46] Annunziata CM, Davis RE, Demchenko Y, *et al.* Frequent engagement of the classical and alternative NF-kappaβ pathways by diverse genetic abnormalities in multiple myeloma. Cancer Cell 2007; 12(2): 115-30.
[http://dx.doi.org/10.1016/j.ccr.2007.07.004] [PMID: 17692804]

[47] Keats JJ, Fonseca R, Chesi M, *et al.* Promiscuous mutations activate the noncanonical NF-kappaβ pathway in multiple myeloma. Cancer Cell 2007; 12(2): 131-44.
[http://dx.doi.org/10.1016/j.ccr.2007.07.003] [PMID: 17692805]

[48] Krappmann D, Vincendeau M. Mechanisms of NF-κB deregulation in lymphoid malignancies. Semin Cancer Biol 2016; 39: 3-14.
[http://dx.doi.org/10.1016/j.semcancer.2016.05.002] [PMID: 27262792]

[49] Jost PJ, Ruland J. Aberrant NF-kappaβ signaling in lymphoma: mechanisms, consequences, and therapeutic implications. Blood 2007; 109(7): 2700-7.
[http://dx.doi.org/10.1182/blood-2006-07-025809] [PMID: 17119127]

[50] Matsuoka M, Jeang KT. Human T-cell leukaemia virus type 1 (HTLV-1) infectivity and cellular transformation. Nat Rev Cancer 2007; 7(4): 270-80.
[http://dx.doi.org/10.1038/nrc2111] [PMID: 17384582]

[51] Young LS, Rickinson AB. Epstein-Barr virus: 40 years on. Nat Rev Cancer 2004; 4(10): 757-68.
[http://dx.doi.org/10.1038/nrc1452] [PMID: 15510157]

[52] Reuther JY, Reuther GW, Cortez D, Pendergast AM, Baldwin AS Jr. A requirement for NF-kappaβ activation in Bcr-Abl-mediated transformation. Genes Dev 1998; 12(7): 968-81.
[http://dx.doi.org/10.1101/gad.12.7.968] [PMID: 9531535]

[53] Perkins ND. NF-kappaβ: tumor promoter or suppressor? Trends Cell Biol 2004; 14(2): 64-9.
[http://dx.doi.org/10.1016/j.tcb.2003.12.004] [PMID: 15102437]

[54] Erstad DJ, Cusack JC Jr. Targeting the NF-κB pathway in cancer therapy. Surg Oncol Clin N Am 2013; 22(4): 705-46.
[http://dx.doi.org/10.1016/j.soc.2013.06.011] [PMID: 24012396]

[55] Gupta SC, Sundaram C, Reuter S, Aggarwal BB. Inhibiting NF-κB activation by small molecules as a therapeutic strategy. Biochim Biophys Acta 2010; 1799(10-12): 775-87.
[http://dx.doi.org/10.1016/j.bbagrm.2010.05.004] [PMID: 20493977]

[56] Durand JK, Baldwin AS. Targeting IKK and NF-κB for Therapy. Adv Protein Chem Struct Biol 2017; 107: 77-115.
[http://dx.doi.org/10.1016/bs.apcsb.2016.11.006] [PMID: 28215229]

[57] de Castro Barbosa ML, da Conceicao RA, Fraga AGM, *et al.* Nf-kappaβ signaling pathway inhibitors as anticancer drug candidates. Anticancer Agents Med Chem 2017; 17(4): 483-90.
[http://dx.doi.org/10.2174/1871520616666160729112854] [PMID: 27481554]

[58] Sethi G, Sung B, Kunnumakkara AB, Aggarwal BB. Targeting TNF for Treatment of Cancer and Autoimmunity. Adv Exp Med Biol 2009; 647: 37-51.
[http://dx.doi.org/10.1007/978-0-387-89520-8_3] [PMID: 19760065]

[59] Balak DM, van Doorn MB, Arbeit RD, *et al.* IMO-8400, a toll-like receptor 7, 8, and 9 antagonist, demonstrates clinical activity in a phase 2a, randomized, placebo-controlled trial in patients with moderate-to-severe plaque psoriasis. Clin Immunol 2017; 174: 63-72.
[http://dx.doi.org/10.1016/j.clim.2016.09.015] [PMID: 27876460]

[60] Novero A, Ravella PM, Chen Y, Dous G, Liu D. Ibrutinib for B cell malignancies. Exp Hematol Oncol 2014; 3(1): 4-4.
[http://dx.doi.org/10.1186/2162-3619-3-4] [PMID: 24472371]

[61] Awasthee N, Rai V, Chava S, *et al.* Targeting ikappaappab kinases for cancer therapy. Semin Cancer Biol 2019; 56: 12-24.
[PMID: 29486318]

[62] Begalli F, Bennett J, Capece D, *et al.* Unlocking the nf-kappaβ conundrum: Embracing complexity to achieve specificity. Biomedicines 2017; 5(3): 5.
[PMID: 28829404]

[63] Swinney DC, Xu Y-Z, Scarafia LE, *et al.* A small molecule ubiquitination inhibitor blocks NF-κ B-dependent cytokine expression in cells and rats. J Biol Chem 2002; 277(26): 23573-81.
[http://dx.doi.org/10.1074/jbc.M200842200] [PMID: 11950839]

[64] Mateos MV, Richardson PG, Dimopoulos MA, *et al.* Effect of cumulative bortezomib dose on survival in multiple myeloma patients receiving bortezomib-melphalan-prednisone in the phase III VISTA study. Am J Hematol 2015; 90(4): 314-9.
[http://dx.doi.org/10.1002/ajh.23933] [PMID: 25557740]

[65] Stewart AK, Rajkumar SV, Dimopoulos MA, *et al.* Carfilzomib, lenalidomide, and dexamethasone for relapsed multiple myeloma. N Engl J Med 2015; 372(2): 142-52.
[http://dx.doi.org/10.1056/NEJMoa1411321] [PMID: 25482145]

[66] Groll M, Potts BC. Proteasome structure, function, and lessons learned from beta-lactone inhibitors. Curr Top Med Chem 2011; 11(23): 2850-78.
[http://dx.doi.org/10.2174/156802611798281320] [PMID: 21824111]

[67] Gilmore TD, Herscovitch M. Inhibitors of NF-kappaβ signaling: 785 and counting. Oncogene 2006; 25(51): 6887-99.
[http://dx.doi.org/10.1038/sj.onc.1209982] [PMID: 17072334]

[68] Zhang S, Won YK, Ong CN, Shen HM. Anti-cancer potential of sesquiterpene lactones: bioactivity

and molecular mechanisms. Curr Med Chem Anticancer Agents 2005; 5(3): 239-49.
[http://dx.doi.org/10.2174/1568011053765976] [PMID: 15992352]

[69] Kobayashi T, Yoshimori A, Kino K, Komori R, Miyazawa H, Tanuma SI. A new small molecule that directly inhibits the DNA binding of NF-kappaβ. Bioorg Med Chem 2009; 17(14): 5293-7.
[http://dx.doi.org/10.1016/j.bmc.2009.05.030] [PMID: 19539480]

[70] Kang H, Lee M, Choi KC, Shin DM, Ko J, Jang SWN. N-(4-hydroxyphenyl)retinamide inhibits breast cancer cell invasion through suppressing NF-KB activation and inhibiting matrix metalloproteinase-9 expression. J Cell Biochem 2012; 113(9): 2845-55.
[http://dx.doi.org/10.1002/jcb.24159] [PMID: 22488409]

[71] Marzaro G, Guiotto A, Borgatti M, *et al.* Psoralen derivatives as inhibitors of NF-κB/DNA interaction: synthesis, molecular modeling, 3D-QSAR, and biological evaluation. J Med Chem 2013; 56(5): 1830-42.
[http://dx.doi.org/10.1021/jm3009647] [PMID: 23414143]

[72] Yin MJ, Yamamoto Y, Gaynor RB. The anti-inflammatory agents aspirin and salicylate inhibit the activity of I(kappa)B kinase-beta. Nature 1998; 396(6706): 77-80.
[http://dx.doi.org/10.1038/23948] [PMID: 9817203]

[73] Yamamoto Y, Yin MJ, Lin KM, Gaynor RB. Sulindac inhibits activation of the NF-kappaβ pathway. J Biol Chem 1999; 274(38): 27307-14.
[http://dx.doi.org/10.1074/jbc.274.38.27307] [PMID: 10480951]

[74] Ghanghas P, Jain S, Rana C, Sanyal SN. Chemopreventive action of non-steroidal anti-inflammatory drugs on the inflammatory pathways in colon cancer. Biomed Pharmacother 2016; 78: 239-47.

[75] Rao NA, McCalman MT, Moulos P, *et al.* Coactivation of GR and NFKB alters the repertoire of their binding sites and target genes. Genome Res 2011; 21(9): 1404-16.
[http://dx.doi.org/10.1101/gr.118042.110] [PMID: 21750107]

[76] Shanmugam MK, Lee JH, Chai EZ, *et al.* Cancer prevention and therapy through the modulation of transcription factors by bioactive natural compounds. Semin Cancer Biol 2016; 40-41: 35-47.
[http://dx.doi.org/10.1016/j.semcancer.2016.03.005] [PMID: 27038646]

[77] Deorukhkar A, Krishnan S, Sethi G, Aggarwal BB. Back to basics: how natural products can provide the basis for new therapeutics. Expert Opin Investig Drugs 2007; 16(11): 1753-73.
[http://dx.doi.org/10.1517/13543784.16.11.1753] [PMID: 17970636]

[78] Yang SF, Weng CJ, Sethi G, Hu DN. Natural bioactives and phytochemicals serve in cancer treatment and prevention. Evid Based Complement Alternat Med 2013; 698190.

[79] Siveen KS, Mustafa N, Li F, *et al.* Thymoquinone overcomes chemoresistance and enhances the anticancer effects of bortezomib through abrogation of NF-κB regulated gene products in multiple myeloma xenograft mouse model. Oncotarget 2014; 5(3): 634-48.
[http://dx.doi.org/10.18632/oncotarget.1596] [PMID: 24504138]

[80] Shanmugam MK, Kannaiyan R, Sethi G. Targeting cell signaling and apoptotic pathways by dietary agents: role in the prevention and treatment of cancer. Nutr Cancer 2011; 63(2): 161-73.
[http://dx.doi.org/10.1080/01635581.2011.523502] [PMID: 21294053]

[81] Shanmugam MK, Ahn KS, Lee JH, *et al.* Celastrol attenuates the invasion and migration and augments the anticancer effects of bortezomib in a xenograft mouse model of multiple myeloma. Front Pharmacol 2018; 9: 365.
[http://dx.doi.org/10.3389/fphar.2018.00365] [PMID: 29773987]

[82] Sethi G, Shanmugam MK, Warrier S, *et al.* Pro-apoptotic and anti-cancer properties of diosgenin: A comprehensive and critical review. Nutrients 2018; 10(5): 645.
[http://dx.doi.org/10.3390/nu10050645] [PMID: 29783752]

[83] Liu L, Ahn KS, Shanmugam MK, *et al.* Oleuropein induces apoptosis *via* abrogating nf-kappaβ activation cascade in estrogen receptor-negative breast cancer cells. J Cell Biochem 2019; 120(3):

4504-13.
[PMID: 30260018]

[84] Shrimali D, Shanmugam MK, Kumar AP, *et al.* Targeted abrogation of diverse signal transduction cascades by emodin for the treatment of inflammatory disorders and cancer. Cancer Lett 2013; 341(2): 139-49.
[http://dx.doi.org/10.1016/j.canlet.2013.08.023] [PMID: 23962559]

[85] Li F, Shanmugam MK, Siveen KS, *et al.* Garcinol sensitizes human head and neck carcinoma to cisplatin in a xenograft mouse model despite downregulation of proliferative biomarkers. Oncotarget 2015; 6(7): 5147-63.
[http://dx.doi.org/10.18632/oncotarget.2881] [PMID: 25762616]

[86] Sethi G, Ahn KS, Sung B, Aggarwal BB. Pinitol targets nuclear factor-kappaβ activation pathway leading to inhibition of gene products associated with proliferation, apoptosis, invasion, and angiogenesis. Mol Cancer Ther 2008; 7(6): 1604-14.
[http://dx.doi.org/10.1158/1535-7163.MCT-07-2424] [PMID: 18566231]

[87] Aggarwal BB, Shishodia S. Molecular targets of dietary agents for prevention and therapy of cancer. Biochem Pharmacol 2006; 71(10): 1397-421.
[http://dx.doi.org/10.1016/j.bcp.2006.02.009] [PMID: 16563357]

[88] Shanmugam MK, Warrier S, Kumar AP, Sethi G, Arfuso F. Potential role of natural compounds as anti-angiogenic agents in cancer. Curr Vasc Pharmacol 2017; 15(6): 503-19.
[http://dx.doi.org/10.2174/1570161115666170713094319] [PMID: 28707601]

[89] Bishayee A, Sethi G. Bioactive natural products in cancer prevention and therapy: Progress and promise. Semin Cancer Biol 2016; 40-41: 1-3.
[http://dx.doi.org/10.1016/j.semcancer.2016.08.006] [PMID: 27565447]

[90] Venkateswararao E, Sharma VK, Yun J, Kim Y, Jung SH. Anti-proliferative effect of chalcone derivatives through inactivation of NF-κB in human cancer cells. Bioorg Med Chem 2014; 22(13): 3386-92.
[http://dx.doi.org/10.1016/j.bmc.2014.04.045] [PMID: 24835787]

[91] Zhao B, Ma Y, Xu Z, *et al.* Hydroxytyrosol, a natural molecule from olive oil, suppresses the growth of human hepatocellular carcinoma cells *via* inactivating AKT and nuclear factor-kappa B pathways. Cancer Lett 2014; 347(1): 79-87.
[http://dx.doi.org/10.1016/j.canlet.2014.01.028] [PMID: 24486741]

[92] Hasanpourghadi M, Looi CY, Pandurangan AK, Sethi G, Wong WF, Mustafa MR. Phytometabolites targeting the warburg effect in cancer cells: A mechanistic review. Curr Drug Targets 2017; 18(9): 1086-94.
[http://dx.doi.org/10.2174/1389450117666160401124842] [PMID: 27033190]

[93] Qiu X, Du Y, Lou B, *et al.* Synthesis and identification of new 4-arylidene curcumin analogues as potential anticancer agents targeting nuclear factor-κB signaling pathway. J Med Chem 2010; 53(23): 8260-73.
[http://dx.doi.org/10.1021/jm1004545] [PMID: 21070043]

[94] Olivera A, Moore TW, Hu F, *et al.* Inhibition of the NF-κB signaling pathway by the curcumin analog, 3,5-Bis(2-pyridinylmethylidene)-4-piperidone (EF31): anti-inflammatory and anti-cancer properties. Int Immunopharmacol 2012; 12(2): 368-77.
[http://dx.doi.org/10.1016/j.intimp.2011.12.009] [PMID: 22197802]

CHAPTER 7

Bruton's Tyrosine Kinase Signaling and Advancement in Multiple Myeloma Therapy

Krishne Gowda[1,*], **Max Von Suskil**[2], **Omar Al-Adat**[2], **Jennifer Dang**[2], **Kuntal Bhowmick**[2], **Prachi S. Narayan**[2], **Shantu G Amin**[1] and **Manoj K. Pandey**[2,*]

[1] *Department Pharmacology, Penn State College of Medicine, Hershey, PA, USA*

[2] *Department of Biomedical Sciences, Cooper Medical School of Rowan University, Camden, NJ 08103, USA*

Abstract: The Bruton's tyrosine kinase (BTK) is a non-receptor protein-tyrosine kinase (PTK) required for the growth and differentiation of B-lymphocytes, which play a critical role in the progression of numerous neoplasms. Therefore, BTK has emerged as an exciting and attractive target for inhibition of hematological malignancies. Various BTK inhibitors have already proved remarkable tumor suppressing ability in clinical studies. Ibrutinib was the trail blazing BTK inhibitor that first showed exceptional tumor inhibition in patients, this molecule showed excellent response in refractory/relapsed (R/R) conditions with high-risk genetic lesions patients, particularly among chronic lymphocytic leukemia (CLL) and mantle cell lymphoma (MCL). Based on ibrutinib's efficacy and tolerability, in 2016, the Food and Drug Administration (FDA) approved it as a first-line treatment for CLL patients. Ibrutinib occupies the ATP-binding active site of BTK, making salt bridges within the hinge that connects the two enzyme lobes followed by the unsaturated acrylamide group of ibrutinib covalently bonding with the BTK cysteine 481 residue to irreversibly form an inactive adduct. However, ibrutinib's irreversible binding mechanism leads to acquired resistance to the medication. Both resistance arising due to mutations that impair the affinity of ibrutinib for BTK and the undesirable side effects of the drug have led to the development of numerous second-generation inhibitors. The efficacy and specificity of novel BTK inhibiting agents such as Acalabrutinib, ONO/GS-4059, KS99, and other small molecules have substantiated solutions to ibrutinib's shortcomings. The detailed role of BTK signaling pathways, and its cross-talk between other signaling pathways, the significance of BTK inhibition in hematological malignancies, and the current progress in the discovery of small molecule BTK inhibitors are presented in this chapter.

Keywords: Multiple myeloma, Hematological malignancies, Bruton's tyrosine kinase, Myeloma stem cells, Drug development.

* **Corresponding author Krishne Gowda**: Department Pharmacology, Penn State College of Medicine, Hershey, PA, USA; Tel: 717-531-0003 Ext 285014; Fax: 717-531-0244; E-mail: kxg21@psu.edu
* **Corresponding author Manoj K Pandey**: Department of Biomedical Sciences, Cooper Medical School of Rowan University, Camden, NJ 08103, USA; Tel: 856-956-2751; E-mail: pandey@rowan.edu

Manoj K. Pandey & Vijay P. Kale (Eds.)

INTRODUCTION

Protein kinases (PKs) are enzymes that regulate the biological activities of proteins through mediating phosphorylation and play an essential role in every aspect of cellular functions [1]. PKs regulate cellular metabolism, transcription, division, migration, and apoptosis, as well as participate in immune responses and nervous system function. Protein phosphorylation involves the balanced action of PKs and phosphatases [2]. Phosphorylation plays a critical role in increasing or decreasing enzyme activities through post-transcriptional modification, thereby controlling signal transduction, gene expression, protein stabilization, enzyme affinity, and cellular location. Thus, the aberrant activation of PKs is associated with various disorders, especially neoplasms [3, 4].

BTK signaling was first discovered as the functional defect in the immune system condition X-linked agammaglobulinemia (XLA) in 1993. People with XLA suffer from marginal populations of B cells due to mutations in the BTK gene preventing either BTK production or function. Following the discovery of BTK in XLA, a number of studies have demonstrated conclusively that BTK is required for B-cell development, differentiation, and survival [5 - 8]. BTK knockdown studies in animal models suggest that B-lymphocytes deficient in BTK showed impaired signal transduction resulting in functional defects, inability to reach a mature state, and ultimately, high rates of apoptosis.

The B cell receptor (BCR) stimulation induces BTK phosphorylation and signal transduction [9, 10]. The BCR is a trans-membrane protein complex comprised of multiple subunits, including an immunoglobulin heavy chain (IgHC) covalently linked by disulfide bonds to an immunoglobulin light chain (IgLC) [11]. The B cell surface expresses BCR, which mediates antigen recognition. Besides the BCR pathway, BTK activation modulates various other receptor pathways vital to B cells, including chemokine-X-chemokine receptors (CXCR4 and CXCR5], toll-like receptor (TLR), and signaling mediated by Fc receptors [12 - 15]. Though in some cell types, such as in myeloid lineages, BTK acts as a downstream target of TLRs, FcεR, and FcγRI signaling pathways [16 - 19]. Furthermore, BTK is shown to be linked in numerous additional signaling pathways, including receptor activator of nuclear factor-κB (RANK) in osteoclasts, collagen/CD32 signaling in platelets, and the NLRP3 (NOD-, LRR- and Pryin Domain-containing protein 3] inflammasome signaling in macrophages and neutrophils [20 - 22]. Based on various scientific reports, it is now established that most hematopoietic cells, including myeloid cells, express BTK, which has created significant interest among drug discovery and development groups in using BTK inhibition as an anti-cancer therapy against various malignancies (Fig. 1) [23 - 25].

This chapter describes the significance of BTK signaling as well as the pathway cross talks. Also, how the small molecule inhibitors have clinical benefits of targeting BTK in B cell malignancies is described.

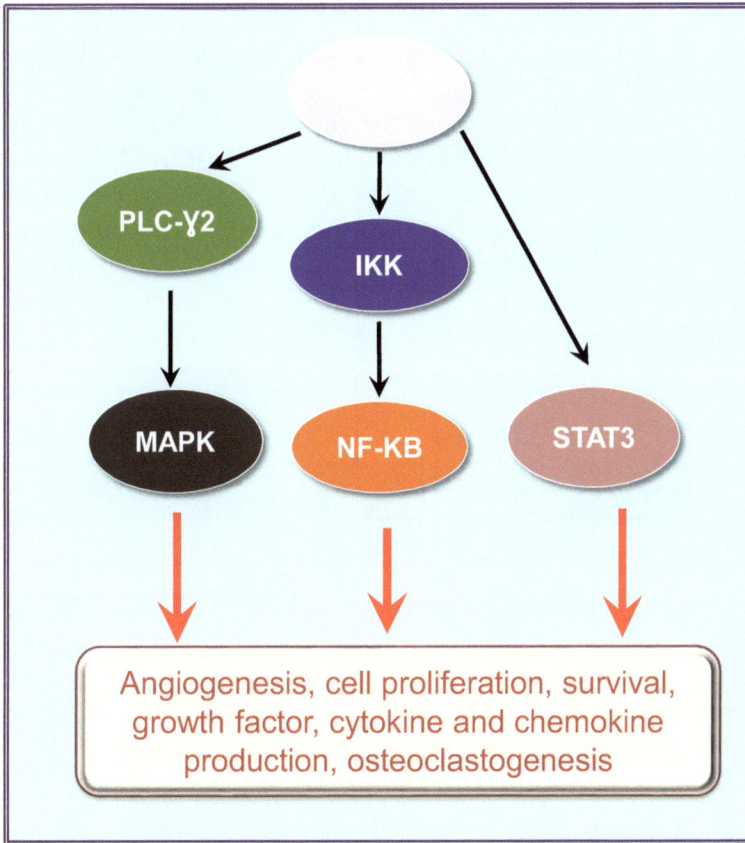

Fig. (1). The signaling of BTK pathways regulates various intermediate signaling. These signaling pathways individually contribute in the pathogenesis of malignancies.

THE BTK SIGNALING PATHWAY

Structure and Activation of BTK

BTK is one of the five members of TEC (Tec protein tyrosine kinase) family and consists of 659 amino acid residues [10]. The BTK domain structure is similar to that of the SRC family kinases in containing a C-terminal catalytic domain and the SRC homology domains (SH2 and SH3] (Fig. **2**). As compared to SRC, BTK lacks a negative regulatory tyrosine residue at the C-terminal and an N-terminal myristoylation signal [10]. Instead, BTK contains a proline-rich TEC homology (TH) domain and an N-terminal pleckstrin homology (PH) domain, which facilitates interaction with phosphatidylinositol lipids and membrane recruitment (Fig. **2**). Because of these structural characteristics, BTK remains cytoplasmic and is only transiently recruited to the plasma membrane when the PH domain binds with phosphatidylinositol 3,4,5-triphosphate (PIP3], following its activation by phosphoinositide 3-kinase (PI3K) [11]. The activation of BTK is mediated in large part by its interaction with the B-cell receptor (BCR). Either spleen associated tyrosine kinase (SYK) or SRC family kinases trans-phosphorylate the BTK tyrosine 551 (Y551] residues in the kinase domain of BTK, which consequently results in its auto-phosphorylation at position Y223 residues in the SH3 domain [26, 27]. Phosphorylation of the Y223 residues is believed to stabilize the kinase conformation and further induces the kinase activity [28]. However, *in vivo* studies revealed that the function of BTK was not significantly affected by a Y223F mutation [29]. Therefore, the role of auto-phosphorylation of Y223 is still unclear.

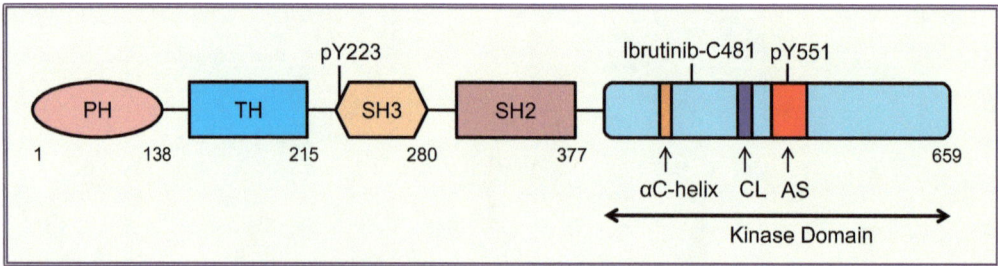

Fig. (2). Schematic presentation of BTK protein showing various domains and activation sites. The various tyrosine sites are targets of kinases.

Role of BTK in B Cell Receptor Signaling

B-lymphocytes express BCR on the cell membrane, which recognizes foreign body antigens and initiates an intercellular cascade, which plays a critical role in protective antibody responses. It is essential for the survival of B cells expressing BCR isotypes IgM-BCR to encounter an antigen of a pathogen because, without the activity of BTK, B cells undergo apoptosis negatively regulated by anti-apoptotic protein B cell lymphoma extra-large (Bcl-xL). This interaction between BCR and B cell apoptosis, regulated by Bcl-xL, indicates that Bcl-xL is the first downstream target of BTK [30, 31]. Upon antigen binding to the BCR, cell size enlargement and degradation of the cyclin dependent kinase inhibitor 1B (CDKN1B) occurs, demonstrating that BTK is not crucial for several G1 events [32]. An abnormal cell cycle has been demonstrated in BTK-deficient B cells, these cells enter an early G1 phase, but cannot enter the S phase, because they fail to induce cyclin D2 expression [33]. Apart from B cell development and function, the BCR controls integrin subunit alpha 4 (ITGA4 or VLA-4] - mediated adhesion to vascular cell adhesion molecule-1 (VCAM-1] and fibronectin *via* BTK [34]. Additionally, the signal transducers of non-receptor PTKs, namely phospholipase Cγ (PLCγ), nuclear factor kappa-B cells (NF-κB), mitogen-activated protein kinase (MAPK), and serine/threonine kinase AKT, are also activated by cross-linking with BCR (Fig. 1).

BCR signaling needs a network of PKs and adaptors that mediate intercellular responses to antigen stimulation. The BCR complex consists of the receptor itself, which is associated with the disulfide-linked Igα/Igβ (CD79a/CD79b) heterodimers. After stimulation of the receptor, LYN proto-oncogene, an Src family kinase, phosphorylates the Igα and Igβ immune-receptor tyrosine-based activation motifs (ITAMs), thereby creating a docking site for the two SH2 domains of SYK [35]. SYK activates PI3Kδ and catalyzes the conversion of membrane-associated phosphatidylinositol 4,5 bis-phosphate (PIP2] to phosphatidylinositol 3,4,5-trisphosphate (PIP3]. PIP3 recruits the amino-terminal PH lipid-interaction component of BTK, thereby permitting SYK and LYN to catalyze the trans-phosphorylation of BTK at Y551, resulting in enzymes activation. Additionally, PIP3 molecules, within the membrane, can directly facilitate trans-phosphorylation of BTK as well [36].

BTK catalyzes the phosphorylation of phospholipase C gamma 2 (PLCγ2] at Y753 and Y759, which is critical for its lipase activity [11]. PLCγ2 catalyzes the hydrolysis of PIP2 into inositol trisphosphate (IP3] and diacylglycerol (DAG). IP3 is required for calcium ion (Ca^{2+}) flux from intracellular stores. Consecutively, DAG and Ca^{2+} activate protein kinase C beta (PKC β), which initiates the MAPK kinases signaling pathway promoting cell growth, proliferation, and survival (Fig. 1) [37, 38]. Additionally, PKCβ activates the NF-κB signaling pathway through a scaffold complex including CARD11 (caspase recruitment domain-containing protein 11], BCL10 (B cell lymphoma protein 10], and MALT1 (mucosa-associated lymphoid tissue lymphoma translocation protein 1], thereby BTK links the BCR to NF-κB activation [38, 39].

BTK in Other Signaling Pathways

Chemokine Receptors

BTK participates in many pathways, including TLR and chemokine receptor signaling in B cells. Chemokine receptors are guanine nucleotide-binding protein (G-protein) coupled receptors composed of seven trans-membrane bridging domains and intracellular hetero-trimeric G-proteins consisting of Gα, Gβ, and Gγ subunits [40]. BTK is one of the crucial signaling molecules for the chemokine receptors, CXCR4 and CXCR5 (Fig. 3) [41]. B-cells express CXCR4 and CXCR5 during several developmental phases. These receptors are required for trafficking, homing, and homeostasis [42]. Studies have illustrated that CXCL12, or stromal derived factor 1 (SDF-1], a chemokine primarily secreted by stromal cells in the bone marrow, readily activates BTK. The chemokine ligands bind to the extracellular domains of its respective receptors (*e.g.* binding of CXCL12 to CXCR4] and induce conformational modifications in the receptor resulting in dissociation of the coupled Gα and Gβγ subunits. The Gα and Gβγ subunits can individually stimulate PI3K leading to activation of BTK, AKT, and MAPK signaling pathways [12, 43]. Additionally, both Gα and Gβγ subunits can directly bind BTK *via* the PH and TH domain and the Gα subunit can directly stimulate the activity of BTK as well [12, 44, 45]. The downstream signaling of BTK through CXCR4 and CXCR5 is essential for the movement of B cells in various lymphoid tissues. *In vivo* experiments have validated chemokine signaling in BTK using conditional BTK-deficient mice and revealed that the homing of B cells to lymph nodes were directly dependent on BTK activation [41].

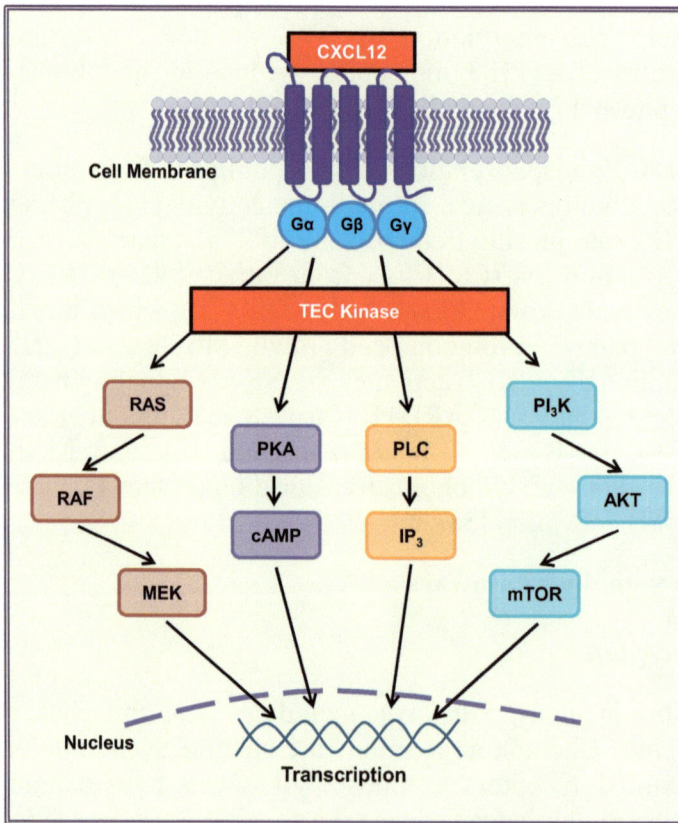

Fig. (3). The signaling cross-talk of CXCR4 and BTK.

Toll-like Receptors

A number of studies indicated that BTK and toll-like receptors (TLRs) cross-talk, for example, it has been demonstrated that BTK- deficient cells do not respond to lipopolysaccharides, which is a ligand of TLRs [46]. The common cross point of TLR and BTK signaling is the adaptor myeloid differentiation primary response 88 protein (MYD88] [47]. MYD88 activates interleukin-1- receptor-associated kinase 1 (IRAK1] in combination with another adaptor protein called TIR domain -containing adaptor protein (TIRAP, also known as MyD88 adapter-like, MAL). It has been demonstrated that BTK interacts with these intermediate TIR, MYD88, IRAK1, and TIRAP/MAL proteins downstream of the TLR [13, 14, 48]. TLR signaling also induces several transcription factors, including activator protein-1 (AP-1], interferon regulatory factor 3 (IRF3], and NF-κB. These transcription factors regulate a number of proteins involved in antibody secretion, class switch recombination, pro-inflammatory cytokine production, and proliferation in B cells. Furthermore, studies have shown synergy between TLR and BCR signaling in the secretion of IL-6, as well as generation of auto-phagosomes- like compartments [49]. Because of BCR's unique position at the cell surface and its connection with intracellular compartments, it can regulate a variety of signaling, thus making it a unique signaling component and the connection of TLR and BCR further make this signaling even more important [50].

Fc Receptor Signaling

The cross-talk between BTK and Fc receptors has been reported by several investigators [16]. BTK is one of the main components of both ITAM (Immunoreceptor tyrosine-based activation motif)-activating and ITIM (Immunoreceptor tyrosine-based inhibitory motif)-inhibitory Fc-receptors. The delicate balance between these two receptors regulates several biological activities, such as processing, activation, polarization, and phagocytosis of myeloid cells [15, 51]. In parallel to BCR signaling, following activating Fc-receptor cross-linking, SRC-kinases, SYK, PI3K-γ, and BTK are activated [15]. In contrast, inhibitory Fc-receptors (FcγRIIB) containing ITIM domains recruit phosphatases and reduce BTK activation.

Role of BTK Signaling in Hematological Malignancies

Chronic Lymphocytic Leukemia

Chronic lymphocytic leukemia (CLL) is the most prevalent adult leukemia in Western countries. Predominantly affecting the elderly, this condition is categorized by the increase of non-proliferating monoclonal low-level IgM, CD5+ mature B cells in the blood and hyper-activation of anti-apoptotic signaling pathways [52]. Several genetic abnormalities comprise CLL, including the loss of the chromosomal sections 17p13 (containing the TP53 tumor suppressor gene), 11q23 (containing DNA damage checkpoint protein ATM), or 13q14 (miR-15a, miR-16-1], and trisomy of chromosome 12 [53, 54]. Furthermore, above 80% of cases have a deletion of 17p and commonly carry TP53 mutations in the residual allele [55]. Patients with TP53 faults are classified as 'high-risk' and show poor responses to therapy [56]. Furthermore, a major fraction of CLL patients have TP53 mutation in the absence of a 17p deletion [57, 58].

Based on the somatic hyper mutation (SHM) status of Ig heavy variable (IGHV), CLL can be classified into mutated (M-CLL) and un-mutated CLL (U-CLL). Though the origin of U-CLL is not well understood yet [59 - 62], the gene profiling studies have demonstrated that M-CLL and U-CLL are quite homogeneous and related to memory B cells derived from T-cell dependent and T-cell independent [60], respectively. Though more studies have counter opinions and suggest that M-CLL and U-CLL have different origins [61]. The studies by Seifert *et al.* show that U-CLL derives from un-mutated mature CD5+ B cells and M-CLL originates from a distinct and previously unrecognized post germinal center (GC) B cell subset with a CD5+ CD27+ surface phenotype.

Numerous findings mentioned that the initiation or maintenance of CLL requires BTK signaling. The overexpression and constitutively phosphorylated BTK in CLL B cell patient samples is noteworthy [63]. In a CLL mouse model, BTK deficit revoked tumor development, whereas transgenic BTK overexpression amplified tumor occurrence and inclusive mortality [64, 65]. *In vitro* studies have demonstrated that ibrutinib reduced cell survival and propagation of CLL cells [63, 66]. Moreover, ibrutinib eliminated BCR-stimulated AKT, ERK phosphorylation, VCAM1 mediated adhesion [66, 67] and also reduced the expression of lymphocyte cytosolic protein 1 (LCP1; also known as plastic 2], which is filamentous actin (F-actin) cross-linking molecule and crucial for CXCL12 mediated migration [68]. The *in vitro* treatment of ibrutinib of CLL cells revealed an efficient blocking of CXCL12 and CXCL13 induced migration, indicating that BTK signaling controls CLL cell movement to propagative sites in lymph nodes [66, 67]. Also, the potential for disrupting the co-stimulatory feedback in the lymph node microenvironments was shown by reduced CLL cell survival, proliferation, and C-C motif chemokine ligand 3 (CCL3: also known as MIP1α) and C-C motif chemokine ligand 4 (CCL4] production when CLL cells were co-cultured with nurse-like cells (NLCs) [66]. Furthermore, ibrutinib treated patients with CLL had an overall decline in serum CCL3 and CCL4 levels [13], which are particularly very important because serum CCL3 is a strong marker of disease progression [69].

In vivo, BTK inhibition affects the overall survival of CLL cells showing cytotoxic effects. Ibrutinib treatment prompted lymphocytosis in CLL patients and mouse CLL adoptive transfer models [66, 70]. Also, BTK inhibition was effective in the removal of CLL cells from the protective lymph nodes environment [71].

Mantle Cell Lymphoma

Mantle cell lymphoma (MCL) is a type of B cell non-Hodgkin lymphoma in which its name "Mantle Cell Lymphoma" comes from the fact that the abnormal B cells originate in the mantle zone (the outer edge) of the lymph node [72]. A majority of MCL patients harbor the chromosomal translocation of t[11:14) (q13; 32) and more than 90 percent of MCL patient's lymphoma cells overexpress cyclin D1 [73]. While diagnosing MCL, the measurement of excess cyclin D1 from the biopsy is one of the most sensitive tools. The expression of sry box transcription factor 11 (SOX11] has also been observed to be high in MCL patients, indicating it as one of the specific markers for MCL independent of CCND1 positivity, suggesting a diagnostic role of SOX11 expression in t [11;14)-negative MCLs [74, 75]. Primary MCL cells show high expression phosphorylated BTK [76] and a subset of the patient also shows constitutive phosphorylation of LYN, SLP65, SYKs and PKCβ [77, 78]. Similar to CLL, the tumor microenvironment plays an essential role in the pathogenesis of MCL. To retain MCL cells in lymphoid tissues, BTK is essential since BTK inhibition departs malignant cells into the peripheral blood [79].

Waldenström's Macroglobulinemia

Waldenstrom macroglobulinemia (WM) is a kind of non-Hodgkin lymphoma (NHL). WM cells produce the IgM antibody in excess quantities. MYD88 L265P is a commonly recurring mutation in patients with WM that can be helpful in distinguishing WM and non-IgM lymphoplasmacytic lymphoma (LPL) from B-cell illnesses, as they have certain similar factors [80]. Additionally, it shows the role BTK has in this condition, as the mutated MyD88 L265P protein activates NF-κB signaling through binding with phosphorylated BTK [81]. Additionally, about 30% of WM patients show a somatic mutation of CXCR4 S338X and induce the activation of AKT and ERK under the influence of CXCL12. The CXCR4/CXCL12 axis plays critical role in the interaction of WM cells to bone marrow. Thus any mutation in the axis or modulation with drugs, such as ibrutinib, may disrupt the interaction of WM cells and overall survival [82, 83].

Diffuse Large B-cell Lymphoma

The diffuse large B-cell lymphoma (DLBCL) is one of the most common subtypes of B cell non-Hodgkin lymphoma (B-NHL) as it represents about 30-40% of all cases. The DLBLC patients develop tumors at various sites and it can be classified as either multiple or nodal or extra nodal. Based on the gene expressions, DLBCL can be further divided into three major groups: germinal center B-cell (GCB-DLBLCL), activated-B-cell-like (ABC-DLBCL), and primary mediastinal B-cell lymphoma (PMBL) [84]. The majority of cases are GCB-DLBCL and ABC-DLBCL, arising in similar incidence, whereas PMBL occurs in only 10% of cases of DLBCL [85]. ABC-DLBCL tumors primarily express IgM+, similar to that of antigen-activated plasmablasts, whereas gene expression in GCB-DLBCL is comparable to GC B-cells [86, 87]. ABC-DLBCL has less favorable clinical results than GCB-DLBCL with a three-year survival of only ~45% [88]. However, the survival and proliferation of ABC-DLBCL are essentially dependent on active NF-κB [89, 90]. Almost 50% of ABC-DLBCL populations show mutations in NF-κB signaling pathway, CARD11 and MyD88 through L265P mutation [91] and nearly 20% of patients have a mutation in BCR component CD79A/B. The knockdown of BCR components, CD79A/B, and related signaling modules with unmutated CARD11, leads to apoptosis in ABC-DLBCL cell lines confirming the role of NF-κB downstream of the BCR [92]. Moreover, NF-κB components in the TLR pathway and MyD88 and its associated kinase IRAK1, are shown to be essential for the survival of ABC-DLBCL. Furthermore, upregulation of SYK and loss of phosphatase and tensin homolog (PTEN, a phosphatase that targets PIP3], are also selective genetic modifications recognized in ABC-DLBCL [93]. In comparison with ABC-DLBCL, GCB DLBCLs do not harbor frequent mutations in CD79A/B or NF-κB modules. However, BTK inhibition leads to ABC-DLBCL reduction, whereas it does not have any effect on the survival of GCB-DLBCL patients [94].

Multiple Myeloma

Normal plasma cells are mainly found in the bone marrow and play an important part in the immune system. The overproduction of malignant monoclonal plasma cells in the bone marrow is the hallmark of multiple myeloma (MM) and results in altered bone homeostasis and hence osteolytic bone disease. Accumulation and uncontrolled proliferation of plasma cells disrupt the balance of osteoblast bone formation and osteoclast bone resorption, producing altered bone remodeling forces. The survival and proliferation of MM cells are encouraged by these altered signals generated within the bone marrow microenvironment (BMM) [95, 96]. The activation and proliferation of MM cells are governed by the ligands from the BMM, including key players such as osteoclasts, osteoblasts, endothelial cells, macrophages and bone marrow stromal cells (BMSCs) [97], producing chemicals such as APRIL (A Proliferation-Induction Ligand; aka TNFα), IL-6 and CXCL12 [98]. These signals create a protective niche within the bone marrow of patients with MM, resulting in a resilient and deadly disease. Thus, therapies that are in the process of development are targeting the pro-survival signals that are produced from the BMM [99].

Published mice studies have validated that NF-κB ligand (RANKL; also known as TNFSF11] prompts BTK and TEC, which are crucial for osteoclast development [22, 100]. By measuring bone contraction activity, it has been shown that ibrutinib inhibited *in vitro* osteoclast function by preventing RANKL-induced phosphorylation of BTK and downstream PLCγ activation. After the treatment of ibrutinib, an MM clinical study showed that osteoclasts and BMSCs reduced the secretion of tumor-supporting factors like APRIL, CCL3, CXCL12, and TGF-β. Additionally, ibrutinib abrogated CXCL12-induced adhesion and relocation of MM cells and reduced the proliferation that was initiated by IL-6 [101]. In an MM transplantation mouse model study, ibrutinib strongly abolished tumor development. Another study showed that ibrutinib repressed the *in vitro* colony-forming abilities of MM stem-like cells (MMSCs); it is, therefore, plausible that this drug might have significant effects in the signaling of MM stem-like cells (MMSCs) [101]. BTK inhibition in MM cells can also block additional pathways involved in disease progressions, such as TLR signaling, which, in MM, can exasperate disease progression [102] and protein products that are involved in NF-κB signaling [103 - 105].

THE DEVELOPMENT OF BTK INHIBITORS

Ibrutinib

Ibrutinib is a specific inhibitor of BTK developed by Pharmacyclics (Fig. **4**). It is an orally bioavailable, and irreversible BTK inhibitor that is highly competitive to endogenous ATP and covalently binds to Cys481 in the ATP binding domain [106]. Ibrutinib inhibits BTK catalytic activity, but is unable to block phosphorylation at Y551 by SYK. In the United States, ibrutinib was first approved to treat MCL patients in 2013, and later in 2014 was approved for CLL treatment. The European Union countries recommended the use of ibrutinib to treat resistant MCL and previously treated CLL patients with genetic mutations of del17p or TP53. Later in 2015, both the United States (U.S.) and European Union (E.U.) allowed physicians to treat WM patients with ibrutinib. The European Medicines Agency (EMA) and the FDA also approved ibrutinib for the treatment of R/R CLL and small lymphocytic lymphoma in combination with bendamustine and rituximab [107 - 109]. In a clinical study examing the efficacy of ibrutinib, the drug showed significant activity, and clinical safety was reported in patients with B-cell NHL and B-cell CLL. Mainly, the total response rate was ~71%, irrespective of clinical or genomic risk factors [110]. In a phase II study, patients with R/R MCL were treated orally with ibrutinib and had an overall response rate (ORR) of ~68% [111]. Ibrutinib was extremely active, related to strong responses, and non-toxic in pretreated patients with WM, but this drug is not responsive to the mutated MYD88 and CXCR4 neoplasms [112].

Several investigators reported the therapeutic mode of action of ibrutinib. Ibrutinib inhibits BTK tyrosine phosphorylation, along with blockade of downstream pathways regulated by this kinase, such as ERK1/2, PI3K, and NF-κB [63]. Ibrutinib also reduces the level of expression of BCR-dependent chemokines (CCL3, CCL4] in the CLL cells [66]. Ibrutinib inhibits cell interaction with the tumor microenvironment by blocking integrin α4β1-mediated adhesion of CLL cells to fibronectin and VCAM1 [67]. Thus, ibrutinib inhibits cell growth and the interaction with the tumor microenvironment.

Even though ibrutinib proved to be clinically successful in B cell malignancy treatment, there is a relapse in a minor fraction of patients. The development of resistance to ibrutinib is due to cysteine to serine mutation (C481S) occurring in the binding site of BTK, thus, allowing the protein to bypass ibrutinib binding. Besides two additional mutations in PLCγ2 (R665W, S707Y, and L845F) that are downstream to BTK, this drug resistance mechanism emphasizes the prominence of the BCR pathway in the mechanism of action of ibrutinib in CLL [113, 114]. More recently, an additional BTK mutation occurs at T316A in the SH2 domain and led to both clonal and primary leukemia progression in patients with ibrutinib-relapsed CLL [115]. Also, an initiating mutation has been reported in the L528W residue that confers resistance to ibrutinib in CLL patients [116]. The constant development of resistant clones has led to the discovery of the second generation of ibrutinib-like drugs [117]. Along these lines, several attempts have been made. The following section discusses the notable development.

Acalabrutinib (ACP-196]

Acalabrutinib is an irreversible BTK inhibitor, which is developed by Acerta Pharma. As shown in Fig. (**4**), it is structurally similar to ibrutinib, and covalently binds to the same amino acid residue (C481). However, it exhibits better selectivity and inhibitory potency to BTK and has less off-target kinase activity than ibrutinib [118]. Interestingly, acalabrutinib suppresses several other downstream targets, such as ERK, IKB, and AKT, in primary human CLL cells. On the other hand, it does not inhibit the kinase activities of ITK, EGFR, ERBB2, ERBB4, JAK3, BLK, FGR, FYN, HCK, LCK, LYN, SRC, and YES1 [119 - 121]. The overall response rate was ~ 95% in phase I and II clinical trials with R/R CLL patients, and it was 100% in patients having del [17] (p13.1) under the median follow-up up of ~ 14 months [122]. Additionally, thrombus formation was considerably repressed in platelets following ibrutinib treatment; however, no such effect on thrombus creation was recognized in patients treated with acalabrutinib. To date, there are no complaints related to bleeding, atrial fibrillation, or dose-limiting toxicity (DLT) issues. These discoveries strongly show that acalabrutinib has an enhanced care outline with marginal adverse effects compared with ibrutinib [123]. Currently, a phase III clinical trial is underway for R/R CLL patients to evaluate whether this molecule is better than ibrutinib (NCT02477696). Moreover, acalabrutinib insisted on a total response of ~ 81% in phase II clinical trial in patients with R/R MCL, and ~ 40% of patients succeeding a complete response [124]. These results prompted the FDA authorization for acalabrutinib in MCL treatment (2018).

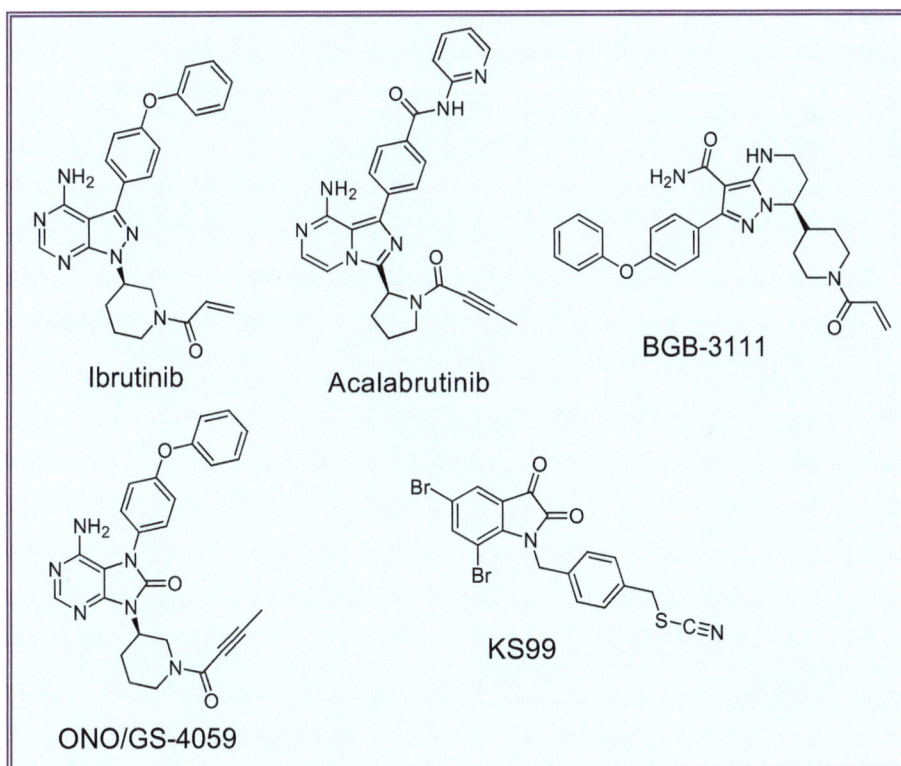

Fig. (4). The structure of various BTK inhibitors

BGB-3111

BGB-3111 is another specific BTK kinase inhibitor for various MCL and DLBCL cell lines (Fig. **4**). It has demonstrated oral bioavailability and binding selectivity superior to ibrutinib [125]. BGB-3111 exhibited more controlled off-target actions against a panel of kinases. Together with ITK in preclinical studies, BGB-3111 showed weaker activity than ibrutinib in preventing off-target antibody-dependent cell-mediated cytotoxicity (ADCC) induced by rituximab, because of comparatively less action against interleukin-2-inducible T cell kinase (ITK). Among advanced B cell malignancies, the first-in-human open-label phase 1 trial of BGB3111 is ongoing as a modified 3 + 3 dose-escalation (40, 80, 160, 320 mg PO QD; 160 mg PO BID). In this study, the pharmacokinetics, efficiency, and safety of BGB-3111 will be assessed. At the last update from the 2015 ASH annual meeting, 25 patients were enrolled in five cohorts: 40 mg (n = 4), 80 mg (n = 5), 160 mg (n = 6), 320 mg (n = 6) QD, and 160 mg BID (n = 4). Sixty-four percentage (16/25) of the patients had objective responses, including 1 CR and 6 SD. So far, no adverse effects and dose limited toxicities have been reported. These results indicate that this inhibitor is clinically secure, and acceptable as demonstrated in the early phase 1 trial. On the other hand, it was an initial study report, and its toxicity perception and clinical efficiency need to be assessed. Interestingly, phase I and II clinical studies on 45 CLL patients showed it was well tolerated and patients had a 90% recovery rate in a follow up of 7.5 months [126].

Tirabrutinib (Ono/GS-4059]

Tirabrutinib is another second-generation BTK inhibitor. It is an advanced version, a selective and more effective drug for B-cell malignancies (Fig. **4**). It could block auto-phosphorylation at Tyr223 of BTK through the signaling pathways of ERK, AKT, and PKD. In preclinical models and phase I clinical trials, this drug reveals remarkable antitumor activity. The success of ibrutinib against hematological malignancies inspired the researchers to develop many novel agents. Although novel BTK inhibitors have better potency and specificity than ibrutinib, they are in the initial stage of clinical studies. Importantly, now tirabrutinib is under phase II clinical trial for lymphoma patients with central nervous system complications [127, 128]. In 2014, Gilead got the approval for the development and commercialization of tirabrutinib for the treatment of B cell malignancies. Gilead has been exploring to improve the efficacy of this molecule by adding either obinutuzumab or idellalisib. Remarkably, in 2017, tirabrutinib was labeled as an orphan drug for the treatment of CLL in the U.S.

KS99

The research group of this study recently showed that KS99, a dual inhibitor of BTK and tubulin polymerization, inhibits the cell proliferation of MM cells [129]. They synthesized this novel molecule from the backbone of the natural agent isatin [130] and showed that KS99 modulates phosphorylation and expression of BTK, inhibits constitutive NF-κB activation, suppresses RANKL- induced osteoclastogenesis, and MM tumor growth in athymic nude mice and significantly suppressed the survival of MMSCs, which are key mediators of relapse [129]. It was shown, for the first time, that KS99 inhibits 50% kinase activities (IC_{50} at much lower concentration (0.5μM) than the concentrations required to inhibit phosphorylation of BTK (2.5μM) [129]. It was also confirmed that inhibition of BTK further inhibits one of the downstream substrates of BTK, PLCγ2 [131]. Thus, it was shown that KS99 not only interacts with BTK, but also inhibits the BTK mediated signaling pathways.

CONCLUSIONS AND FUTURE DIRECTIONS

This chapter presents a thorough summary of the present facts about the roles BTK plays in B cell malignancy. BTK is a critical component in B cell growth and differentiation, thus, targeting of BTK function forms a rational therapeutic approach in many B cell-related cancers. BTK inhibition also presents as a fantastically promising point of entry for modulating and regulating the tumor microenvironment as well as to dampen the tumor's capacity to induce immunotolerance. This, along with its effect on stem cells, has great potential in numerous neoplasms, including MM. Small molecule inhibitors are gaining traction as a smart curative approach for patients with B cell malignancies. Considerable progress has also been made in the therapeutic strategy for BTK inhibition. However, ibrutinib and acalabrutinib represent long-awaited therapies for patients with high-risk CLL or B cell lymphoma. Clinical trials with ibrutinib in patients with B cell malignancies confirmed that BTK inhibition by ibrutinib was well tolerated but it may be more helpful to use BTK inhibitors that show a broad range of kinases inhibition related to specific malignancies. Even though the worth of BTK inhibition as a single agent therapy is important, the resistance may develop. Therefore, to overcome this problem, a wide variety of studies focus on the effective combination of therapies to enhance clinical outcomes. A combination of BTK inhibitors and other specific inhibitors (new CD19 and CD20 antibodies, BCL-2 inhibitors, PI3 kinase inhibitors, ALK inhibitors, *etc.*) for B cell malignancies show great promise to enhance therapeutic responses. The summaries of difference in efficacy and toxicity between existing inhibitors of BTK predict an authentic clinical practice. Therefore, in conclusion, other selective BTK inhibitors, like ONO/GS-4059, ARQ-531, and BGB-3111 that are currently in clinical studies are leading to keep the door open for even more innovative treatment options, currently under development, to become accessible for B cell malignancies.

CONSENT FOR PUBLICATION

Not applicable.

CONFLICT OF INTEREST

The authors declare no conflict of interest, financial or otherwise.

ACKNOWLEDGEMENTS

This work was supported by the departmental fund from Cooper Medical School of Rowan University, Camden, NJ (M.K.P.), and partially from the Camden Research Initiative grant of Rowan University (M.K.P.).

ABBREVIATIONS

ABC-DLBCL	Activated B-cell-like Diffuse Large B-cell Lymphoma
ADCC	Antibody-Dependent Cell-Mediated Cytotoxicity
AEs	adverse effects
ALK	ALK Receptor Tyrosine Kinase
AP-1	Activator Protein-1
APRIL	A Proliferation-Induction Ligand
ASEAN	Association of Southeast Asian Nations
ASH	American Society of Hematology
ATP	Adenosine Tri-Phosphate
B-NHL	B cell Non-Hodgkin Lymphoma
BCL10	B cell Lymphoma Protein 10
BCL-XL	B Cell Lymphoma-Extra Large
BCR	B Cell Receptor
BID	Bi-daily
BLK	BLK Proto-Oncogene, Src Family Tyrosine Kinase
BTK	Bruton's Tyrosine Kinase
CARD11	Caspase Recruitment Domain-Containing Protein 11
CCL	C-C Motif Chemokine Ligand
CLL	Chronic Lymphocytic Leukemia
CR	Complete Remission
CXCR	Chemokine Receptor
CXCL	Chemokine Ligand
DAG	Diacylglycerol
DLBCL	Diffuse Large B-cell Lymphoma
DLTs	Dose Limited Toxicities
EU	European Union

EGFR	Epidermal Growth Factor Receptor
EMA	European Medicine Agency
ERBB	Erb-B2 Receptor Tyrosine Kinase
ERK	Extracellular-Signal-Related Kinase
F-actin	Filamentous Actin
FDA	Food and Drug Administration
FGR	FGR Proto-oncogene, Src Family Tyrosine Kinase
FYN	FYN Proto-oncogene, Src Family Tyrosine Kinase
GC	Germinal Center
GCB-DLBCL	Germinal Center B-cell-like Diffuse Large B-cell Lymphoma
HCK	Hematopoietic Cell Kinase
IgHC	Immunoglobulin Heavy Chain
IGHV	Immunoglobulin Heavy Variable
IgLC	Immunoglobulin Light Chain
IL	Interleukin
IP3	Inositol Triphosphate
IRAK1	Interleukin-1 Receptor-Associated Kinase 1
IRF	Interferon Regulatory Factor
ITAM	Immunoreceptor Tyrosine-based Activation Motif
ITIM	Immunoreceptor Tyrosine-based Inhibitory Motif
ITK	Intereukin-2-Inducible T cell Kinase
JAK3	Janus Kinase 3
LCK	LCK Proto-oncogene, Src Family Tyrosine Kinase
LCP1	Lymphocyte Cytosolic Protein 1
LPL	Lymphoplasmacytic Lymphoma
LPS	Lipopolysaccharide
LYN	LYN Proto-oncogene, Src Family Tyrosine Kinase
M-CLL	Mutated-Chronic Lymphocytic Leukemia
MAL	MYD88-adaptor-like
MALT1	MALT1 Paracaspase
MAPK	Mitogen-Activated Protein Kinase
MCL	Mantel Cell Lymphoma
MM	Multiple Myeloma
MTD	Maximum Tolerated Dose
MYD88	MYD88 Innate Immune Signal Transduction Adaptor

MZ	Marginal Zone
NFAT	Nuclear Factor of Activated T cells
NFκB	Nuclear Factor Kappa B
NHL	Non-Hodgkin Lymphoma
NK	Natural Killer
NLCs	Nurse-Like Cells
NLRP3	NOD-,LRR- and Pryin Domain-Containing Protein 3
PCNSL	Primary Central Nervous System Lymphoma
PH	Pleckstrin Homology
PI3K	Phosphoinositide 3-Kinase
PIP2	Phosphatidylinositol 4,5-bisphosphate
PIP3	Phosphatidylinositol 3,4,5-trisphosphate
PKC	Protein Kinase C
PLCγ	Phospholipase Cγ
PMBL	Primary Mediastinal B-cell Lymphoma
PO	Oral Administration
PTEN	Phosphatase and Tensin Homolog
PTKs	Protein Kinases
QD	Once Daily
RANK	Receptor Activator of Nuclear Factor-κB
RANKL	Receptor Activator of Nuclear Factor-κB Ligand
SD	Standard Deviation
SHM	Somatic Hyper Mutation
SOX11	SRY-Box Transcription Factor 11
SRC	SRC Proto-oncogene, Non-receptor Tyrosine Kinase
SYK	Spleen Associated Tyrosine Kinase
TEC	TEC Protein Tyrosine Kinase
TH	Tec Homology
TIRAP	TIR Domain Containing Adaptor Protein
TLR	Toll Like Receptor
U-CLL	Unmutated-Chronic Lymphocytic Leukemia
US	United States
VCAM-1	Vascular Cell Adhesion Molecule-1
WM	Waldenström's Macroglobulinemia

| XLA | X-Linked Agammaglobulinemia |
| YES1 | YES Proto-oncogene, Src Family Tyrosine Kinase |

REFERENCES

[1] Manning G, Whyte DB, Martinez R, Hunter T, Sudarsanam S. The protein kinase complement of the human genome. Science 2002; 298(5600): 1912-34.
[http://dx.doi.org/10.1126/science.1075762] [PMID: 12471243]

[2] Alonso A, Sasin J, Bottini N, *et al.* Protein tyrosine phosphatases in the human genome. Cell 2004; 117(6): 699-711.
[http://dx.doi.org/10.1016/j.cell.2004.05.018] [PMID: 15186772]

[3] Gross S, Rahal R, Stransky N, Lengauer C, Hoeflich KP. Targeting cancer with kinase inhibitors. J Clin Invest 2015; 125(5): 1780-9.
[http://dx.doi.org/10.1172/JCI76094] [PMID: 25932675]

[4] Hanahan D, Weinberg RA. Hallmarks of cancer: the next generation. Cell 2011; 144(5): 646-74.
[http://dx.doi.org/10.1016/j.cell.2011.02.013] [PMID: 21376230]

[5] Vetrie D, Vorechovský I, Sideras P, *et al.* The gene involved in X-linked agammaglobulinaemia is a member of the src family of protein-tyrosine kinases. Nature 1993; 361(6409): 226-33.
[http://dx.doi.org/10.1038/361226a0] [PMID: 8380905]

[6] Tsukada S, Saffran DC, Rawlings DJ, *et al.* Deficient expression of a B cell cytoplasmic tyrosine kinase in human X-linked agammaglobulinemia. Cell 1993; 72(2): 279-90.
[http://dx.doi.org/10.1016/0092-8674(93)90667-F] [PMID: 8425221]

[7] Thomas JD, Sideras P, Smith CI, Vorechovský I, Chapman V, Paul WE. Colocalization of X-linked agammaglobulinemia and X-linked immunodeficiency genes. Science 1993; 261(5119): 355-8.
[http://dx.doi.org/10.1126/science.8332900] [PMID: 8332900]

[8] Rawlings DJ, Saffran DC, Tsukada S, *et al.* Mutation of unique region of Bruton's tyrosine kinase in immunodeficient XID mice. Science 1993; 261(5119): 358-61.
[http://dx.doi.org/10.1126/science.8332901] [PMID: 8332901]

[9] Hyvönen M, Saraste M. Structure of the PH domain and Btk motif from Bruton's tyrosine kinase: molecular explanations for X-linked agammaglobulinaemia. EMBO J 1997; 16(12): 3396-404.
[http://dx.doi.org/10.1093/emboj/16.12.3396] [PMID: 9218782]

[10] Bradshaw JM. The Src, Syk, and Tec family kinases: distinct types of molecular switches. Cell Signal 2010; 22(8): 1175-84.
[http://dx.doi.org/10.1016/j.cellsig.2010.03.001] [PMID: 20206686]

[11] Hendriks RW, Yuvaraj S, Kil LP. Targeting Bruton's tyrosine kinase in B cell malignancies. Nat Rev Cancer 2014; 14(4): 219-32.
[http://dx.doi.org/10.1038/nrc3702] [PMID: 24658273]

[12] Lowry WE, Huang XYG. G Protein beta gamma subunits act on the catalytic domain to stimulate Bruton's agammaglobulinemia tyrosine kinase. J Biol Chem 2002; 277(2): 1488-92.
[http://dx.doi.org/10.1074/jbc.M110390200] [PMID: 11698416]

[13] Jefferies CA, Doyle S, Brunner C, *et al.* Bruton's tyrosine kinase is a Toll/interleukin-1 receptor domain-binding protein that participates in nuclear factor kappaB activation by Toll-like receptor 4. J Biol Chem 2003; 278(28): 26258-64.
[http://dx.doi.org/10.1074/jbc.M301484200] [PMID: 12724322]

[14] Gray P, Dunne A, Brikos C, Jefferies CA, Doyle SL, O'Neill LA. MyD88 adapter-like (Mal) is phosphorylated by Bruton's tyrosine kinase during TLR2 and TLR4 signal transduction. J Biol Chem 2006; 281(15): 10489-95.
[http://dx.doi.org/10.1074/jbc.M508892200] [PMID: 16439361]

[http://dx.doi.org/10.1038/nri2206] [PMID: 18064051]

[16]   Kawakami Y, Yao L, Miura T, Tsukada S, Witte ON, Kawakami T. Tyrosine phosphorylation and activation of Bruton tyrosine kinase upon Fc epsilon RI cross-linking. Mol Cell Biol 1994; 14(8): 5108-13.
[http://dx.doi.org/10.1128/MCB.14.8.5108] [PMID: 7518558]

[17]   Hata D, Kawakami Y, Inagaki N, *et al.* Involvement of Bruton's tyrosine kinase in FcepsilonRI-dependent mast cell degranulation and cytokine production. J Exp Med 1998; 187(8): 1235-47.
[http://dx.doi.org/10.1084/jem.187.8.1235] [PMID: 9547335]

[18]   Jongstra-Bilen J, Puig Cano A, Hasija M, Xiao H, Smith CI, Cybulsky MI. Dual functions of Bruton's tyrosine kinase and Tec kinase during Fcgamma receptor-induced signaling and phagocytosis. J Immunol 2008; 181(1): 288-98.
[http://dx.doi.org/10.4049/jimmunol.181.1.288] [PMID: 18566394]

[19]   Wang D, Feng J, Wen R, *et al.* Phospholipase Cgamma2 is essential in the functions of B cell and several Fc receptors. Immunity 2000; 13(1): 25-35.
[http://dx.doi.org/10.1016/S1074-7613(00)00005-4] [PMID: 10933392]

[20]   Ito M, Shichita T, Okada M, *et al.* Bruton's tyrosine kinase is essential for NLRP3 inflammasome activation and contributes to ischaemic brain injury. Nat Commun 2015; 6: 7360.
[http://dx.doi.org/10.1038/ncomms8360] [PMID: 26059659]

[21]   Oda A, Ikeda Y, Ochs HD, *et al.* Rapid tyrosine phosphorylation and activation of Bruton's tyrosine/Tec kinases in platelets induced by collagen binding or CD32 cross-linking. Blood 2000; 95(5): 1663-70.
[PMID: 10688822]

[22]   Shinohara M, Koga T, Okamoto K, *et al.* Tyrosine kinases Btk and Tec regulate osteoclast differentiation by linking RANK and ITAM signals. Cell 2008; 132(5): 794-806.
[http://dx.doi.org/10.1016/j.cell.2007.12.037] [PMID: 18329366]

[23]   Kokabee L, Wang X, Sevinsky CJ, *et al.* Bruton's tyrosine kinase is a potential therapeutic target in prostate cancer. Cancer Biol Ther 2015; 16(11): 1604-15.
[http://dx.doi.org/10.1080/15384047.2015.1078023] [PMID: 26383180]

[24]   Grassilli E, Pisano F, Cialdella A, *et al.* A novel oncogenic BTK isoform is overexpressed in colon cancers and required for RAS-mediated transformation. Oncogene 2016; 35(33): 4368-78.
[http://dx.doi.org/10.1038/onc.2015.504] [PMID: 26804170]

[25]   Zucha MA, Wu AT, Lee WH, *et al.* Bruton's tyrosine kinase (Btk) inhibitor ibrutinib suppresses stem-like traits in ovarian cancer. Oncotarget 2015; 6(15): 13255-68.
[http://dx.doi.org/10.18632/oncotarget.3658] [PMID: 26036311]

[26]   Rawlings DJ, Scharenberg AM, Park H, *et al.* Activation of BTK by a phosphorylation mechanism initiated by SRC family kinases. Science 1996; 271(5250): 822-5.
[http://dx.doi.org/10.1126/science.271.5250.822] [PMID: 8629002]

[27]   Park H, Wahl MI, Afar DE, *et al.* Regulation of Btk function by a major autophosphorylation site within the SH3 domain. Immunity 1996; 4(5): 515-25.
[http://dx.doi.org/10.1016/S1074-7613(00)80417-3] [PMID: 8630736]

[28]   Marcotte DJ, Liu YT, Arduini RM, *et al.* Structures of human Bruton's tyrosine kinase in active and inactive conformations suggest a mechanism of activation for TEC family kinases. Protein Sci 2010; 19(3): 429-39.
[http://dx.doi.org/10.1002/pro.321] [PMID: 20052711]

[29]   Middendorp S, Dingjan GM, Maas A, Dahlenborg K, Hendriks RW. Function of Bruton's tyrosine kinase during B cell development is partially independent of its catalytic activity. J Immunol 2003; 171(11): 5988-96.
[http://dx.doi.org/10.4049/jimmunol.171.11.5988] [PMID: 14634110]

[30]   Anderson JS, Teutsch M, Dong Z, Wortis HH. An essential role for Bruton's [corrected] tyrosine kinase in the regulation of B-cell apoptosis. Proc Natl Acad Sci USA 1996; 93(20): 10966-71.
[http://dx.doi.org/10.1073/pnas.93.20.10966] [PMID: 8855292]

[31]   Solvason N, Wu WW, Kabra N, *et al.* Transgene expression of bcl-xL permits anti-immunoglobulin (Ig)-induced proliferation in xid B cells. J Exp Med 1998; 187(7): 1081-91.
[http://dx.doi.org/10.1084/jem.187.7.1081] [PMID: 9529324]

[32]   Brorson K, Brunswick M, Ezhevsky S, *et al.* xid affects events leading to B cell cycle entry. J Immunol 1997; 159(1): 135-43.
[PMID: 9200448]

[33]   Glassford J, Soeiro I, Skarell SM, *et al.* BCR targets cyclin D2 *via* Btk and the p85alpha subunit of PI3-K to induce cell cycle progression in primary mouse B cells. Oncogene 2003; 22(15): 2248-59.
[http://dx.doi.org/10.1038/sj.onc.1206425] [PMID: 12700661]

[34]   Spaargaren M, Beuling EA, Rurup ML, *et al.* The B cell antigen receptor controls integrin activity through Btk and PLCgamma2. J Exp Med 2003; 198(10): 1539-50.
[http://dx.doi.org/10.1084/jem.20011866] [PMID: 14610042]

[35]   Mócsai A, Ruland J, Tybulewicz VL. The SYK tyrosine kinase: a crucial player in diverse biological functions. Nat Rev Immunol 2010; 10(6): 387-402.
[http://dx.doi.org/10.1038/nri2765] [PMID: 20467426]

[36]   Saito K, Scharenberg AM, Kinet JP. Interaction between the Btk PH domain and phosphatidylinositol-3,4,5-trisphosphate directly regulates Btk. J Biol Chem 2001; 276(19): 16201-6.
[http://dx.doi.org/10.1074/jbc.M100873200] [PMID: 11279148]

[37]   Okada H, Bolland S, Hashimoto A, *et al.* Role of the inositol phosphatase SHIP in B cell receptor-induced Ca2+ oscillatory response. J Immunol 1998; 161(10): 5129-32.
[PMID: 9820480]

[38]   Petro JB, Rahman SM, Ballard DW, Khan WN. Bruton's tyrosine kinase is required for activation of IkappaB kinase and nuclear factor kappaB in response to B cell receptor engagement. J Exp Med 2000; 191(10): 1745-54.
[http://dx.doi.org/10.1084/jem.191.10.1745] [PMID: 10811867]

[39]   Bajpai UD, Zhang K, Teutsch M, Sen R, Wortis HH. Bruton's tyrosine kinase links the B cell receptor to nuclear factor kappaB activation. J Exp Med 2000; 191(10): 1735-44.
[http://dx.doi.org/10.1084/jem.191.10.1735] [PMID: 10811866]

[40]   Ritter SL, Hall RA. Fine-tuning of GPCR activity by receptor-interacting proteins. Nat Rev Mol Cell Biol 2009; 10(12): 819-30.
[http://dx.doi.org/10.1038/nrm2803] [PMID: 19935667]

[41]   de Gorter DJ, Beuling EA, Kersseboom R, *et al.* Bruton's tyrosine kinase and phospholipase Cgamma2 mediate chemokine-controlled B cell migration and homing. Immunity 2007; 26(1): 93-104.
[http://dx.doi.org/10.1016/j.immuni.2006.11.012] [PMID: 17239630]

[42]   Okada T, Ngo VN, Ekland EH, *et al.* Chemokine requirements for B cell entry to lymph nodes and Peyer's patches. J Exp Med 2002; 196(1): 65-75.
[http://dx.doi.org/10.1084/jem.20020201] [PMID: 12093871]

[43]   Servant G, Weiner OD, Herzmark P, Balla T, Sedat JW, Bourne HR. Polarization of chemoattractant receptor signaling during neutrophil chemotaxis. Science 2000; 287(5455): 1037-40.
[http://dx.doi.org/10.1126/science.287.5455.1037] [PMID: 10669415]

[44]   Tsukada S, Simon MI, Witte ON, Katz A. Binding of beta gamma subunits of heterotrimeric G proteins to the PH domain of Bruton tyrosine kinase. Proc Natl Acad Sci USA 1994; 91(23): 11256-60.
[http://dx.doi.org/10.1073/pnas.91.23.11256] [PMID: 7972043]

[45]   Bence K, Ma W, Kozasa T, Huang XY. Direct stimulation of Bruton's tyrosine kinase by G(q)-protein alpha-subunit. Nature 1997; 389(6648): 296-9.
[http://dx.doi.org/10.1038/38520] [PMID: 9305846]

[46]   Khan WN, Alt FW, Gerstein RM, *et al.* Defective B cell development and function in Btk-deficient mice. Immunity 1995; 3(3): 283-99.
[http://dx.doi.org/10.1016/1074-7613(95)90114-0] [PMID: 7552994]

[47]   Rawlings DJ, Schwartz MA, Jackson SW, Meyer-Bahlburg A. Integration of B cell responses through Toll-like receptors and antigen receptors. Nat Rev Immunol 2012; 12(4): 282-94.
[http://dx.doi.org/10.1038/nri3190] [PMID: 22421786]

[48]   Liu X, Zhan Z, Li D, *et al.* Intracellular MHC class II molecules promote TLR-triggered innate immune responses by maintaining activation of the kinase Btk. Nat Immunol 2011; 12(5): 416-24.
[http://dx.doi.org/10.1038/ni.2015] [PMID: 21441935]

[49]   Kenny EF, Quinn SR, Doyle SL, Vink PM, van Eenennaam H, O'Neill LA. Bruton's tyrosine kinase mediates the synergistic signalling between TLR9 and the B cell receptor by regulating calcium and calmodulin. PLoS One 2013; 8(8): e74103.
[http://dx.doi.org/10.1371/journal.pone.0074103] [PMID: 23967355]

[50]   Chaturvedi A, Dorward D, Pierce SK. The B cell receptor governs the subcellular location of Toll-like receptor 9 leading to hyperresponses to DNA-containing antigens. Immunity 2008; 28(6): 799-809.
[http://dx.doi.org/10.1016/j.immuni.2008.03.019] [PMID: 18513998]

[51]   Bournazos S, Wang TT, Ravetch JV. The Role and Function of Fcγ Receptors on Myeloid Cells. Microbiol Spectr 2016; 4(6).
[PMID: 28087938]

[52]   Ammann EM, Shanafelt TD, Wright KB, McDowell BD, Link BK, Chrischilles EA. Updating survival estimates in patients with chronic lymphocytic leukemia or small lymphocytic lymphoma (CLL/SLL) based on treatment-free interval length. Leuk Lymphoma 2018; 59(3): 643-9.
[http://dx.doi.org/10.1080/10428194.2017.1349905] [PMID: 28718694]

[53]   Kil LP, Yuvaraj S, Langerak AW, Hendriks RW. The role of B cell receptor stimulation in CLL pathogenesis. Curr Pharm Des 2012; 18(23): 3335-55.
[http://dx.doi.org/10.2174/138161212801227041] [PMID: 22591389]

[54]   Zenz T, Eichhorst B, Busch R, *et al.* TP53 mutation and survival in chronic lymphocytic leukemia. J Clin Oncol 2010; 28(29): 4473-9.
[http://dx.doi.org/10.1200/JCO.2009.27.8762] [PMID: 20697090]

[55]   Gonzalez D, Martinez P, Wade R, *et al.* Mutational status of the TP53 gene as a predictor of response and survival in patients with chronic lymphocytic leukemia: results from the LRF CLL4 trial. J Clin Oncol 2011; 29(16): 2223-9.
[http://dx.doi.org/10.1200/JCO.2010.32.0838] [PMID: 21483000]

[56]   Robak P, Robak T. Novel synthetic drugs currently in clinical development for chronic lymphocytic leukemia. Expert Opin Investig Drugs 2017; 26(11): 1249-65.
[http://dx.doi.org/10.1080/13543784.2017.1384814] [PMID: 28942659]

[57]   Zenz T, Kröber A, Scherer K, *et al.* Monoallelic TP53 inactivation is associated with poor prognosis in chronic lymphocytic leukemia: results from a detailed genetic characterization with long-term follow-up. Blood 2008; 112(8): 3322-9.
[http://dx.doi.org/10.1182/blood-2008-04-154070] [PMID: 18689542]

[58]   Malcikova J, Smardova J, Rocnova L, *et al.* Monoallelic and biallelic inactivation of TP53 gene in chronic lymphocytic leukemia: selection, impact on survival, and response to DNA damage. Blood 2009; 114(26): 5307-14.
[http://dx.doi.org/10.1182/blood-2009-07-234708] [PMID: 19850740]

[59]   Chiorazzi N, Ferrarini M. Cellular origin(s) of chronic lymphocytic leukemia: cautionary notes and

additional considerations and possibilities. Blood 2011; 117(6): 1781-91.
[http://dx.doi.org/10.1182/blood-2010-07-155663] [PMID: 21148333]

[60] Klein U, Tu Y, Stolovitzky GA, *et al.* Gene expression profiling of B cell chronic lymphocytic leukemia reveals a homogeneous phenotype related to memory B cells. J Exp Med 2001; 194(11): 1625-38.
[http://dx.doi.org/10.1084/jem.194.11.1625] [PMID: 11733577]

[61] Seifert M, Sellmann L, Bloehdorn J, *et al.* Cellular origin and pathophysiology of chronic lymphocytic leukemia. J Exp Med 2012; 209(12): 2183-98.
[http://dx.doi.org/10.1084/jem.20120833] [PMID: 23091163]

[62] DiLillo DJ, Weinberg JB, Yoshizaki A, *et al.* Chronic lymphocytic leukemia and regulatory B cells share IL-10 competence and immunosuppressive function. Leukemia 2013; 27(1): 170-82.
[http://dx.doi.org/10.1038/leu.2012.165] [PMID: 22713648]

[63] Herman SE, Gordon AL, Hertlein E, *et al.* Bruton tyrosine kinase represents a promising therapeutic target for treatment of chronic lymphocytic leukemia and is effectively targeted by PCI-32765. Blood 2011; 117(23): 6287-96.
[http://dx.doi.org/10.1182/blood-2011-01-328484] [PMID: 21422473]

[64] ter Brugge PJ, Ta VB, de Bruijn MJ, *et al.* A mouse model for chronic lymphocytic leukemia based on expression of the SV40 large T antigen. Blood 2009; 114(1): 119-27.
[http://dx.doi.org/10.1182/blood-2009-01-198937] [PMID: 19332766]

[65] Kil LP, de Bruijn MJ, van Hulst JA, Langerak AW, Yuvaraj S, Hendriks RW. Bruton's tyrosine kinase mediated signaling enhances leukemogenesis in a mouse model for chronic lymphocytic leukemia. Am J Blood Res 2013; 3(1): 71-83.
[PMID: 23359016]

[66] Ponader S, Chen SS, Buggy JJ, *et al.* The Bruton tyrosine kinase inhibitor PCI-32765 thwarts chronic lymphocytic leukemia cell survival and tissue homing *in vitro* and *in vivo.* Blood 2012; 119(5): 1182-9.
[http://dx.doi.org/10.1182/blood-2011-10-386417] [PMID: 22180443]

[67] de Rooij MF, Kuil A, Geest CR, *et al.* The clinically active BTK inhibitor PCI-32765 targets B-cell receptor- and chemokine-controlled adhesion and migration in chronic lymphocytic leukemia. Blood 2012; 119(11): 2590-4.
[http://dx.doi.org/10.1182/blood-2011-11-390989] [PMID: 22279054]

[68] Dubovsky JA, Chappell DL, Harrington BK, *et al.* Lymphocyte cytosolic protein 1 is a chronic lymphocytic leukemia membrane-associated antigen critical to niche homing. Blood 2013; 122(19): 3308-16.
[http://dx.doi.org/10.1182/blood-2013-05-504597] [PMID: 24009233]

[69] Sivina M, Hartmann E, Kipps TJ, *et al.* CCL3 (MIP-1α) plasma levels and the risk for disease progression in chronic lymphocytic leukemia. Blood 2011; 117(5): 1662-9.
[http://dx.doi.org/10.1182/blood-2010-09-307249] [PMID: 21115978]

[70] Byrd JC, Furman RR, Coutre SE, *et al.* Targeting BTK with ibrutinib in relapsed chronic lymphocytic leukemia. N Engl J Med 2013; 369(1): 32-42.
[http://dx.doi.org/10.1056/NEJMoa1215637] [PMID: 23782158]

[71] Herishanu Y, Pérez-Galán P, Liu D, *et al.* The lymph node microenvironment promotes B-cell receptor signaling, NF-kappaB activation, and tumor proliferation in chronic lymphocytic leukemia. Blood 2011; 117(2): 563-74.
[http://dx.doi.org/10.1182/blood-2010-05-284984] [PMID: 20940416]

[72] Cheah CY, Seymour JF, Wang ML. Mantle Cell Lymphoma. J Clin Oncol 2016; 34(11): 1256-69.
[http://dx.doi.org/10.1200/JCO.2015.63.5904] [PMID: 26755518]

[73] Bertoni F, Rinaldi A, Zucca E, Cavalli F. Update on the molecular biology of mantle cell lymphoma.

Hematol Oncol 2006; 24(1): 22-7.
[http://dx.doi.org/10.1002/hon.767] [PMID: 16402392]

[74]   Meggendorfer M, Kern W, Haferlach C, Haferlach T, Schnittger S. SOX11 overexpression is a specific marker for mantle cell lymphoma and correlates with t(11;14) translocation, CCND1 expression and an adverse prognosis. Leukemia 2013; 27(12): 2388-91.
[http://dx.doi.org/10.1038/leu.2013.141] [PMID: 23648671]

[75]   Navarro A, Clot G, Royo C, *et al.* Molecular subsets of mantle cell lymphoma defined by the IGHV mutational status and SOX11 expression have distinct biologic and clinical features. Cancer Res 2012; 72(20): 5307-16.
[http://dx.doi.org/10.1158/0008-5472.CAN-12-1615] [PMID: 22915760]

[76]   Cinar M, Hamedani F, Mo Z, Cinar B, Amin HM, Alkan S. Bruton tyrosine kinase is commonly overexpressed in mantle cell lymphoma and its attenuation by Ibrutinib induces apoptosis. Leuk Res 2013; 37(10): 1271-7.
[http://dx.doi.org/10.1016/j.leukres.2013.07.028] [PMID: 23962569]

[77]   Pighi C, Gu TL, Dalai I, *et al.* Phospho-proteomic analysis of mantle cell lymphoma cells suggests a pro-survival role of B-cell receptor signaling. Cell Oncol (Dordr) 2011; 34(2): 141-53.
[http://dx.doi.org/10.1007/s13402-011-0019-7] [PMID: 21394647]

[78]   Boyd RS, Jukes-Jones R, Walewska R, Brown D, Dyer MJ, Cain K. Protein profiling of plasma membranes defines aberrant signaling pathways in mantle cell lymphoma. Mol Cell Proteomics 2009; 8(7): 1501-15.
[http://dx.doi.org/10.1074/mcp.M800515-MCP200] [PMID: 19346216]

[79]   Chang BY, Francesco M, De Rooij MF, *et al.* Egress of CD19(+)CD5(+) cells into peripheral blood following treatment with the Bruton tyrosine kinase inhibitor ibrutinib in mantle cell lymphoma patients. Blood 2013; 122(14): 2412-24.
[http://dx.doi.org/10.1182/blood-2013-02-482125] [PMID: 23940282]

[80]   Treon SP, Xu L, Yang G, *et al.* MYD88 L265P somatic mutation in Waldenström's macroglobulinemia. N Engl J Med 2012; 367(9): 826-33.
[http://dx.doi.org/10.1056/NEJMoa1200710] [PMID: 22931316]

[81]   Yang G, Zhou Y, Liu X, *et al.* A mutation in MYD88 (L265P) supports the survival of lymphoplasmacytic cells by activation of Bruton tyrosine kinase in Waldenström macroglobulinemia. Blood 2013; 122(7): 1222-32.
[http://dx.doi.org/10.1182/blood-2012-12-475111] [PMID: 23836557]

[82]   Ngo HT, Leleu X, Lee J, *et al.* SDF-1/CXCR4 and VLA-4 interaction regulates homing in Waldenstrom macroglobulinemia. Blood 2008; 112(1): 150-8.
[http://dx.doi.org/10.1182/blood-2007-12-129395] [PMID: 18448868]

[83]   Hunter ZR, Xu L, Yang G, *et al.* The genomic landscape of Waldenstrom macroglobulinemia is characterized by highly recurring MYD88 and WHIM-like CXCR4 mutations, and small somatic deletions associated with B-cell lymphomagenesis. Blood 2014; 123(11): 1637-46.
[http://dx.doi.org/10.1182/blood-2013-09-525808] [PMID: 24366360]

[84]   Iqbal J, Shen Y, Huang X, *et al.* Global microRNA expression profiling uncovers molecular markers for classification and prognosis in aggressive B-cell lymphoma. Blood 2015; 125(7): 1137-45.
[http://dx.doi.org/10.1182/blood-2014-04-566778] [PMID: 25498913]

[85]   Dunleavy K, Wilson WH. Primary mediastinal B-cell lymphoma and mediastinal gray zone lymphoma: do they require a unique therapeutic approach? Blood 2015; 125(1): 33-9.
[http://dx.doi.org/10.1182/blood-2014-05-575092] [PMID: 25499450]

[86]   Alizadeh AA, Eisen MB, Davis RE, *et al.* Distinct types of diffuse large B-cell lymphoma identified by gene expression profiling. Nature 2000; 403(6769): 503-11.
[http://dx.doi.org/10.1038/35000501] [PMID: 10676951]

[87]   Lenz G, Nagel I, Siebert R, *et al.* Aberrant immunoglobulin class switch recombination and switch translocations in activated B cell-like diffuse large B cell lymphoma. J Exp Med 2007; 204(3): 633-43. [http://dx.doi.org/10.1084/jem.20062041] [PMID: 17353367]

[88]   Roschewski M, Staudt LM, Wilson WH. Diffuse large B-cell lymphoma-treatment approaches in the molecular era. Nat Rev Clin Oncol 2014; 11(1): 12-23. [http://dx.doi.org/10.1038/nrclinonc.2013.197] [PMID: 24217204]

[89]   Davis RE, Brown KD, Siebenlist U, Staudt LM. Constitutive nuclear factor kappaB activity is required for survival of activated B cell-like diffuse large B cell lymphoma cells. J Exp Med 2001; 194(12): 1861-74. [http://dx.doi.org/10.1084/jem.194.12.1861] [PMID: 11748286]

[90]   Compagno M, Lim WK, Grunn A, *et al.* Mutations of multiple genes cause deregulation of NF-kappaB in diffuse large B-cell lymphoma. Nature 2009; 459(7247): 717-21. [http://dx.doi.org/10.1038/nature07968] [PMID: 19412164]

[91]   Lenz G, Davis RE, Ngo VN, *et al.* Oncogenic CARD11 mutations in human diffuse large B cell lymphoma. Science 2008; 319(5870): 1676-9. [http://dx.doi.org/10.1126/science.1153629] [PMID: 18323416]

[92]   Davis RE, Ngo VN, Lenz G, *et al.* Chronic active B-cell-receptor signalling in diffuse large B-cell lymphoma. Nature 2010; 463(7277): 88-92. [http://dx.doi.org/10.1038/nature08638] [PMID: 20054396]

[93]   Chen L, Monti S, Juszczynski P, *et al.* SYK inhibition modulates distinct PI3K/AKT- dependent survival pathways and cholesterol biosynthesis in diffuse large B cell lymphomas. Cancer Cell 2013; 23(6): 826-38. [http://dx.doi.org/10.1016/j.ccr.2013.05.002] [PMID: 23764004]

[94]   Havranek O, Xu J, Köhrer S, *et al.* Tonic B-cell receptor signaling in diffuse large B-cell lymphoma. Blood 2017; 130(8): 995-1006. [http://dx.doi.org/10.1182/blood-2016-10-747303] [PMID: 28646116]

[95]   Kuehl WM, Bergsagel PL. Molecular pathogenesis of multiple myeloma and its premalignant precursor. J Clin Invest 2012; 122(10): 3456-63. [http://dx.doi.org/10.1172/JCI61188] [PMID: 23023717]

[96]   Raje N, Roodman GD. Advances in the biology and treatment of bone disease in multiple myeloma. Clin Cancer Res 2011; 17(6): 1278-86. [http://dx.doi.org/10.1158/1078-0432.CCR-10-1804] [PMID: 21411443]

[97]   Abe M, Kido S, Hiasa M, *et al.* BAFF and APRIL as osteoclast-derived survival factors for myeloma cells: a rationale for TACI-Fc treatment in patients with multiple myeloma. Leukemia 2006; 20(7): 1313-5. [http://dx.doi.org/10.1038/sj.leu.2404228] [PMID: 16617317]

[98]   Alsayed Y, Ngo H, Runnels J, *et al.* Mechanisms of regulation of CXCR4/SDF-1 (CXCL12)- dependent migration and homing in multiple myeloma. Blood 2007; 109(7): 2708-17. [http://dx.doi.org/10.1182/blood-2006-07-035857] [PMID: 17119115]

[99]   Hideshima T, Mitsiades C, Tonon G, Richardson PG, Anderson KC. Understanding multiple myeloma pathogenesis in the bone marrow to identify new therapeutic targets. Nat Rev Cancer 2007; 7(8): 585-98. [http://dx.doi.org/10.1038/nrc2189] [PMID: 17646864]

[100]   Lee SH, Kim T, Jeong D, Kim N, Choi Y. The tec family tyrosine kinase Btk Regulates RANKL-induced osteoclast maturation. J Biol Chem 2008; 283(17): 11526-34. [http://dx.doi.org/10.1074/jbc.M708935200] [PMID: 18281276]

[101]   Tai YT, Chang BY, Kong SY, *et al.* Bruton tyrosine kinase inhibition is a novel therapeutic strategy targeting tumor in the bone marrow microenvironment in multiple myeloma. Blood 2012; 120(9):

1877-87.
[http://dx.doi.org/10.1182/blood-2011-12-396853] [PMID: 22689860]

[102] Bao H, Lu P, Li Y, *et al.* Triggering of toll-like receptor-4 in human multiple myeloma cells promotes proliferation and alters cell responses to immune and chemotherapy drug attack. Cancer Biol Ther 2011; 11(1): 58-67.
[http://dx.doi.org/10.4161/cbt.11.1.13878] [PMID: 21248470]

[103] Chapman MA, Lawrence MS, Keats JJ, *et al.* Initial genome sequencing and analysis of multiple myeloma. Nature 2011; 471(7339): 467-72.
[http://dx.doi.org/10.1038/nature09837] [PMID: 21430775]

[104] Keats JJ, Fonseca R, Chesi M, *et al.* Promiscuous mutations activate the noncanonical NF-kappaB pathway in multiple myeloma. Cancer Cell 2007; 12(2): 131-44.
[http://dx.doi.org/10.1016/j.ccr.2007.07.003] [PMID: 17692805]

[105] Annunziata CM, Davis RE, Demchenko Y, *et al.* Frequent engagement of the classical and alternative NF-kappaB pathways by diverse genetic abnormalities in multiple myeloma. Cancer Cell 2007; 12(2): 115-30.
[http://dx.doi.org/10.1016/j.ccr.2007.07.004] [PMID: 17692804]

[106] Regan JA, Cao Y, Dispenza MC, Ma S, Gordon LI, Petrich AM, *et al.* Ibrutinib, a Bruton's tyrosine kinase inhibitor used for treatment of lymphoproliferative disorders, eliminates both aeroallergen skin test and basophil activation test reactivity. J Allergy Clin Immunol 2017; 140(3): 875-9. e1.

[107] Guha M. Imbruvica--next big drug in B-cell cancer--approved by FDA. Nat Biotechnol 2014; 32(2): 113-5.
[http://dx.doi.org/10.1038/nbt0214-113] [PMID: 24509736]

[108] Akinleye A, Chen Y, Mukhi N, Song Y, Liu D. Ibrutinib and novel BTK inhibitors in clinical development. J Hematol Oncol 2013; 6: 59.
[http://dx.doi.org/10.1186/1756-8722-6-59] [PMID: 23958373]

[109] Aalipour A, Advani RH. Bruton's tyrosine kinase inhibitors and their clinical potential in the treatment of B-cell malignancies: focus on ibrutinib. Ther Adv Hematol 2014; 5(4): 121-33.
[http://dx.doi.org/10.1177/2040620714539906] [PMID: 25360238]

[110] Advani RH, Buggy JJ, Sharman JP, *et al.* Bruton tyrosine kinase inhibitor ibrutinib (PCI-32765) has significant activity in patients with relapsed/refractory B-cell malignancies. J Clin Oncol 2013; 31(1): 88-94.
[http://dx.doi.org/10.1200/JCO.2012.42.7906] [PMID: 23045577]

[111] Wang ML, Rule S, Martin P, *et al.* Targeting BTK with ibrutinib in relapsed or refractory mantle-cell lymphoma. N Engl J Med 2013; 369(6): 507-16.
[http://dx.doi.org/10.1056/NEJMoa1306220] [PMID: 23782157]

[112] Treon SP, Tripsas CK, Meid K, *et al.* Ibrutinib in previously treated Waldenström's macroglobulinemia. N Engl J Med 2015; 372(15): 1430-40.
[http://dx.doi.org/10.1056/NEJMoa1501548] [PMID: 25853747]

[113] Woyach JA, Furman RR, Liu TM, *et al.* Resistance mechanisms for the Bruton's tyrosine kinase inhibitor ibrutinib. N Engl J Med 2014; 370(24): 2286-94.
[http://dx.doi.org/10.1056/NEJMoa1400029] [PMID: 24869598]

[114] Furman RR, Cheng S, Lu P, *et al.* Ibrutinib resistance in chronic lymphocytic leukemia. N Engl J Med 2014; 370(24): 2352-4.
[http://dx.doi.org/10.1056/NEJMc1402716] [PMID: 24869597]

[115] Kadri S, Lee J, Fitzpatrick C, *et al.* Clonal evolution underlying leukemia progression and Richter transformation in patients with ibrutinib-relapsed CLL. Blood Adv 2017; 1(12): 715-27.
[http://dx.doi.org/10.1182/bloodadvances.2016003632] [PMID: 29296715]

[116] Maddocks KJ, Ruppert AS, Lozanski G, *et al.* Etiology of Ibrutinib Therapy Discontinuation and

Outcomes in Patients With Chronic Lymphocytic Leukemia. JAMA Oncol 2015; 1(1): 80-7.
[http://dx.doi.org/10.1001/jamaoncol.2014.218] [PMID: 26182309]

[117] Janda E, Palmieri C, Pisano A, *et al.* Btk regulation in human and mouse B cells *via* protein kinase C phosphorylation of IBtkγ. Blood 2011; 117(24): 6520-31.
[http://dx.doi.org/10.1182/blood-2010-09-308080] [PMID: 21482705]

[118] Herman SEM, Montraveta A, Niemann CU, *et al.* The bruton tyrosine kinase (BTK) inhibitor acalabrutinib demonstrates potent on-target effects and efficacy in two mouse models of chronic lymphocytic leukemia. Clin Cancer Res 2017; 23(11): 2831-41.

[119] Fraietta JA, Beckwith KA, Patel PR, *et al.* Ibrutinib enhances chimeric antigen receptor T-cell engraftment and efficacy in leukemia. Blood 2016; 127(9): 1117-27.
[http://dx.doi.org/10.1182/blood-2015-11-679134] [PMID: 26813675]

[120] Harrington BK, Gardner HL, Izumi R, *et al.* Preclinical Evaluation of the Novel BTK Inhibitor Acalabrutinib in Canine Models of B-Cell Non-Hodgkin Lymphoma. PLoS One 2016; 11(7): e0159607.
[http://dx.doi.org/10.1371/journal.pone.0159607] [PMID: 27434128]

[121] Wu J, Zhang M, Liu D. Acalabrutinib (ACP-196): a selective second-generation BTK inhibitor. J Hematol Oncol 2016; 9: 21.
[http://dx.doi.org/10.1186/s13045-016-0250-9] [PMID: 26957112]

[122] Byrd JC, Harrington B, O'Brien S, *et al.* Acalabrutinib (ACP-196) in Relapsed Chronic Lymphocytic Leukemia. N Engl J Med 2016; 374(4): 323-32.
[http://dx.doi.org/10.1056/NEJMoa1509981] [PMID: 26641137]

[123] Herman SE, Sun X, McAuley EM, *et al.* Modeling tumor-host interactions of chronic lymphocytic leukemia in xenografted mice to study tumor biology and evaluate targeted therapy. Leukemia 2013; 27(12): 2311-21.
[http://dx.doi.org/10.1038/leu.2013.131] [PMID: 23619564]

[124] Wang M, Rule S, Zinzani PL, *et al.* Acalabrutinib in relapsed or refractory mantle cell lymphoma (ACE-LY-004): a single-arm, multicentre, phase 2 trial. Lancet 2018; 391(10121): 659-67.
[http://dx.doi.org/10.1016/S0140-6736(17)33108-2] [PMID: 29241979]

[125] Tam C, Grigg AP, Opat S, *et al.* The BTK inhibitor, Bgb-3111, is safe, tolerable, and highly active in patients with relapsed/ refractory b-cell malignancies: Initial report of a phase 1 first-in-human trial. Blood 2015; 126(23): 832-2.
[http://dx.doi.org/10.1182/blood.V126.23.832.832]

[126] Thompson PA, Burger JA. Bruton's tyrosine kinase inhibitors: first and second generation agents for patients with Chronic Lymphocytic Leukemia (CLL). Expert Opin Investig Drugs 2018; 27(1): 31-42.
[http://dx.doi.org/10.1080/13543784.2018.1404027] [PMID: 29125406]

[127] Walter HS, Rule SA, Dyer MJ, *et al.* A phase 1 clinical trial of the selective BTK inhibitor ONO/GS-4059 in relapsed and refractory mature B-cell malignancies. Blood 2016; 127(4): 411-9.
[http://dx.doi.org/10.1182/blood-2015-08-664086] [PMID: 26542378]

[128] Walter HS, Jayne S, Rule SA, *et al.* Long-term follow-up of patients with CLL treated with the selective Bruton's tyrosine kinase inhibitor ONO/GS-4059. Blood 2017; 129(20): 2808-10.
[http://dx.doi.org/10.1182/blood-2017-02-765115] [PMID: 28377400]

[129] Pandey MK, Gowda K, Sung SS, *et al.* A novel dual inhibitor of microtubule and Bruton's tyrosine kinase inhibits survival of multiple myeloma and osteoclastogenesis. Exp Hematol 2017; 53: 31-42.
[http://dx.doi.org/10.1016/j.exphem.2017.06.003] [PMID: 28647392]

[130] Krishnegowda G, Prakasha Gowda AS, Tagaram HR, *et al.* Synthesis and biological evaluation of a novel class of isatin analogs as dual inhibitors of tubulin polymerization and Akt pathway. Bioorg Med Chem 2011; 19(20): 6006-14.
[http://dx.doi.org/10.1016/j.bmc.2011.08.044] [PMID: 21920762]

[131] Kim YJ, Sekiya F, Poulin B, Bae YS, Rhee SG. Mechanism of B-cell receptor-induced phosphorylation and activation of phospholipase C-gamma2. Mol Cell Biol 2004; 24(22): 9986-99. [http://dx.doi.org/10.1128/MCB.24.22.9986-9999.2004] [PMID: 15509800]

CHAPTER 8

The Tumor Microenvironment Mediated Signaling Pathways in the Progression of Acute Myeloid Leukemia

Anup S. Pathania[1], Rachel Weber[2] and Kishore B. Challagundla[1,3,*]

[1] *Department of Biochemistry and Molecular Biology & The Fred and Pamela Buffett Cancer Center; University of Nebraska Medical Center, Omaha, NE, USA*

[2] *Department of Biochemistry and Molecular Biology, University of Nebraska Medical Center, Omaha, NE, USA*

[3] *The Children's Health Research Institute, University of Nebraska Medical Center, Omaha, NE, USA*

Abstract: Acute myeloid leukemia (AML) is a cancer of blood and bone marrow, caused by abnormal production of white blood cells. According to the recent 2020 statistics, an estimated number of 19,940 people in the United States will be diagnosed with AML. The hematologic tumor microenvironment plays a critical role in the progression of AML. Emerging evidence indicates that chemotherapy resistance and disease relapse are linked through the signaling pathways associated with the tumor microenvironment in AML. The leukemia cells communicate with the other non-cancerous cells of the tumor microenvironment through small vesicles that are within the size of 30-120nm called exosomes, a type of extracellular vesicles. Exosomes contain genetic information in their cargo, in the form of either protein, DNA, or non-coding RNAs and communicate to the distinct cells through various signaling pathways. The c-Myc oncogenic transcription factor protein is a master regulator of oncogenic signaling pathways in various cancers, including AML. C-Myc has been associated with the development of therapy resistance in AML, representing a key target. The interconnection between exosomes, tumor microenvironment, c-Myc and the development of progression, therapy resistance are discussed in this chapter and thus, represents a fundamental knowledge of the recent advances in cancer signal transduction and therapy.

Keywords: Acute myeloid leukemia, C-Myc, Drug resistance, Exosomes, Oncogene, Tumor microenvironment, Tumor suppressor gene.

*****Correspondence author Kishore B. Challagundla:** Department of Biochemistry & Molecular Biology, The Fred and Pamela Buffet Cancer Center, FPBCC 6.12.320, University of Nebraska Medical Center, 985870 Nebraska Medical Center, Omaha, NE 68198-5870, USA; Tel: 402.559.9032; Fax: 402.559.6650;
E-mail: kishore.challagundla@unmc.edu
# Anup S. Pathania & Rachel Weber share equal contribution

Manoj K. Pandey & Vijay P. Kale (Eds.)

INTRODUCTION

Leukemia is a type of cancer that forms in the blood and is typically characterized by an abnormal number of aberrant leukocytes. The bone marrow and lymphatic system are affected as that are where white blood cells are produced and found after maturation. Leukemia made up 30.4% of all blood cancers in 2017 and accounts for 2.9% of cancer cases overall [1]. This cancer is divided into two categories: acute and chronic. From there, it can be separated into subcategories based on the cell it affects, myeloid or lymphocytic. The five main types are acute myeloid leukemia (AML), chronic myeloid leukemia (CML), chronic myelomonocytic leukemia (CMML), acute lymphoblastic leukemia (ALL), and chronic lymphocytic leukemia (CLL) [2]. Leukemia is the highest occurring cancer in children, with ALL making up the majority and AML is the second most common [3]. Acute leukemias tend to affect pediatric patients, whereas adults are more often seen with chronic leukemia. Major risk factors include smoking, family history, genetic disorders, exposure to chemicals, and other environmental factors [4, 5]. Chemotherapy, radiation, or bone marrow transplantation are typical treatment options, although most of these therapies are used in conjunction with another [6]. Cancer type and patient age affect the outcome of the treatment. It can be unsuccessful due to the leukemia cells communicating with the bone marrow microenvironment they reside in. During this exchange, cancer cells are able to develop the ability of self-renewal and chemoresistance [7 - 9]. Bone marrow is where hematopoietic stem cells (HSC) are located, which aids in the stemness of leukemia cells, thus leading to increased resistance to treatment [10, 11].

THE TUMOR MICROENVIRONMENT AND ACUTE MYELOID LEUKEMIA

The microenvironment cells, such as surrounding the blood, and lymph vessels, extracellular matrix, fibroblasts, and tumor-infiltrating immune cells, including B and T lymphocytes, natural killer cells, macrophages, neutrophils, dendritic cells, and mast cells are called tumor microenvironment. The tumor microenvironment plays a crucial role in the initiation and progression of leukemia. Many studies have extensively addressed the role of microenvironment in hematologic malignancies, including AML. One of the examples is retinoic acid receptor γ deficiency in bone marrow microenvironment, which can induce the development of myeloproliferative disorders, a group of slow-growing blood cancers in the bone marrow [12]. The genetic changes in specific mesenchymal cells of the hematopoietic microenvironment can induce myelodysplasia, a condition in which immature blood cells do not mature and later may progress to leukemia. Deletion of *Dicer1*, an RNAse III endonuclease essential for miRNA biogenesis and RNA processing in mesenchymal osteolineage cells, induces myelodysplasia that later progression into AML. The transplantation of hematopoietic cells from *Dicer1* knock out mice into healthy mice does not induce myelodysplastic symptoms. Conversely, transplantation of hematopoietic cells from healthy mice into lethally irradiated mutant mice results in the development of leukemia like symptoms suggesting the role of microenvironment in determining leukemia induction [13]. Moreover, a constitutively active β-catenin mutation in mouse osteoblasts alters differentiation in myeloid and lymphoid progenitors, that can lead to the development of AML. β-catenin is the critical effector molecule that transduces Wnt singling to the nucleus and activate the transcription of Wnt specific genes involved in cell fate decisions [14].

Transplantation of bone marrow cells from constitutively active β-catenin mice into lethally irradiated wild-type mice induces hematopoietic dysfunction and AML [15]. β-catenin activation in osteoblasts stimulates expression of the Jagged 1, a Notch ligand that contributes to the deregulation of hematopoietic stem cells (HSC) lineage differentiation and AML development. Interestingly, β-catenin mutant and Jagged 1 knockdown mice do not show deregulated hematopoietic differentiation and AML development, suggesting that Notch signaling is required in β-catenin induced AML development. In patients with myelodysplastic syndrome or AML, 38.3% have increased β-catenin signaling and nuclear localization in osteoblasts. These patients also show a two-fold increase in NOTCH signaling in their hematopoietic cells compared to healthy controls. Mesenchymal stromal cells (MSCs) from AML patients have a higher level of Notch1 and jagged 1 expression compared to healthy controls. Pharmacological inhibitors of Notch significantly abrogate the survival effects of bonemarrow-derived stromal cells on leukemia cells from chemotherapy-induced apoptosis [16].

Activating mutations in *Ptpn11* gene (encodes protein tyrosine phosphatase SHP2) in the mouse bone marrow microenvironment hyperactivates cell proliferating pathways, including ERK, AKT, and NF-κB in HSCs that drives myeloproliferative neoplasm (NPM) development. Interestingly, *Ptpn11* mutations in mesenchymal stem/progenitor cells and osteoprogenitors and not in differentiated osteoblasts, or endothelial cells induces the development of NPM. *Ptpn11* mutated mesenchymal stem/progenitor cells, or osteoprogenitors secrete an excessive amount of inflammatory CC chemokine CCL3 and matrix metalloproteinase inhibitor TIMP-1 that attracts monocytes in the area. Activated monocytes secrete proinflammatory cytokines, including interleukin-1β, which hyperactivates HSCs residing in that area, resulting in the development of MPN [17]. Bone marrow MSCs secrete chemokine CXCL8 (also known as IL-8) that promotes AML cell proliferation and survival by activating the PI3/AKT survival pathway in leukemic cells [18]. CXCL8 is a CXC-type chemokine that acts as a leukocyte chemoattractant and binds with C-X-C motif chemokine receptors, CXCR1, and CXCR2 present on tumor cells [19]. Overall, these studies show that the microenvironment has a significant contribution to leukemia initiation and development.

LEUKEMIC CELLS AND THE MODULATION OF THE TUMOR MICROENVIRONMENT

Conversely, leukemic cells can also modulate tumor microenvironment that favors their growth and progression of the disease. During the development of myeloproliferative neoplasia (MPN), the endosteal bone marrow niche is progressively remolded into leukemia, supporting a niche that comprises high HSCs activity and rapidly expanding endosteal osteoblastic lineage cells (OBC), the derivatives of multipotent stromal cells [20]. MPN myeloid cells stimulate multipotent stromal cells to produce more OBCs that impairs normal hematopoiesis, promotes myeloid differentiation, and enhances leukemic stem cell functions (LSCs). Multipotent stromal cells co-culture with bone marrow cells isolated from chronic myelogenous leukemia (CML) mice have large size OBC colonies with a high proliferation rate compared to healthy controls. These OBC derivatives show changes in tumor growth factor β (TGF-β), Notch, and inflammatory signaling, including increased expression of interleukin 1 (IL-1) receptor, tumor necrosis factor-α (TNF-α), and IκBα that are associated with MPN induced OBCs expansion and leads to inflammatory myelofibrosis and leukemia development. MPN expanded OBCs do not maintain normal HSCs but support LSCs due to the downregulation of essential HSC retention and upregulation of myeloid differentiation-promoting proteins [20].

AML blasts induce senescence in stromal cells present within the bone marrow microenvironment and transform into tumor supporting cells that promote AML survival and proliferation. The bone marrow stromal cells consist of a heterogeneous population of cells that support hematopoietic cells like adipocytes and osteoblasts and cells with stem-cell-like characters that later differentiate into bones, cartilages, adipocytes, and hematopoietic supporting tissues. AML blasts induce reactive oxygen species (ROS) in bone marrow stromal cells by activating NADPH oxidase, NOX2. The generation of oxidative stress due to NOX2 activation induces cell cycle inhibitor, p16INK4a expression. Stromal cells expressing p16INK4a have the senescence-associated secretory phenotype, including reduced cell proliferation followed by irreversible cell cycle arrest and secreting high levels of inflammatory cytokines, chemokines, proteases, growth factors, and immune-modulatory signals that further potentiate AML development. Pharmacological inhibition of NOX2 significantly reduces bone marrow stromal cell senescence, and therefore, AML cell proliferation [21]. Furthermore, MSCs isolated from myelodysplastic syndrome and AML patients bone marrow show reduced proliferative capacity compared to healthy controls, support leukemic cell viability, proliferation and tumor supportive T regulatory cells activity [20]. MSCs from myelodysplastic syndrome instruct healthy MSCs to acquire myelodysplastic MSC, like phenotype, to support their growth [22]. The orthotropic intra-femoral transplantation of stem-like CD34+ cells with MSCs, both isolated from myelodysplastic syndrome patients into sub-lethally irradiated NOD/SCID mice, results in significantly higher and efficient engraftment compared to CD34+ cells alone. The co-transplanted engrafted mice show a high percentage of dysplastic cells, one of the main clinical features of myelodysplastic syndrome. Moreover, the engrafted MSC expansion is associated with the overproduction of N-Cadherin (CDH2), insulin-like growth factor-binding protein 2 (IGFBP2), vascular endothelial growth factor A (VEGFA), and leukemia inhibitory factor (LIF) that contributes to myelodysplastic expansion [22].

THE TUMOR MICROENVIRONMENT AND ACUTE MYELOID LEUKEMIA THERAPY RESPONSE

The role of tumor microenvironment in the leukemia chemoresistance is well documented in the literature. The changes in the tumor microenvironment support leukemic cells to resists chemotherapy and contribute to disease relapse. Bone marrow MSCs protect leukemic cells from chemotherapy-induced apoptosis and promotes their survival [23, 24]. Co-culture of human-derived bone marrow MSCs with AML cells activates NF-κB and its target genes, including IL-8, IL-6, CCL2 (C-C motif chemokine ligand 2) and VCAM-1 (Vascular cell adhesion protein 1) [25]. Inhibition of NF-κB activation blocks MSCs mediated resistance of leukemia cells to chemotherapy drugs. Leukemic cells express integrin receptor very late antigen 4 (VLA-4) on their cell surface that binds with VCAM on MSCs and activates the NF-κB survival pathway in both leukemic and stromal cells. The activation of the NF-κB pathway contributes to the microenvironment mediated chemoresistance in leukemia [25].

VLA-4 on AML cells also interacts with fibronectin on stromal cells and activate the PI3Kinase/AKT/Bcl2 signaling pathway resulting in resistance to anoikis and drug-induced apoptosis. Importantly, anti-VLA4 treatment, in combination with Ara-C (also known as cytarabine, chemotherapy drug for leukemia treatment) in mice transplanted with human leukemia shows a 100% survival rate [26]. Anti-VLA-4 agents AS101 (ammonium trichloro (dioxoethylene-o,o') tellurate) and natalizumab are proven pre-clinically effective against patient-derived leukemia xenografts [27, 28]. Furthermore, bone marrow MSCs can transfer functional mitochondria to AML cells through endocytosis. During chemotherapy, this transfer increases and provides a survival advantage to leukemic blasts and leukemic initiating cells [29]. Chemotherapy-resistant AML cells are enriched in quiescent CD34+CD38- leukemic stem (LS) cells that reside and expand within the osteoblast-rich endosteal area. The majority of these cells are in the G0 phase of the cell cycle and are resistant to chemotherapy that acts on fast-growing AML cells present in the center of bone marrow. Intravenous injection of human LS cells into AML mice xenograft model NOD/SCID/IL2rg[null] (nonobese diabetic/severe combined immunodeficient/interleukin null) reveals that LS cells reside preferentially at the endosteal surface of bone marrow near murine osteoblasts suggesting the role of microenvironment in the localization and adhesion of LS cells [30].

Signaling molecules like CD44 that are highly expressed on leukocytes, HSCs, and leukemia-initiating cells and its associate CD49d, play a crucial role in the homing of leukemic cells in the bone marrow and other locations [31]. Both molecules are involved in trans-endothelial cell adhesion, migration, mobilization, hematopoietic cell proliferation, and apoptosis resistance [32]. Another critical signaling molecule is CXCL12 (C-X-C motif chemokine 12), also known as stromal cell-derived factor 1 (SDF1), that is secreted by bone marrow stroma and regulates LSCs activity. T cell acute lymphoblastic leukemia (T-ALL) cells form direct and stable contact with CXCL12, producing vascular endothelial cells. CXCL12 produced by vascular endothelial cells is necessary for T-ALL progression, and its absence significantly reduces tumor burden in leukemic mice [33]. CXCL12 receptor CXCR4 is expressed in all T cells, and its deletion affects leukemic cell localization and function. Also, CXCR4 silencing affects key T-ALL regulators, including a decrease in MYC expression and leukemia-initiating cell activity in T-ALL primary xenografts. Moreover, pharmacological inhibition of CXCR4 using highly selective CXCR4 antagonist AMD3465 controls primary human T-ALL progression in a xenograft model [33].

From the above discussion, it is clear that leukemic cells need microenvironment reconstruction that favors their survival, progression, and chemotherapy resistance. Thus, targeting continued crosstalk between cancer cells and the surrounding microenvironment may be an attractive approach to enhance responsiveness to therapies.

ACUTE MYELOID LEUKEMIA AND EXOSOMES

Exosomes are extracellular vesicles produced and secreted from eukaryotic cells, such as endothelial cells, epithelial cells, lymphocytes, neuronal cells, and dendritic cells [34, 35]. They are of 30-100 nm in diameter and can be found all over the body within the plasma, serum, urine, cerebrospinal fluid, and even tears [36, 37]. They are secreted into body fluids by many different cell types to mediate intercellular communication [38]. Some examples of what they transport include lipids, proteins, mRNA, microRNA, and long non-coding RNA. Exosomes have markers on their surface that help characterize them. Common markers include CD9, CD63, CD81, major histocompatibility proteins (MHC), heat shock proteins 70 and 90 (HSC70 and HSC90), ALIX, syndecan-1, and tumor susceptibility gene 101 (TSC 101) [39]. Exosomes carry signals for growth, migration, differentiation, and immune responses [40]. Within the immune system, they can present antigens and transport foreign peptides to dendritic cells to boost the immune response [41]. Exosomes have been shown to function in many types of cancers, including AML. Studies have reported a high presence of exosomes in the body fluids of cancer patients [42]. Exosomes may function in mediating signaling pathways that can lead to chemoresistance or tumor cell aggression, and also regulate the tumor microenvironment. Chemotherapy has been shown to decrease levels of exosomes in patients with AML [43]. Any form of a ruptured blood vessel may cause exosome levels to be elevated in the plasma and can contribute to the malignancy of leukemia [44]. AML-derived exosomes may carry some of the following molecules: FMS-like tyrosine kinase 3 (FLT 3), CXCR 4, insulin-like growth factor 1 receptor (IGF-1R), nucleophosmin 1 (NPM 1), and matrix metalloproteinase 9 (MMP 9) [45]. These molecules play an important role in influencing the microenvironment that can favor growth and evolution of cancerous cells. They may be used as biomarkers in identifying AML and may contribute to the pathogenesis. A recent study found that AML exosome trafficking changed the growth, migratory, and angiogenic properties of surrounding stroma and hematopoietic progenitor cell lines [45]. These demonstrate the ability of exosomes to regulate leukemia progression. Additionally, mouse studies have shown that exosomes originating from melanoma have been found in the bone marrow, which leads to the development of pre-malignant cells within a tumor-promoting niche, suggesting that cancer-derived exosomes can alter the bone marrow microenvironment [46].

EXOSOMES WITHIN THE ACUTE MYELOID LEUKEMIA MICROENVIRONMENT

Exosomes act as communicating molecules between cancer cells and the surrounding microenvironment cells. Cancer derived exosomes play a crucial role in the modulation of tumor-infiltrating immune cells, tend to target and kill the cancer cells. A recent study found that exosomes played a role in immunosuppression in patient-derived AML mouse models [47]. Exosomes isolated from AML PDX mice downregulated NK-cell activated receptor NKG2D expression in normal human NK cells and induces apoptosis in CD8$^+$ T cells [48].

The sera of AML patients contain higher levels of exosomes compared to healthy controls and enriched with transforming growth factor (TGF)-β1, MHC class I molecules, MICA/MICB, and myeloid blast markers, CD34, CD33, and CD117, suggesting that the exosomes are derived from leukemic blasts. Co-incubation of these exosomes with NK cells inhibits NK cell activity by blocking NK-cell activating receptor, NKG2D (Natural Killer Group 2D). This inhibitory effect is rescued by anti-TGF-β1 antibody and IL-15, an NK cell homeostatic cytokine implying the role of exosomal TGF-β1 in NK cells suppression and immune invasion [49]. Chang-Sook Hong et al. reported that exosomes might also interfere with the immune cell functions in immunotherapy treatment and limit their therapeutic benefits. Exosomes isolated from plasma of AML patients, receiving NK-92 cells (an NK cell type) therapy, inhibits the cytolytic activity of NK-92 cells and significantly reduces the expression of NKG2D receptor present on their surface. Activation of the NKG2D receptor stimulates both innate and adaptive immune response and is regulated by different NKG2D ligands that play an important role in NKG2D activation or inhibition. AML-derived exosomes deliver TGFβ on NK-92 cell surface that activate TGFβ receptors, causing increased phosphorylation of SMAD 2/3 and decreased TGFβ expression levels that result in the loss of NKG2D expression and cytolytic functions [50].

Exosomes enhanced the recruitment of regulatory T cells (Tregs) [51]. Tregs inhibit the function of the immune system when the response needs to be turned off, thus maintaining homeostasis and stopping autoimmunity [52, 53]. CD4+CD39+ Tregs are found in tissues and peripheral blood of patients with cancer and differ from natural Tregs present in normal individuals. Tregs incubated with exosomes isolated from cancer patients in the presence of ATP produces adenosine, an immune suppressor in inflammatory environments [54]. Moreover, exosomes interfere with the differentiation of immune cells, including the development of dendritic cells. Exosomes isolated from tumor cells block the differentiation of CD11b+ myeloid precursor cells into dendritic cells in vitro [55].

As exosomes can carry genetic information, they may cause a normal hematopoietic cell to develop a malignant phenotype. Exosomes isolated from AML cell line, K562, that has a breakpoint cluster region-Abelson leukemia gene human homolog 1 (*BCR-ABL1*) gene contains *BCR-ABL1* mRNA. Incubation of these exosomes with mononuclear cells isolated from normal hematopoietic transplants induces leukemia-like malignant phenotype and genomic instability. The recipient cells have DNA hypermethylation in the promoter region of tumor suppressor genes p53 and RIZ1, and increased expression of oncogene Myc. Additionally, these cells have high levels of reactive oxygen species and overexpressed activation-induced cytidine deaminase (AICDA), an enzyme that creates mutations in DNA by deamination of cytosine bases. This suggests that exosome-mediated transfer of BCR-ABL from leukemic to mononuclear cells can transform normal hematopoietic cells by inducing genomic instability [56]. A model is demonstrating the functions of leukemia-derived exosomes within the tumor microenvironment is given in Fig. (**1**).

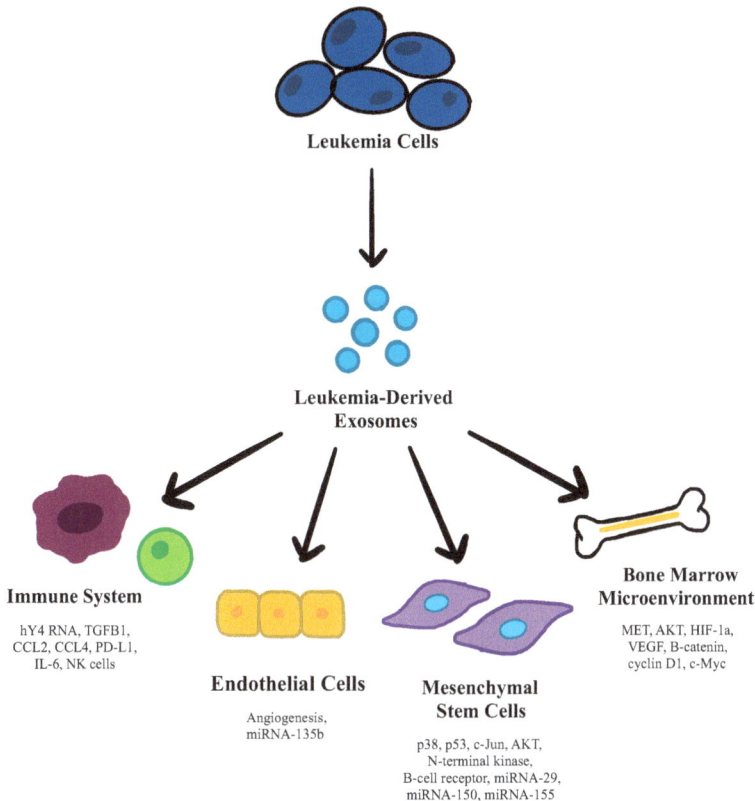

Fig. (1).   **A model represents the functions of leukemia-derived exosomes within the tumor microenvironment.** Leukemia-derived exosomes induce oncogenic signaling pathways through interaction with the cells of the tumor microenvironment. Various proteins involved in the education process of the surrounding cells are given.

AML exosomes can alter the normal bone marrow function, directly or indirectly through stromal components causing leukemic invasion of the bone marrow. This can create an environment in the stroma that's more conducive to leukemia growth [45]. The engraftment of human AML blasts or cell lines into irradiated immunodeficient mice develops leukemia and modifies the hematopoietic and non-hematopoietic compartments in the bone marrow niche through exosome secretion. Inhibition of Rab27, an essential regulator of exosomes secretion, significantly delayed leukemia development in AML engrafted mice. Moreover, injection of AML-derived exosomes in mice induces significant changes in the cellular composition of bone-marrow niche, including an increase in Sca+ and CD146+ stromal cells, and bone marrow multipotent long-term hematopoietic cells (LT-HSC) cells. These stromal cells have decreased expression of genes involved in normal hematopoiesis or bone development whereas, DKK1 expression, a suppressor of normal hematopoiesis with an increase of osteoblast development. Treatment of AML-engrafted mice with DKK inhibitor delays AML progression and prolongs survival. This suggests that AML-derived exosomes could suppress osteoblast differentiation and supports leukemia through the induction of DKK [8]. In AML xenografts, exosomes are taken by hematopoietic stem and progenitor cells (HSPC) and bone marrow stromal cells. The recipient bone marrow stromal cells show reduced growth and downregulation in HSPC retention factors Scf and Cxcl12. Moreover, murine bone marrow stromal cells cultured with exosomes derived from AML cell lines Molm-14 or HL-60 shows intake of human transcripts, including FMS-like tyrosine kinase 3 (*FLT3)* and *CXCR4*. The exosomal transfer of these transcripts affects the expression of genes important for stromal regulation of hematopoiesis, including Scf, Cxcl2, Angpt1, and Tgfb1. AML derived exosomes can also regulate HSPC directly and suppress its functions. These exosomes inhibit HSPC clonogenicity and affect the expression of transcription factors involved in HSPC functions, including *c-Kit, c-Myb, Dnmt1, Pcna, Cebp-β Hoxa-9, E2f3, Paics, NF-kB*. This all suggests that AML cells trafficked transcripts through exosomes to bone marrow cells to deregulate hematopoietic functions and favors leukemia development [57]. Hornick et al. reported the presence of micro RNAs (miR) such as miR-150 and miR-155 in AML exosomes that target cMYB in the recipient HSPC cells and inhibit their clonogenicity. cMYB is a transcription factor involved in HSPC differentiation and proliferation [58].

Wang et al., reported that AML cell lines derived exosomes enhance glycolysis in human umbilical vein endothelial cells (HUVECs) and promote its proliferation, migration and tube-forming activity. The exosomes contain high amounts of vascular endothelial growth factor (VEGF) and vascular endothelial growth factor receptor (VEGFR) mRNA, and can induce VEGFR mRNA in HUVECs. Co-culturing of HUVECs with AML cells protect the latter from leukemia drug cytarabine induced apoptosis [59]. Exosomes secreted from human bone marrow mesenchymal stem cells contain miR-222-3P that inhibits proliferation and induces apoptosis in AML cell lines by inhibiting IRF2/NPP4B signaling [60]. Moreover, exosomal transfer of micro RNA miR-711 from AML cell line K562 to human bone marrow mesenchymal stem cells inhibits CD44 expression in these cells and weakens their adhesive properties [61 - 64]. These studies show that exosomes are essential players in communication between cancer and microenvironment. Therefore, a better understanding of this communication may help in the development of promising anti-leukemia therapy. The effect of leukemia–derived exosomes on the function of various immune cells is depicted in Fig. (**2**).

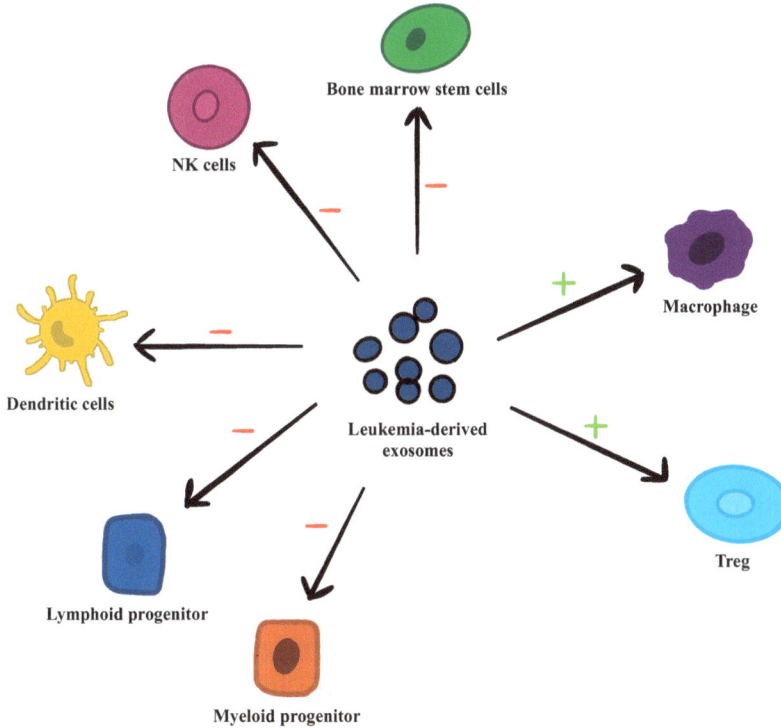

Fig. (2). Leukemia-derived exosomes and the function of the immune cells. The effect of leukemia–derived exosomes on various immune cells is indicated as – and +, respectively.

THE CMYC AND ACUTE MYELOID LEUKEMIA

c-Myc is a transcription factor that can act as an oncogene, and studies have found it to be upregulated in cancers, which may lead to tumor progression [65, 66]. The proto-oncogene c-Myc functions as a master transcriptional regulator and encodes the c-terminal basic helix-loop-helix-leucine zipper domain-containing MYC protein that forms a heterodimer with MYC associated protein X or MAX to exert biological activities [67]. Impairment of MYC/MAX axis plays an important role in the development of aggressive neural tumors [68]. The c-MYC overexpression is observed in many human hematopoietic malignancies and plays an essential role in leukemogenesis [69]. C-MYC overexpression is associated with remission after drug treatment and is an important prognostic factor in AML patients having a higher risk for relapse [70]. The c-Myc mRNA is very short-lived and is tightly regulated at transcriptional and translational levels by mitogenic signals. Normal cells express very low levels of c-Myc compared to cancer cells. Phosphorylation plays an important role in cMYC regulation and stability. There are two phosphorylation sites, Threonine 58 and Serine 62, in the N-terminus of c-MYC, and both are regulated by growth signals. The stability of c-MYC is differentially regulated by these two phosphorylation sites, where Serine 62 phosphorylation stabilizes the c-MYC protein, and threonine 58 phosphorylation destabilizes it [71]. Stimulatory signals promote c-MYC protein stabilization through ERK-mediated phosphorylation of Serine 62. However, these signals also activate Ras or PI3 Kinase/AKT pathway, which inhibits GSK3β, further stabilizing c-MYC protein levels. After signals end, Ras/PI3Kinase/Akt signaling terminates, which leads to GSK3β reactivation and c-MYC threonine 58 phosphorylation. Thus, phosphorylation events are essential for c-MYC regulation and stability. The majority of acute lymphoblastic leukemia (ALL) cell lines have high c-MYC stability due to abnormal phosphorylation at Threonine 50 and Serine 62 residues [72]. Inhibition of c-MYC overcomes cytotoxic drug resistance and inhibits colony-forming ability in AML cells [73].

One of the important regulators of c-Myc stability is GSK3β. This kinase has tumor-suppressive properties and has been associated with cancer pathogenesis [74]. GSK3β phosphorylates number of pro-oncogenic molecules, including c-MYC [75], cyclin D1 [76], cAMP response element-binding protein (CREB) [77], c-Jun [78], heat shock factor-1 (HSF-1) [79], and Nuclear factor of activated cells (NFATc) [80]. GSK3β dependent phosphorylation induces ubiquitin-dependent proteasomal degradation in these molecules. GSK3β itself is regulated by kinases that phosphorylate its serine 9 residue and inhibit its activity [81]. A recent study measured GSK3β/β phosphorylation in 511 patients with AML using reverse-phase protein analysis [82]. FOXO3β and β-catenin had a negative correlation with phosphorylated GSK3, while p-AKT, BAD, and P70S6K all demonstrated a positive correlation. The study hypothesized that AKT phosphorylation of GSK3β/β was essential for the survival of AML cells and thus, could be used as a prognostic factor [82].

GSK3β deficiency leads to the development of aggressive AML in mice. GSK3β null mice have impaired hematopoiesis and show symptoms of myelodysplasia that are morphologically similar to human myelodysplastic syndrome. Transplantation of bone marrow cells from GSK3β null mice showing myelodysplasia symptoms into secondary mice that display similar dysplastic features and lethality. This suggests that GSK3β deletion may allow the generation of self-renewing cells that functions like myelodysplasia initiating cells and are capable of sustaining the disease in mice. Additionally, GSK3α and

GSK3β double knock out mice show an increase in Wnt/Akt/mTOR signaling that contributes to AML development [83]. GSK3β phosphorylation is elevated in AML patients and correlates with the poor survival outcome. GSK3β phosphorylation is associated with the high levels of survival proteins that phosphorylate GSK3 kinases, including phospho-S6K1 (T389) and phospho-AKT (S473) in AML patients [82]. Contrary to the above findings, Wang et al. reported that proto-oncogene mixed-lineage leukemia (MLL) associated leukemia depends on GSK3 activity for its growth and proliferation. MLL transformed cells require GSK3 for their proliferation and maintenance of transformed phenotypes. GSK3 inhibition induces CDK inhibitor (CDKI) p27 expression whose knockdown prevents growth arrest induced by GSK3 inhibitors in human leukemia cell lines and MLL-transformed myeloid progenitors [84]. GSK3 regulates Homeobox (HOX) proteins that are involved in cell differentiation, organ, and tissue formation, and stem cell functions [85]. Dysregulation of the HOX pathway affecting normal hematopoiesis and HSC functions has been observed in acute leukemia [86]. HOX-transformed leukemia cells are generally sensitive to GSK3 inhibitors. GSK3 phosphorylates cAMP-response element-binding protein (CREB) and promotes its association with MEIS1, an evolutionarily conserved Hox family transcription factor. Phosphorylated CREB and its co-activators, including CREB-binding protein (CBP) and Transducer of regulated CREB-binding proteins (TORC), form a functional association with HOX/PBS/MEIS transcriptional complex to facilitate HOX mediated functions. One of the target genes of this complex is proto-oncogene Fos [87]. Overexpression of FOS in MLL leukemia cells increases resistance to GSK-3 inhibition. FOS regulation is crucial in myeloid cell differentiation in AML [88].

Another important c-Myc regulator is protein phosphatase 2A (PP2A), a serine-threonine phosphatase that acts as a tumor suppressor. PP2A has been found silenced in many solid tumors and leukemias. Deregulation of the c-MYC and the functional inactivation of PP2A plays a synergistic role in the initiation and progression of AML [89, 90]. PP2A activity is regulated by its interacting partners, such as SET (I2PP2A, inhibitor 2 of PP2A) and cancerous inhibitor of PP2A (CIP2A). SET oncoprotein binds with PP2A through its N and C-terminus regions and inhibits PP2A phosphatase activity [91]. SET is regulated by kinase p38β that directly binds to and stabilizes p38β by inhibiting its degradation in AML cells [92]. p38β activates casein kinase 2 (CK2) and promotes CK2-mediated phosphorylation of SET. SET is mainly localized in the nucleus, but its phosphorylation makes it stay in the cytoplasm and inhibits its degradation. AML cells overexpressing SET shows strong cytoplasmic localization with decreased PP2A activity [92]. Furthermore, SET overexpression restores PP2A induced inhibition of AML cell proliferation and is associated with a poor outcome in AML. The type 3 receptor kinase and proto-oncogene c-KIT regulates PP2A in

AML cells. c-KIT inhibits the PP2A activity by altering the expression of PP2A subunits, PP2A-Aα, and PP2A-Aβ. The gain-of-function mutations in c-KIT are frequently observed in AML patients [93]. The overexpression of PP2A dephosphorylates c-KIT and induces apoptosis in mutant c-KIT cells [94]. This suggests that the reactivation of PP2A by PP2A activators could be a novel therapy for AML with c-kit mutations. The model represents the phosphorylation of GSK-3 and PP2A in the progression of leukemia through various signaling pathways is given in Fig. (**3**).

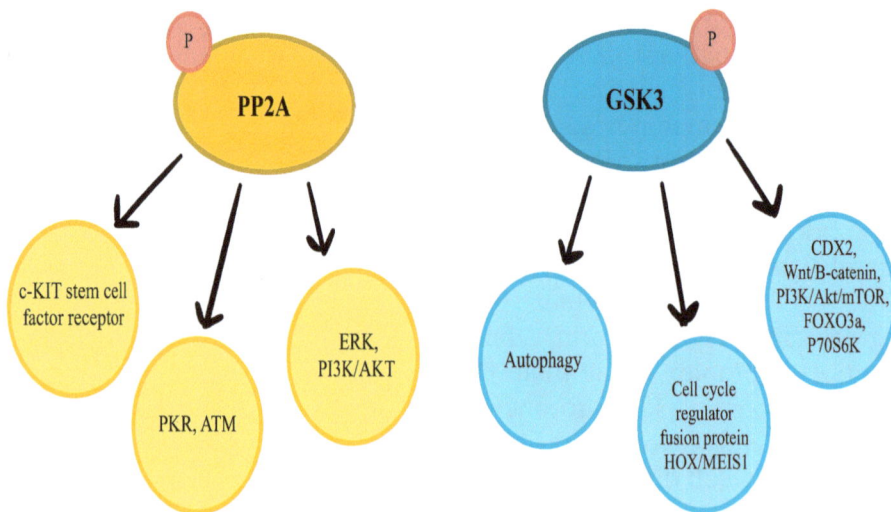

Fig. (3). The model represents the phosphorylation of GSK-3 and PP2A in the progression of leukemia through various signaling pathways.

THE EXOSOMES AND C-MYC IN THE PROGRESSION OF ACUTE MYELOID LEUKEMIA

AML derived exosomes are enriched in c-Myc that is an important prognostic factor in AML [95]. Exosomal c-Myc is taken by myeloid-derived suppressor cells (MDSCs) in the tumor microenvironment and promotes their proliferation and expansion. Co-culture of MDSCs with T cells inhibits their proliferation and activation, suggesting the role of exosomal c-Myc in altering tumor microenvironment and the promotion of immune suppression. The oncoprotein Mucin1 or MUC1 regulates cMyc in AML cells and affects its exosomal release in the tumor microenvironment. The MUC1 silencing decreases c-Myc expression in exosomes and downregulates c-Myc and its downstream targets, including cyclin E1 and cyclin D1 in the recipient MDSC cells. MUC1 regulates c-Myc through the inhibition of cMyc regulator miRNA34a that binds with c-myc 3'UTR and suppresses its expression at a post-transcriptional level [96]. Micro RNA profiling of exosomes from bone marrow-derived MSCs in patients with AML reveals the presence of miR-26a-5p that inhibits cMyc downstream target gene GSK3β in MSCs and AML cells. This suggests that GSK3β expression in AML cells can be inhibited by miR-26a-5p that is increased in MSC-derived exosomes in patients with AML [97].

The direct inhibition of c-MYC has been a challenge for decades due to its undruggable protein structure. Therefore, targeting c-MYC regulation provides a better alternative to treat c-Myc amplified cancers. Leukemia cells can undergo chemosensitization by GSK3 and PP2A-based drugs. As GSK3 and PP2A both regulate c-Myc through phosphorylation, tyrosine kinase inhibitors are essential for therapeutic methods in leukemia. The deletion of GSK3β in hematopoietic stem cells leads to pre-tumor growth conditions similar to human myelodysplastic syndrome (MDS), which can evolve into AML. GSK3β can then be used as a marker for MDS in the absence of HSCs. Both GSK3β and GSK3β regulate the Wnt/Akt/mTOR pathway as well, therefore, these pathways may also be targeted in new therapies [83]. One study explored the resistance to FLT3 inhibitor quizartinib (AC220) mediated by GSK3 inhibition in patients with AML. The study found that GSK3 expression is significantly decreased, whereas its downstream pathways, including FGF/Ras/ERK and Wnt, are upregulated in AC220-resistant AML cells. Inhibition of these pathways desensitizes resistant AML cells to AC220 [98]. Pre-clinical studies have shown the potential of using GSK3 inhibitors like 6-bromoindirubin-30oxime (BIO) in not only AML but ALL and CML as well [99]. GS-87 is another GSK3-specific inhibitor that has been tested in AML cells [100]. A phase II clinical trial analyzed an inhibitor termed LY2090314, and downregulation of GSK3 was observed [101]. This drug shows potential benefits if used in conjunction with others. Another potential treatment option for leukemia is to inhibit the P13K/AKT pathway, which will activate GSK3. Receptor tyrosine kinase inhibitor ABT-869 (linifanib) can suppress AKT while activating GSK3 [102]. ABT-869 reduces the phosphorylation of AKT and GSK3β in FLT3 internal tandem duplication (ITD) mutant AML cells. Inhibition of GSK3β phosphorylation activates it and is synergetic to the apoptotic effect of ABT-869 due to AKT inhibition [102]. Furthermore, dual inhibition of PI3kinase and Bcl-2/Bcl-xL significantly enhanced apoptosis in resistant AML cells through GSK3 activation [103].

Another pro-survival molecule regulated by c-Myc and essential for therapy response is myeloid cell leukemia-1 (MCL-1). In AML, MCL-1 is crucial for its development and often associated with cancer cell survival and resistance to chemotherapy. Activation of GSK3β phosphorylates MCL-1 and causes its proteasomal mediated degradation [104]. Leukemia drug arsenic trioxide inhibits MCL-1 protein expression by promoting its degradation and induces apoptosis in AML cells. GSK3β activation is required for arsenic trioxide induced MCL-1 degradation and apoptosis induction in AML cells [105]. Moreover, the combination of MCL-1 inhibitors with BCL2 inhibitors shows synergistic effects in the treatment of AML models' resistance to MCL-1 therapy [106].

PP2A based drug and sphingosine analog FTY720 acts as a potent PP2A activator in AML. FTY720 mediated apoptosis in AML cells partially depends on PP2A activation [107]. FTY720 restores PP2A activity in AML cells harboring C-KIT/TKD mutation that potentiates FTY720 induced toxicity. PP2A activity is restored due to the downregulation of PP2A inhibitor SET and decreases inhibitory PP2A phosphorylation at tyrosine 307 after FTY720 treatment. SET was identified in acute undifferentiated leukemia as oncogene fused with nucleoporin NUP214 and has been reported in DNA repair, chromatin remodeling, differentiation, transcription, and cell cycle regulation [108, 109]. Overexpression of SET is a recurrent event associated with poor outcome in AML patients and is a key mechanism in the inhibition of PP2A in AML. SET is regulated by p38β that binds and stabilizes SET in AML cells. SET is mainly localized in the nucleus. p38β activates casein kinase 2 (CK2), which phosphorylates SET at serine 9 residue and promotes its cytoplasmic localization and stability. SET stability leads to PP2A inactivation. Pharmacological inhibition of CK2 enhances the anti-leukemic effects of FTY720, suggesting that combination therapy may give a better outcome [92]. Another PP2A inhibitor that shows promising results in AML treatment is OP449. It is physiologically stable, cell-penetrating small peptide that specially binds to SET and inhibits its activity. AML patient samples having overexpressed SET are sensitive to OP449 and show increased activity of PP2A after OP449 treatment [110]. Thus, PP2A could be considered as a promising target for AML. More studies are needed to examine the efficacy of GSK-3 and PP2A based inhibitors for the treatment of AML.

CONCLUSIONS AND OUTLOOK

It is clear that communication with the tumor microenvironmental cells through exosomes and other oncogenic signaling pathways mediated by c-Myc contribute to the development of therapy response in AML. Developing therapy resistance is a significant obstacle for the treatment failure in not only AML but also various other cancers. It is extremely important to find the pathways behind the development of therapy resistance pathways. Extracellular vesicles, including exosomes, mediate the communication between the tumor cells and the other cells of the tumor microenvironment. Furthermore, exosomes also interact with immune cells within the tumor tissue regulating the anti-tumor immune response. The precise molecular mechanisms involved in the regulation of exosomes should be addressed. Extensive feature investigations are required to block the communication with tumor microenvironmental cells to make cancer cells respond to various treatments. C-Myc is known to play a significant role in regulating the anti-tumor immune response. Therapeutically targeting c-Myc is not successful so far, and therefore, the development of dual or triple small molecule inhibitors will provide new strategies to target c-Myc associated oncogenic signaling pathways.

CONSENT FOR PUBLICATION

Not applicable.

CONFLICT OF INTEREST

The author declares that there is no conflict of interest in this chapter.

ACKNOWLEDGEMENTS

Dr.Challagundla's laboratory is supported in whole or part from the NIH/NCI grant (K22CA197074-01); Leukemia Research Foundation (LRF) grant, the Nebraska State DHHS (LB506); UNMC Pediatric Cancer Research Center; Fred and Pamela Buffett Cancer Center's pilot grant (P30 CA036727) in conjunction with the UNMC Pediatric Cancer Research Center; and the Department of Biochemistry and Molecular Biology start-up.

REFERENCES

[1]   Buckley SA, Kirtane K, Walter RB, Lee SJ, Lyman GH. Patient-reported outcomes in acute myeloid leukemia: Where are we now? Blood Rev 2018; 32(1): 81-7.
[http://dx.doi.org/10.1016/j.blre.2017.08.010] [PMID: 28888621]

[2]   Vardiman JW, Thiele J, Arber DA, *et al.* The 2008 revision of the World Health Organization (WHO) classification of myeloid neoplasms and acute leukemia: rationale and important changes. Blood 2009; 114(5): 937-51.
[http://dx.doi.org/10.1182/blood-2009-03-209262] [PMID: 19357394]

[3]   Disease GBD, Injury I, Prevalence C. Global, regional, and national incidence, prevalence, and years lived with disability for 310 diseases and injuries, 1990-2015: a systematic analysis for the Global Burden of Disease Study 2015. Lancet 2016; 388(10053): 1545-602.
[http://dx.doi.org/10.1016/S0140-6736(16)31678-6] [PMID: 27733282]

[4]   Juliusson G, Hough R. Leukemia. Prog Tumor Res 2016; 43: 87-100.
[http://dx.doi.org/10.1159/000447076] [PMID: 27595359]

[5]   Dahl G, Wiemels J. What causes leukemia? Pediatr Blood Cancer 2015; 62(7): 1123-4.
[http://dx.doi.org/10.1002/pbc.25526] [PMID: 25894591]

[6]   Dombret H, Gardin C. An update of current treatments for adult acute myeloid leukemia. Blood 2016; 127(1): 53-61.

[http://dx.doi.org/10.1182/blood-2015-08-604520] [PMID: 26660429]

[7]   Behrmann L, Wellbrock J, Fiedler W. Acute Myeloid Leukemia and the Bone Marrow Niche-Take a Closer Look. Front Oncol 2018; 8: 444.
[http://dx.doi.org/10.3389/fonc.2018.00444] [PMID: 30370251]

[8]   Kumar B, Garcia M, Weng L, *et al.* Acute myeloid leukemia transforms the bone marrow niche into a leukemia-permissive microenvironment through exosome secretion. Leukemia 2018; 32(3): 575-87.
[http://dx.doi.org/10.1038/leu.2017.259] [PMID: 28816238]

[9]   Wang A, Zhong H. Roles of the bone marrow niche in hematopoiesis, leukemogenesis, and chemotherapy resistance in acute myeloid leukemia. Hematology 2018; 23(10): 729-39.
[http://dx.doi.org/10.1080/10245332.2018.1486064] [PMID: 29902132]

[10]   Holyoake TL, Vetrie D. The chronic myeloid leukemia stem cell: stemming the tide of persistence. Blood 2017; 129(12): 1595-606.
[http://dx.doi.org/10.1182/blood-2016-09-696013] [PMID: 28159740]

[11]   Zhou HS, Carter BZ, Andreeff M. Bone marrow niche-mediated survival of leukemia stem cells in acute myeloid leukemia: Yin and Yang. Cancer Biol Med 2016; 13(2): 248-59.
[http://dx.doi.org/10.20892/j.issn.2095-3941.2016.0023] [PMID: 27458532]

[12]   Walkley CR, Olsen GH, Dworkin S, *et al.* A microenvironment-induced myeloproliferative syndrome caused by retinoic acid receptor gamma deficiency. Cell 2007; 129(6): 1097-110.
[http://dx.doi.org/10.1016/j.cell.2007.05.014] [PMID: 17574023]

[13]   Raaijmakers MH, Mukherjee S, Guo S, *et al.* Bone progenitor dysfunction induces myelodysplasia and secondary leukaemia. Nature 2010; 464(7290): 852-7.
[http://dx.doi.org/10.1038/nature08851] [PMID: 20305640]

[14]   Valenta T, Hausmann G, Basler K. The many faces and functions of β-catenin. EMBO J 2012; 31(12): 2714-36.
[http://dx.doi.org/10.1038/emboj.2012.150] [PMID: 22617422]

[15]   Kode A, Manavalan JS, Mosialou I, *et al.* Leukaemogenesis induced by an activating β-catenin mutation in osteoblasts. Nature 2014; 506(7487): 240-4.
[http://dx.doi.org/10.1038/nature12883] [PMID: 24429522]

[16]   Takam Kamga P, Bassi G, Cassaro A, *et al.* Notch signalling drives bone marrow stromal cell-mediated chemoresistance in acute myeloid leukemia. Oncotarget 2016; 7(16): 21713-27.
[http://dx.doi.org/10.18632/oncotarget.7964] [PMID: 26967055]

[17]   Dong L, Yu WM, Zheng H, *et al.* Leukaemogenic effects of Ptpn11 activating mutations in the stem cell microenvironment. Nature 2016; 539(7628): 304-8.
[http://dx.doi.org/10.1038/nature20131] [PMID: 27783593]

[18]   Cheng J, Li Y, Liu S, *et al.* CXCL8 derived from mesenchymal stromal cells supports survival and proliferation of acute myeloid leukemia cells through the PI3K/AKT pathway. FASEB J 2019; 33(4): 4755-64.
[http://dx.doi.org/10.1096/fj.201801931R] [PMID: 30592634]

[19]   Liu Q, Li A, Tian Y, *et al.* The CXCL8-CXCR1/2 pathways in cancer. Cytokine Growth Factor Rev 2016; 31: 61-71.
[http://dx.doi.org/10.1016/j.cytogfr.2016.08.002] [PMID: 27578214]

[20]   Schepers K, Pietras EM, Reynaud D, *et al.* Myeloproliferative neoplasia remodels the endosteal bone marrow niche into a self-reinforcing leukemic niche. Cell Stem Cell 2013; 13(3): 285-99.
[http://dx.doi.org/10.1016/j.stem.2013.06.009] [PMID: 23850243]

[21]   Abdul-Aziz AM, Sun Y, Hellmich C, *et al.* Acute myeloid leukemia induces protumoral p16INK4a-driven senescence in the bone marrow microenvironment. Blood 2019; 133(5): 446-56.
[http://dx.doi.org/10.1182/blood-2018-04-845420] [PMID: 30401703]

[22]   Medyouf H, Mossner M, Jann JC, *et al.* Myelodysplastic cells in patients reprogram mesenchymal stromal cells to establish a transplantable stem cell niche disease unit. Cell Stem Cell 2014; 14(6): 824-37.
[http://dx.doi.org/10.1016/j.stem.2014.02.014] [PMID: 24704494]

[23]   Corradi G, Baldazzi C, Očadlíková D, *et al.* Mesenchymal stromal cells from myelodysplastic and acute myeloid leukemia patients display in vitro reduced proliferative potential and similar capacity to support leukemia cell survival. Stem Cell Res Ther 2018; 9(1): 271.
[http://dx.doi.org/10.1186/s13287-018-1013-z] [PMID: 30359303]

[24]   Wang W, Bochtler T, Wuchter P, *et al.* Mesenchymal stromal cells contribute to quiescence of therapy-resistant leukemic cells in acute myeloid leukemia. Eur J Haematol 2017; 99(5): 392-8.
[http://dx.doi.org/10.1111/ejh.12934] [PMID: 28800175]

[25]   Jacamo R, Chen Y, Wang Z, *et al.* Reciprocal leukemia-stroma VCAM-1/VLA-4-dependent activation of NF-κB mediates chemoresistance. Blood 2014; 123(17): 2691-702.
[http://dx.doi.org/10.1182/blood-2013-06-511527] [PMID: 24599548]

[26]   Matsunaga T, Takemoto N, Sato T, *et al.* Interaction between leukemic-cell VLA-4 and stromal fibronectin is a decisive factor for minimal residual disease of acute myelogenous leukemia. Nat Med 2003; 9(9): 1158-65.
[http://dx.doi.org/10.1038/nm909] [PMID: 12897778]

[27]   Layani-Bazar A, Skornick I, Berrebi A, *et al.* Redox modulation of adjacent thiols in VLA-4 by AS101 converts myeloid leukemia cells from a drug-resistant to drug-sensitive state. Cancer Res 2014; 74(11): 3092-103.
[http://dx.doi.org/10.1158/0008-5472.CAN-13-2159] [PMID: 24699624]

[28]   Hsieh YT, Gang EJ, Geng H, *et al.* Integrin alpha4 blockade sensitizes drug resistant pre-B acute lymphoblastic leukemia to chemotherapy. Blood 2013; 121(10): 1814-8.
[http://dx.doi.org/10.1182/blood-2012-01-406272] [PMID: 23319569]

[29]   Moschoi R, Imbert V, Nebout M, *et al.* Protective mitochondrial transfer from bone marrow stromal cells to acute myeloid leukemic cells during chemotherapy. Blood 2016; 128(2): 253-64.
[http://dx.doi.org/10.1182/blood-2015-07-655860] [PMID: 27257182]

[30]   Ishikawa F, Yoshida S, Saito Y, *et al.* Chemotherapy-resistant human AML stem cells home to and engraft within the bone-marrow endosteal region. Nat Biotechnol 2007; 25(11): 1315-21.
[http://dx.doi.org/10.1038/nbt1350] [PMID: 17952057]

[31]   Christ O, Kronenwett R, Haas R, Zöller M. Combining G-CSF with a blockade of adhesion strongly improves the reconstitutive capacity of mobilized hematopoietic progenitor cells. Exp Hematol 2001; 29(3): 380-90.
[http://dx.doi.org/10.1016/S0301-472X(00)00674-3] [PMID: 11274767]

[32]   Singh V, Erb U, Zöller M. Cooperativity of CD44 and CD49d in leukemia cell homing, migration, and survival offers a means for therapeutic attack. J Immunol 2013; 191(10): 5304-16.
[http://dx.doi.org/10.4049/jimmunol.1301543] [PMID: 24127558]

[33]   Pitt LA, Tikhonova AN, Hu H, *et al.* CXCL12-Producing Vascular Endothelial Niches Control Acute T Cell Leukemia Maintenance. Cancer Cell 2015; 27(6): 755-68.
[http://dx.doi.org/10.1016/j.ccell.2015.05.002] [PMID: 26058075]

[34]   Johnstone RM, Adam M, Hammond JR, Orr L, Turbide C. Vesicle formation during reticulocyte maturation. Association of plasma membrane activities with released vesicles (exosomes). J Biol Chem 1987; 262(19): 9412-20.
[PMID: 3597417]

[35]   Pan BT, Teng K, Wu C, Adam M, Johnstone RM. Electron microscopic evidence for externalization of the transferrin receptor in vesicular form in sheep reticulocytes. J Cell Biol 1985; 101(3): 942-8.
[http://dx.doi.org/10.1083/jcb.101.3.942] [PMID: 2993317]

[36]   He C, Zheng S, Luo Y, Wang B. Exosome Theranostics: Biology and Translational Medicine. Theranostics 2018; 8(1): 237-55.
[http://dx.doi.org/10.7150/thno.21945] [PMID: 29290805]

[37]   Ludwig AK, Giebel B. Exosomes: small vesicles participating in intercellular communication. Int J Biochem Cell Biol 2012; 44(1): 11-5.
[http://dx.doi.org/10.1016/j.biocel.2011.10.005] [PMID: 22024155]

[38]   Skog J, Würdinger T, van Rijn S, *et al.* Glioblastoma microvesicles transport RNA and proteins that promote tumour growth and provide diagnostic biomarkers. Nat Cell Biol 2008; 10(12): 1470-6.
[http://dx.doi.org/10.1038/ncb1800] [PMID: 19011622]

[39]   Subra C, Grand D, Laulagnier K, *et al.* Exosomes account for vesicle-mediated transcellular transport of activatable phospholipases and prostaglandins. J Lipid Res 2010; 51(8): 2105-20.
[http://dx.doi.org/10.1194/jlr.M003657] [PMID: 20424270]

[40]   Bobrie A, Théry C. Unraveling the physiological functions of exosome secretion by tumors. OncoImmunology 2013; 2(1): e22565.
[http://dx.doi.org/10.4161/onci.22565] [PMID: 23483742]

[41]   Raposo G, Nijman HW, Stoorvogel W, *et al.* B lymphocytes secrete antigen-presenting vesicles. J Exp Med 1996; 183(3): 1161-72.
[http://dx.doi.org/10.1084/jem.183.3.1161] [PMID: 8642258]

[42]   Melo SA, Luecke LB, Kahlert C, *et al.* Glypican-1 identifies cancer exosomes and detects early pancreatic cancer. Nature 2015; 523(7559): 177-82.
[http://dx.doi.org/10.1038/nature14581] [PMID: 26106858]

[43]   Hong CS, Muller L, Whiteside TL, Boyiadzis M. Plasma exosomes as markers of therapeutic response in patients with acute myeloid leukemia. Front Immunol 2014; 5: 160.
[http://dx.doi.org/10.3389/fimmu.2014.00160] [PMID: 24782865]

[44]   Zwicker JI, Liebman HA, Neuberg D, *et al.* Tumor-derived tissue factor-bearing microparticles are associated with venous thromboembolic events in malignancy. Clin Cancer Res 2009; 15(22): 6830-40.
[http://dx.doi.org/10.1158/1078-0432.CCR-09-0371] [PMID: 19861441]

[45]   Huan J, Hornick NI, Shurtleff MJ, *et al.* RNA trafficking by acute myelogenous leukemia exosomes. Cancer Res 2013; 73(2): 918-29.
[http://dx.doi.org/10.1158/0008-5472.CAN-12-2184] [PMID: 23149911]

[46]   Peinado H, Alečković M, Lavotshkin S, *et al.* Melanoma exosomes educate bone marrow progenitor cells toward a pro-metastatic phenotype through MET. Nat Med 2012; 18(6): 883-91.
[http://dx.doi.org/10.1038/nm.2753] [PMID: 22635005]

[47]   Hong CS, Danet-Desnoyers G, Shan X, Sharma P, Whiteside TL, Boyiadzis M. Human acute myeloid leukemia blast-derived exosomes in patient-derived xenograft mice mediate immune suppression. Exp Hematol 2019; 76: 60-66.e2.
[http://dx.doi.org/10.1016/j.exphem.2019.07.005] [PMID: 31369790]

[48]   Hong CS, Danet-Desnoyers G, Shan X, *et al.* Human acute myeloid leukemia blast-derived exosomes in patient-derived xenograft mice mediate immune suppression. Exp Hematol 2019; 76: 60-66.e2.
[http://dx.doi.org/10.1016/j.exphem.2019.07.005]

[49]   Szczepanski MJ, Szajnik M, Welsh A, Whiteside TL, Boyiadzis M. Blast-derived microvesicles in sera from patients with acute myeloid leukemia suppress natural killer cell function via membrane-associated transforming growth factor-beta1. Haematologica 2011; 96(9): 1302-9.
[http://dx.doi.org/10.3324/haematol.2010.039743] [PMID: 21606166]

[50]   Hong CS, Sharma P, Yerneni SS, *et al.* Circulating exosomes carrying an immunosuppressive cargo interfere with cellular immunotherapy in acute myeloid leukemia. Sci Rep 2017; 7(1): 14684.
[http://dx.doi.org/10.1038/s41598-017-14661-w] [PMID: 29089618]

[51]   Lei H, Schmidt-Bleek K, Dienelt A, Reinke P, Volk HD. Regulatory T cell-mediated anti-inflammatory effects promote successful tissue repair in both indirect and direct manners. Front Pharmacol 2015; 6: 184.
[http://dx.doi.org/10.3389/fphar.2015.00184] [PMID: 26388774]

[52]   Grindebacke H, Stenstad H, Quiding-Järbrink M, *et al.* Dynamic development of homing receptor expression and memory cell differentiation of infant CD4+CD25high regulatory T cells. J Immunol 2009; 183(7): 4360-70.
[http://dx.doi.org/10.4049/jimmunol.0901091] [PMID: 19734224]

[53]   Burzyn D, Kuswanto W, Kolodin D, *et al.* A special population of regulatory T cells potentiates muscle repair. Cell 2013; 155(6): 1282-95.
[http://dx.doi.org/10.1016/j.cell.2013.10.054] [PMID: 24315098]

[54]   Schuler PJ, Saze Z, Hong CS, *et al.* Human CD4+ CD39+ regulatory T cells produce adenosine upon co-expression of surface CD73 or contact with CD73+ exosomes or CD73+ cells. Clin Exp Immunol 2014; 177(2): 531-43.
[http://dx.doi.org/10.1111/cei.12354] [PMID: 24749746]

[55]   Yu S, Liu C, Su K, *et al.* Tumor exosomes inhibit differentiation of bone marrow dendritic cells. J Immunol 2007; 178(11): 6867-75.
[http://dx.doi.org/10.4049/jimmunol.178.11.6867] [PMID: 17513735]

[56]   Zhu X, You Y, Li Q, *et al.* BCR-ABL1-positive microvesicles transform normal hematopoietic transplants through genomic instability: implications for donor cell leukemia. Leukemia 2014; 28(8): 1666-75.
[http://dx.doi.org/10.1038/leu.2014.51] [PMID: 24480987]

[57]   Huan J, Hornick NI, Goloviznina NA, *et al.* Coordinate regulation of residual bone marrow function by paracrine trafficking of AML exosomes. Leukemia 2015; 29(12): 2285-95.
[http://dx.doi.org/10.1038/leu.2015.163] [PMID: 26108689]

[58]   Hornick NI, Doron B, Abdelhamed S, *et al.* AML suppresses hematopoiesis by releasing exosomes that contain microRNAs targeting c-MYB. Sci Signal 2016; 9(444): ra88.
[http://dx.doi.org/10.1126/scisignal.aaf2797] [PMID: 27601730]

[59]   Wang B, Wang X, Hou D, *et al.* Exosomes derived from acute myeloid leukemia cells promote chemoresistance by enhancing glycolysis-mediated vascular remodeling. J Cell Physiol 2019; 234(7): 10602-14.
[http://dx.doi.org/10.1002/jcp.27735] [PMID: 30417360]

[60]   Zhang F, Lu Y, Wang M, *et al.* Exosomes derived from human bone marrow mesenchymal stem cells transfer miR-222-3p to suppress acute myeloid leukemia cell proliferation by targeting IRF2/INPP4B. Mol Cell Probes 2020; 51: 101513.
[http://dx.doi.org/10.1016/j.mcp.2020.101513] [PMID: 31968218]

[61]   Jiang YH, Liu J, Lin J, *et al.* K562 cell-derived exosomes suppress the adhesive function of bone marrow mesenchymal stem cells via delivery of miR-711. Biochem Biophys Res Commun 2020; 521(3): 584-9.
[http://dx.doi.org/10.1016/j.bbrc.2019.10.096] [PMID: 31677790]

[62]   Ghosh AK, Secreto CR, Knox TR, Ding W, Mukhopadhyay D, Kay NE. Circulating microvesicles in B-cell chronic lymphocytic leukemia can stimulate marrow stromal cells: implications for disease progression. Blood 2010; 115(9): 1755-64.
[http://dx.doi.org/10.1182/blood-2009-09-242719] [PMID: 20018914]

[63]   Corrado C, Raimondo S, Saieva L, Flugy AM, De Leo G, Alessandro R. Exosome-mediated crosstalk between chronic myelogenous leukemia cells and human bone marrow stromal cells triggers an interleukin 8-dependent survival of leukemia cells. Cancer Lett 2014; 348(1-2): 71-6.
[http://dx.doi.org/10.1016/j.canlet.2014.03.009] [PMID: 24657661]

[64]   Roccaro AM, Sacco A, Maiso P, *et al*. BM mesenchymal stromal cell-derived exosomes facilitate multiple myeloma progression. J Clin Invest 2013; 123(4): 1542-55.
[http://dx.doi.org/10.1172/JCI66517] [PMID: 23454749]

[65]   Luo H, Li Q, O'Neal J, Kreisel F, Le Beau MM, Tomasson MH. c-Myc rapidly induces acute myeloid leukemia in mice without evidence of lymphoma-associated antiapoptotic mutations. Blood 2005; 106(7): 2452-61.
[http://dx.doi.org/10.1182/blood-2005-02-0734] [PMID: 15972450]

[66]   Salvatori B, Iosue I, Djodji Damas N, *et al*. Critical Role of c-Myc in Acute Myeloid Leukemia Involving Direct Regulation of miR-26a and Histone Methyltransferase EZH2. Genes Cancer 2011; 2(5): 585-92.
[http://dx.doi.org/10.1177/1947601911416357] [PMID: 21901171]

[67]   Amati B, Land H. Myc-Max-Mad: a transcription factor network controlling cell cycle progression, differentiation and death. Curr Opin Genet Dev 1994; 4(1): 102-8.
[http://dx.doi.org/10.1016/0959-437X(94)90098-1] [PMID: 8193530]

[68]   Cascón A, Robledo M. MAX and MYC: a heritable breakup. Cancer Res 2012; 72(13): 3119-24.
[http://dx.doi.org/10.1158/0008-5472.CAN-11-3891] [PMID: 22706201]

[69]   Hoffman B, Amanullah A, Shafarenko M, Liebermann DA. The proto-oncogene c-myc in hematopoietic development and leukemogenesis. Oncogene 2002; 21(21): 3414-21.
[http://dx.doi.org/10.1038/sj.onc.1205400] [PMID: 12032779]

[70]   Ohanian M, Rozovski U, Kanagal-Shamanna R, *et al*. MYC protein expression is an important prognostic factor in acute myeloid leukemia. Leuk Lymphoma 2019; 60(1): 37-48.
[http://dx.doi.org/10.1080/10428194.2018.1464158] [PMID: 29741984]

[71]   Sears R, Nuckolls F, Haura E, Taya Y, Tamai K, Nevins JR. Multiple Ras-dependent phosphorylation pathways regulate Myc protein stability. Genes Dev 2000; 14(19): 2501-14.
[http://dx.doi.org/10.1101/gad.836800] [PMID: 11018017]

[72]   Malempati S, Tibbitts D, Cunningham M, *et al*. Aberrant stabilization of c-Myc protein in some lymphoblastic leukemias. Leukemia 2006; 20(9): 1572-81.
[http://dx.doi.org/10.1038/sj.leu.2404317] [PMID: 16855632]

[73]   Pan XN, Chen JJ, Wang LX, *et al*. Inhibition of c-Myc overcomes cytotoxic drug resistance in acute myeloid leukemia cells by promoting differentiation. PLoS One 2014; 9(8): e105381.
[http://dx.doi.org/10.1371/journal.pone.0105381] [PMID: 25127121]

[74]   Miyashita K, Nakada M, Shakoori A, *et al*. An emerging strategy for cancer treatment targeting aberrant glycogen synthase kinase 3 beta. Anticancer Agents Med Chem 2009; 9(10): 1114-22.
[http://dx.doi.org/10.2174/187152009789734982] [PMID: 19925395]

[75]   Gregory MA, Qi Y, Hann SR. Phosphorylation by glycogen synthase kinase-3 controls c-myc proteolysis and subnuclear localization. J Biol Chem 2003; 278(51): 51606-12.
[http://dx.doi.org/10.1074/jbc.M310722200] [PMID: 14563837]   ·

[76]   Diehl JA, Cheng M, Roussel MF, Sherr CJ. Glycogen synthase kinase-3beta regulates cyclin D1 proteolysis and subcellular localization. Genes Dev 1998; 12(22): 3499-511.
[http://dx.doi.org/10.1101/gad.12.22.3499] [PMID: 9832503]

[77]   Tullai JW, Chen J, Schaffer ME, Kamenetsky E, Kasif S, Cooper GM. Glycogen synthase kinase-3 represses cyclic AMP response element-binding protein (CREB)-targeted immediate early genes in quiescent cells. J Biol Chem 2007; 282(13): 9482-91.
[http://dx.doi.org/10.1074/jbc.M700067200] [PMID: 17277356]

[78]   Shao J, Teng Y, Padia R, *et al*. COP1 and GSK3β cooperate to promote c-Jun degradation and inhibit breast cancer cell tumorigenesis. Neoplasia 2013; 15(9): 1075-85.
[http://dx.doi.org/10.1593/neo.13966] [PMID: 24027432]

[79]   Chu B, Zhong R, Soncin F, Stevenson MA, Calderwood SK. Transcriptional activity of heat shock factor 1 at 37 degrees C is repressed through phosphorylation on two distinct serine residues by glycogen synthase kinase 3 and protein kinases Calpha and Czeta. J Biol Chem 1998; 273(29): 18640-6.
[http://dx.doi.org/10.1074/jbc.273.29.18640] [PMID: 9660838]

[80]   Beals CR, Sheridan CM, Turck CW, Gardner P, Crabtree GR. Nuclear export of NF-ATc enhanced by glycogen synthase kinase-3. Science 1997; 275(5308): 1930-4.
[http://dx.doi.org/10.1126/science.275.5308.1930] [PMID: 9072970]

[81]   Fang X, Yu SX, Lu Y, Bast RC Jr, Woodgett JR, Mills GB. Phosphorylation and inactivation of glycogen synthase kinase 3 by protein kinase A. Proc Natl Acad Sci USA 2000; 97(22): 11960-5.
[http://dx.doi.org/10.1073/pnas.220413597] [PMID: 11035810]

[82]   Ruvolo PP, Qiu Y, Coombes KR, *et al.* Phosphorylation of GSK3α/β correlates with activation of AKT and is prognostic for poor overall survival in acute myeloid leukemia patients. BBA Clin 2015; 4: 59-68.
[http://dx.doi.org/10.1016/j.bbacli.2015.07.001] [PMID: 26674329]

[83]   Guezguez B, Almakadi M, Benoit YD, *et al.* GSK3 Deficiencies in Hematopoietic Stem Cells Initiate Pre-neoplastic State that Is Predictive of Clinical Outcomes of Human Acute Leukemia. Cancer Cell 2016; 29(1): 61-74.
[http://dx.doi.org/10.1016/j.ccell.2015.11.012] [PMID: 26766591]

[84]   Wang Z, Smith KS, Murphy M, Piloto O, Somervaille TC, Cleary ML. Glycogen synthase kinase 3 in MLL leukaemia maintenance and targeted therapy. Nature 2008; 455(7217): 1205-9.
[http://dx.doi.org/10.1038/nature07284] [PMID: 18806775]

[85]   Bhatlekar S, Fields JZ, Boman BM. Role of HOX Genes in Stem Cell Differentiation and Cancer. Stem Cells Int 2018; 2018: 3569493.
[http://dx.doi.org/10.1155/2018/3569493] [PMID: 30154863]

[86]   Alharbi RA, Pettengell R, Pandha HS, Morgan R. The role of HOX genes in normal hematopoiesis and acute leukemia. Leukemia 2013; 27(5): 1000-8.
[http://dx.doi.org/10.1038/leu.2012.356] [PMID: 23212154]

[87]   Wang Z, Iwasaki M, Ficara F, *et al.* GSK-3 promotes conditional association of CREB and its coactivators with MEIS1 to facilitate HOX-mediated transcription and oncogenesis. Cancer Cell 2010; 17(6): 597-608.
[http://dx.doi.org/10.1016/j.ccr.2010.04.024] [PMID: 20541704]

[88]   Hwang ES, Hong JH, Bae SC, Ito Y, Lee SK. Regulation of c-fos gene transcription and myeloid cell differentiation by acute myeloid leukemia 1 and acute myeloid leukemia-MTG8, a chimeric leukemogenic derivative of acute myeloid leukemia 1. FEBS Lett 1999; 446(1): 86-90.
[http://dx.doi.org/10.1016/S0014-5793(99)00190-8] [PMID: 10100620]

[89]   Pippa R, Dominguez A, Malumbres R, *et al.* MYC-dependent recruitment of RUNX1 and GATA2 on the SET oncogene promoter enhances PP2A inactivation in acute myeloid leukemia. Oncotarget 2016; 8(33): 53989-4003.
[http://dx.doi.org/10.18632/oncotarget.9840] [PMID: 28903318]

[90]   Pippa R, Odero MD. The Role of MYC and PP2A in the Initiation and Progression of Myeloid Leukemias. Cells 2020; 9(3): E544.
[http://dx.doi.org/10.3390/cells9030544] [PMID. 32110991]

[91]   Arnaud L, Chen S, Liu F, *et al.* Mechanism of inhibition of PP2A activity and abnormal hyperphosphorylation of tau by I2(PP2A)/SET. FEBS Lett 2011; 585(17): 2653-9.
[http://dx.doi.org/10.1016/j.febslet.2011.07.020] [PMID: 21806989]

[92]   Arriazu E, Vicente C, Pippa R, *et al.* A new regulatory mechanism of protein phosphatase 2A activity via SET in acute myeloid leukemia. Blood Cancer J 2020; 10(1): 3.

[http://dx.doi.org/10.1038/s41408-019-0270-0] [PMID: 31913266]

[93]   Malaise M, Steinbach D, Corbacioglu S. Clinical implications of c-Kit mutations in acute myelogenous leukemia. Curr Hematol Malig Rep 2009; 4(2): 77-82.
[http://dx.doi.org/10.1007/s11899-009-0011-8] [PMID: 20425418]

[94]   Dumont AG, Reynoso DG, Trent JC. Essential requirement for PP2A inhibition by the oncogenic receptor c-KIT suggests PP2A reactivation as a strategy to treat c-KIT+ cancers -- Letter. Cancer Res 2011; 71(6): 2403.
[http://dx.doi.org/10.1158/0008-5472.CAN-10-3383] [PMID: 21406406]

[95]   Jiang L, Deng T, Wang D, Xiao Y. Elevated Serum Exosomal miR-125b Level as a Potential Marker for Poor Prognosis in Intermediate-Risk Acute Myeloid Leukemia. Acta Haematol 2018; 140(3): 183-92.
[http://dx.doi.org/10.1159/000491584] [PMID: 30304715]

[96]   Pyzer AR, Stroopinsky D, Rajabi H, et al. MUC1-mediated induction of myeloid-derived suppressor cells in patients with acute myeloid leukemia. Blood 2017; 129(13): 1791-801.
[http://dx.doi.org/10.1182/blood-2016-07-730614] [PMID: 28126925]

[97]   Barrera-Ramirez J, Lavoie JR, Maganti HB, et al. Micro-RNA Profiling of Exosomes from Marrow-Derived Mesenchymal Stromal Cells in Patients with Acute Myeloid Leukemia: Implications in Leukemogenesis. Stem Cell Rev Rep 2017; 13(6): 817-25.
[http://dx.doi.org/10.1007/s12015-017-9762-0] [PMID: 28918518]

[98]   Hou P, Wu C, Wang Y, et al. A Genome-Wide CRISPR Screen Identifies Genes Critical for Resistance to FLT3 Inhibitor AC220. Cancer Res 2017; 77(16): 4402-13.
[http://dx.doi.org/10.1158/0008-5472.CAN-16-1627] [PMID: 28625976]

[99]   Song EY, et al. Glycogen synthase kinase--3beta inhibitors suppress leukemia cell growth Exp Hematol 2010; 38(10): 908-921.: e1.

[100]   Hu S, Ueda M, Stetson L, et al. A Novel Glycogen Synthase Kinase-3 Inhibitor Optimized for Acute Myeloid Leukemia Differentiation Activity. Mol Cancer Ther 2016; 15(7): 1485-94.
[http://dx.doi.org/10.1158/1535-7163.MCT-15-0566] [PMID: 27196775]

[101]   Rizzieri DA, Cooley S, Odenike O, et al. An open-label phase 2 study of glycogen synthase kinase-3 inhibitor LY2090314 in patients with acute leukemia. Leuk Lymphoma 2016; 57(8): 1800-6.
[http://dx.doi.org/10.3109/10428194.2015.1122781] [PMID: 26735141]

[102]   Hernandez-Davies JE, Zape JP, Landaw EM, et al. The multitargeted receptor tyrosine kinase inhibitor linifanib (ABT-869) induces apoptosis through an Akt and glycogen synthase kinase 3β-dependent pathway. Mol Cancer Ther 2011; 10(6): 949-59.
[http://dx.doi.org/10.1158/1535-7163.MCT-10-0904] [PMID: 21471285]

[103]   Rahmani M, Aust MM, Attkisson E, Williams DC Jr, Ferreira-Gonzalez A, Grant S. Dual inhibition of Bcl-2 and Bcl-xL strikingly enhances PI3K inhibition-induced apoptosis in human myeloid leukemia cells through a GSK3- and Bim-dependent mechanism. Cancer Res 2013; 73(4): 1340-51.
[http://dx.doi.org/10.1158/0008-5472.CAN-12-1365] [PMID: 23243017]

[104]   Wakatsuki S, Tokunaga S, Shibata M, Araki T. GSK3B-mediated phosphorylation of MCL1 regulates axonal autophagy to promote Wallerian degeneration. J Cell Biol 2017; 216(2): 477-93.
[http://dx.doi.org/10.1083/jcb.201606020] [PMID: 28053206]

[105]   Wang R, Xia L, Gabrilove J, Waxman S, Jing Y. Downregulation of Mcl-1 through GSK-3β activation contributes to arsenic trioxide-induced apoptosis in acute myeloid leukemia cells. Leukemia 2013; 27(2): 315-24.
[http://dx.doi.org/10.1038/leu.2012.180] [PMID: 22751450]

[106]   Ramsey HE, Fischer MA, Lee T, et al. A Novel MCL1 Inhibitor Combined with Venetoclax Rescues Venetoclax-Resistant Acute Myelogenous Leukemia. Cancer Discov 2018; 8(12): 1566-81.
[http://dx.doi.org/10.1158/2159-8290.CD-18-0140] [PMID: 30185627]

[107] Chen L, Luo LF, Lu J, *et al.* FTY720 induces apoptosis of M2 subtype acute myeloid leukemia cells by targeting sphingolipid metabolism and increasing endogenous ceramide levels. PLoS One 2014; 9(7): e103033.
[http://dx.doi.org/10.1371/journal.pone.0103033] [PMID: 25050888]

[108] Kandilci A, Mientjes E, Grosveld G. Effects of SET and SET-CAN on the differentiation of the human promonocytic cell line U937. Leukemia 2004; 18(2): 337-40.
[http://dx.doi.org/10.1038/sj.leu.2403227] [PMID: 14671643]

[109] Li M, Makkinje A, Damuni Z. The myeloid leukemia-associated protein SET is a potent inhibitor of protein phosphatase 2A. J Biol Chem 1996; 271(19): 11059-62.
[http://dx.doi.org/10.1074/jbc.271.19.11059] [PMID: 8626647]

[110] Agarwal A, MacKenzie RJ, Pippa R, *et al.* Antagonism of SET using OP449 enhances the efficacy of tyrosine kinase inhibitors and overcomes drug resistance in myeloid leukemia. Clin Cancer Res 2014; 20(8): 2092-103.
[http://dx.doi.org/10.1158/1078-0432.CCR-13-2575] [PMID: 24436473]

SUBJECT INDEX

www.ingramcontent.com/pod-product-compliance
Lightning Source LLC
Chambersburg PA
CBHW041659210326
41598CB00007B/462